THEMES IN CULTURAL PSYCHIATRY

THEMES IN CULTURAL PSYCHIATRY
An Annotated Bibliography, 1975–1980

Armando R. Favazza and Ahmed D. Faheem

University of Missouri Press
Columbia & London, 1982

The authors are most thankful to Kathy Spiers for her energetic and efficient work in typing the bulk of the book; to Debby Burnley and to Rosemary McCallister for their assistance in typing; to Dean Schmidt and the staff of the University of Missouri medical library for their patience and assistance in finding many references; to Brian Harpster and to Walter Griffin for their abstracting skills; and to Dr. James M. A. Weiss, Chairman of the Department of Psychiatry, University of Missouri–Columbia, for his support and encouragement.

Library of Congress Cataloging in Publication Data

Favazza, Armando R.
    Themes in cultural psychiatry, an annotated bibliography, 1975–1980.

    Includes index.
    1. Psychiatry, Transcultural—Bibliography.
I. Faheem, Ahmed D.   II. Title.
Z6664.N5F37   [RC454.4]   016.3622   82–2738
ISBN 0–8262–0377–9   AACR2

To Barbara and Najma

Contents

Introduction

Although psychiatry and anthropology are separate disciplines with rich literatures and traditions, they share many common concerns such as child-rearing, language and communication, the family, sexuality, alcohol use, aggression, and healing or therapy. For the first six decades of this century, however, the majority of psychiatrists and psychologists who wrote about cultural issues did not seem to be aware of the anthropological literature. In general, cultural influences were treated as peripheral asides to investigations. Direct collaboration between psychiatrists and anthropologists was quite limited. While many anthropologists made use of psychoanalytic theory, most psychiatrists only flirted with anthropology. There were, of course, some brilliant collaborative efforts during this period (examples include Sapir and Sullivan, Kardiner and DuBois, Redlich and Caudill, Leighton and Kluckhohn), but, in general, psychiatrists were not strongly influenced by anthropological concepts. Except for the innovative transcultural program at McGill University under the leadership of Wittkower, Murphy, and Prince, psychiatric training tended to ignore cultural factors.

The development of the community psychiatry movement in the 1960s led to important changes in psychiatric thinking. The scientific basis of community psychiatry came from epidemiological studies that demonstrated the influence of social class on the prevalence of mental illness. Attention began to shift away from the office-based treatment of middle- and upper-class neurotic patients to the community-based treatment of lower-class patients and from purely intrapsychic theories of etiology to a recognition of the influence of the social environment on behavior and mental functioning. Concepts used by sociologists such as social class, socioeconomic status, mental status, age, and role were easily understood and readily utilized by psychiatrists.

A further shift in traditional psychiatric thinking grew out of the failure of the community mental health movement to fulfill all its early promises. Especially with the influx of Spanish-speaking immigrants, psychiatrists began to perceive that an understanding of culture is at least as important as an understanding of social class for diagnosing, treating, and even preventing mental illness. It is from this perception that modern cultural psychiatry developed.

One of the first tasks of this new interface discipline was to become familiar with the enormous, albeit often anecdotal and unintegrated, literature. Standard bibliographic tools such as *Index Medicus* and *Psychological Abstracts* neither went back far enough in time nor provided the sort of information needed by cultural psychiatrists. Thus, in 1977 Armando Favazza, along with Mary Oman, compiled *Anthropological and Cross-Cultural Themes in Mental Health: An Annotated Bibliography, 1925–1974* (University of Missouri Press). That book contained 3,634 entries culled from English-language journals in psychiatry and psychology.

Reviewers generally regarded the book favorably. A reviewer for the *Canadian Journal of Psychiatry* concluded that it was "highly recommended to those who study and treat human behavior in its cultural context." The *Johns Hopkins Bulletin of the History of Medicine*

1

noted that the authors "have brought a useful degree of self-consciousness to the production of this bibliography which should make it a truly valuable research tool." The *Bulletin of the Menninger Clinic* commented, "The writing is succinct and the job a complete one. The authors will be blessed by many a researcher."

While the authors were unable to ascertain how many blessings might have been offered, they were grateful to learn from colleagues that the book was widely used and that a second volume would be appreciated. One complaint voiced by several reviewers, however, was that the non-English-language literature was not included. The authors had seriously thought of including foreign-language journals but decided against it for several reasons: (1) few (if any) libraries available to us contained complete sets of these journals dating back to 1925; (2) even if the journals were available, the time involved in finding and translating articles would have delayed publication of the book by at least a year; and (3) quite frankly, the quality of the articles, with some important exceptions, was not terribly high. In this volume, however, we have included much non-English-language material, the quality of which has improved greatly.

One of the conclusions of the first book was that while many psychiatrists and psychologists wrote articles with cultural themes, they often seemed to be unaware of complementary articles in the anthropological literature. In order to remedy this situation and because the reference tools most commonly used by psychiatrists and psychologists (*Index Medicus* and *Psychological Abstracts*) are lacking in this area, we have included pertinent material from anthropological journals in this volume.

A third major change is the inclusion of anthropological, psychiatric, and psychological *books* as well as journals. It was not possible to identify and to obtain relevant books from 1925 to 1974, but we have been able to do so for the years 1975–1980.

Thus, by including non-English-language journals, anthropological journals, and books we have added considerably to the completeness and depth of this book.

The Coming of Age of Cultural Psychiatry

From 1975 to 1980 cultural psychiatry has truly blossomed. For the first time in its history the *American Journal of Psychiatry* featured cover articles in the area—Favazza and Oman's "Foundations of Cultural Psychiatry" (404) and Westermeyer and Wintrob's "Folk Criteria for the Diagnosis of Mental Illness in Rural Laos" (1563). Cox's review article "Aspects of Transcultural Psychiatry" (262) appeared in the *British Journal of Psychiatry*. Arthur Kleinman established the scholarly journal *Culture, Medicine and Psychiatry*. *Medical Anthropology* and the *Journal of Psychological Anthropology* were also founded during this period. In addition, the *Journal of Operational Psychiatry* adopted a strong pro-cultural-psychiatry editorial policy.

The cause of cultural psychiatry received a strong boost with the inclusion of Favazza and Oman's chapter on anthropology and psychiatry in the third edition of Kaplan, Freedman, and Sadock's widely used *Comprehensive Textbook of Psychiatry*. In two previous editions the chapter on anthropology was quite brief, and no mention was even made of the field of cultural psychiatry.

The period also witnessed the rapid growth of the discipline of medical anthropology (Maretzki's article on anthropology and mental health [938] comments on interdisciplinary growth) and, more important for cultural psychiatry, the creation of the Society for the Study of Psychiatry and Culture. The society was begun in 1978 by a small group of psychiatrists who organized a steering committee (Armando Favazza, Ed Foulks, Arthur Kleinman, John Spiegel, Joseph Westermeyer, and Ronald Wintrob). With the conclusion of the society's third annual meeting—held in 1981 in conjunction with the University of Oregon—the group members decided that a sufficient number of psychiatrists knowledgeable in cultural psychiatry had been reached and that the society would become a permanent one. In fact, one impetus for the preparation of this book came from society members who noted the utility of the first bibliography. They stressed the need for continual updating since access to much of the material pertinent to cultural psychiatry still requires time-consuming and difficult library research.

Methods and Sources

In order to identify journals, articles, and books for this bibliography, we first consulted the *Index Medicus, Psychological Abstracts,* and the *Social Science Citation Index.* Each appropriate reference was read and annotated.

We then carefully went through every issue of most of the pertinent journals from 1975 to 1980. This process yielded the majority of articles. Many of the non-English-language articles were gathered from *Transcultural Psychiatric Research Review.* The bibliographies of review articles were studied to detect items that we might have missed. Books were further identified by checking publishers' lists, reviews and advertisements in journals, and journal lists of books received. A fair number of articles and books were obtained through an interlibrary loan program. We then checked the shelf collections of the anthropology, psychiatry, and psychology sections of the University of Missouri–Columbia library system. Finally, we asked colleagues to send lists of their own publications as well as bibliographic lists they had prepared for their own use.

We estimate that we read at least 95 percent of all the items listed in the original. Annotations of the few unavailable books and articles were derived from reviews in scholarly journals.

The Annotations and Subject Index

Our goal in preparing the annotations is to inform the reader of the existence of these books and articles and to present their *general content* as briefly as possible. While we could have written lengthy annotations, we felt that an interested reader would still need to consult the original and complete texts. Certainly no reputable scholar would want to cite an item on the basis of an annotation, nor would any reputable clinician make an important decision on the basis of an annotation. Thus, lengthy annotations would have made this book both long and expensive but provided no substantial advantages.

The titles of many items accurately describe the contents; in those instances we tried not to repeat what was stated in the title. In other instances the titles bear little relationship to an item's contents; thus, some annotations may seem to be unrelated to what is promised in the title. The items that gave us the most trouble were those that were either exquisitely detailed or overly general because a focused annotation would be misleading in either case.

The heart of our volume is its Subject Index. We have tried to include all items of importance for each cited book or article. The annotation for Thernstrom's *Harvard Encyclopedia of Ethnic Groups,* for example, indicates the type of information covered (such as migratory state, race, language, religion, shared tradition, institutions, etc.) while each ethnic group discussed in the *Encyclopedia* is listed in our Index (over 100 entries ranging from Acadians and Afghans to West Indians and Zoroastrians). The thoroughness of an index is what really makes a bibliography valuable.

Cultural Areas and Groups

Many references deal with specific populations and with geographically delimitable culture areas. We have divided these into the following categories: Asia, American Subcultures, Africa, Europe, Native North Americans, Middle East, Latin and South America, and Oceania. Articles are cross-referenced between specific nations and specific groups of people. In the following categorical breakdowns, therefore, the number of articles, as noted in parentheses, may contain duplicates, for example, articles listed under Amhara would also be listed under Ethiopia.

Included in the *Asia* category are seventeen general articles as well as articles dealing with the following areas and peoples:

Afghanistan (2)
Ainu (2)
Azerbaijanis (1)
Bali (2)
Bangladesh (4)
Bants (2)
Bauri (1)
Bengali (4)
Brahmin (2)
Burma (3)
China (46)
Chinese Manchu (1)
Evenk (1)
Goa (2)
Himalayas (1)
Hmong (2)
Hong Kong (5)
India (66)
Indochina (2)
Japan (72)
Kalmyks (1)
Ket (1)
Khant (1)
Kirgiz (1)

Korea (9)
Koryak (1)
Kurds (1)
Lao (2)
Laos (15)
Lembu (2)
Manchu (1)
Meo (1)
Mimusa Tartar (1)
Moger (1)
Mongolia (1)
Na-Khi (2)
Nayar (2)
Nepal (8)
Newar (1)
Nisan (1)
Pahari (2)
Pakistan (7)
Philippines (18)
Sagay (1)
Sherpa (1)
Siberia (3)
Sikkim (1)
Southeast Asia (1)

Sri Lanka (10)	Thailand (17)
Subanum (1)	Tibet (2)
Sunuwar (1)	Tulu (1)
Tartars (1)	Vietnam (7)
Temang (2)	Yukagir (1)

Articles on Japan constitute the largest number; many focus on unique forms of psychotherapy as well as on the enormous problem of Japanese suicide. T. S. Lebra's "Japanese Patterns of Behavior" (821) is a wide-ranging survey. Many articles on India were written by anthropologists for whom India with its many castes and rituals holds a special interest. Psychiatry remains relatively underdeveloped in India, where a vast effort must by necessity be devoted to clinical services rather than to research (see A. V. Rav's overview of Indian psychiatry [1181]). Carstairs and Kapur's "The Great Universe of Kota: Stress, Change and Mental Disorder in an Indian Village" (200) merits special mention as a significant study, as do the numerous studies of J. S. Neki (1039–44). Articles on China have proliferated. Among the most impressive are those by Arthur Kleinman, who has emerged as the foremost scholar in the area of Chinese cultural psychiatry. His book *Patients and Healers in the Context of Culture* (758) is a major ethnoscientific contribution. Unfortunately, but as might be expected, a fair number of articles on China are impressionistic.

Included in the *American Subcultures* category are references on the following groups:

Acadians (1)	German-American (1)
Amish (1)	Greek-American (1)
Anglo-American (1)	Hispanic (17)
Anglo-Saxon (1)	Hutterite (2)
Appalachia (3)	Irish-American (2)
Arab-American (1)	Italian-American (7)
Armenian-American (1)	Japanese-American (12)
Asian-American (8)	Mennonite (1)
Black-American (89)	Mexican-American (57)
Chinese-American (9)	Pennsylvania German (1)
Chinese-Canadian (1)	Polish-American (2)
Creole (1)	Portuguese-American (1)
Cuban-American (3)	Puerto Rican (20)
Doukhobor (1)	Slovak-American (4)
Filipino-American (1)	Southerner (1)
Franco-American (1)	Yankee (1)
French Canadian (2)	

Many of the articles on black Americans were not written with a cultural focus (with exceptions such as Snow's "Sorcerers, Saints and Charlatans: Black Folk Healers in Urban America" [1364]). The paucity of publications on black Americans by cultural psychiatrists reflects in part the notion that the term *black* is not necessarily linked with a particular cultural group but instead reflects a variable physical characteristic; the American black population is vast and vastly heterogeneous. From the perspective of cultural psychiatry, references on Mexican-Americans and Puerto Ricans (two very distinct groups) have greatly improved in quality since 1975. Among the highly recommended references are articles by Vincente Abad (1), Vivian Garrison (476, 477), Joan Koss (778, 779), Cervando Martinez (954, 955), Pedro Ruiz (1247), R. T. Trotter (1468), and M. Gaviria and R. Wintrob (479, 480). Among the psychiatric leaders calling attention to the Asian-American subcultural groups are Joe Yamamoto and Lindbergh Sata.

Included in the *Africa* category are forty-seven general references as well as references dealing with the following areas and peoples:

Akan (1)
Aleta (1)
Amhara (4)
Angola (1)
Anyi (2)
Badyaranke (1)
Baganda (3)
Bakango (1)
Bambara (2)
Bantu (4)
Baralong boo Ratshidi (1)
Bedouin (1)
Bini (1)
Bono (1)
Buganda (3)
Bushman (3)
Cape Verdeans (1)
Chagga (1)
Dahomey (1)
Dogon (1)
East Africa (1)
Ebrie (1)
Ethiopia (13)
Evuzok (1)
Liberia (2)
Lovedu (1)
Luvale (1)
Maasi (1)
Malagasy (2)
Malawi (1)
Mali (1)
Mbuti (2)
Merina (1)
Meru (1)
Morocco (10)
Mpondo (1)
Nandi (2)
Ndembu (4)
Nganga (1)
Niger (1)
Nigeria (38)
North Africans (3)
Nyakyusa-Nyonde (1)
Onitsha (1)
Rwanda (1)
Sadama (1)
Sebei (1)
Senegal (12)

Fang (1)
Fipi (1)
Fon (1)
Fore (1)
Ga (1)
Ganda (1)
Ghana (9)
Gusii (2)
Hausa (2)
Hehe (1)
Ibo (2)
Irigwe (1)
Kalahari Desert San (1)
Kamba (1)
Karimojong (1)
Kenya (9)
Ko Bushman (1)
Kofyar (1)
Kom (1)
Kongo (2)
Kpelle (1)
Kung (1)
Lebou (1)
Serer (1)
Shana (1)
Sidamo (1)
Sierra Leone (3)
Soli (1)
South Africa (8)
Sudan (7)
Swaziland (1)
Taita (1)
Tanzania (8)
Temne (1)
Tunisia (4)
Uganda (13)
Ugandan-Asians (1)
Wapagoro (1)
Washo (1)
Wolof (3)
Xhosa (1)
Yoruba (13)
Zaire (4)
Zambia (8)
Zaramo (1)
Zimbabwe (1)
Zulu (3)

It is no surprise that articles on Nigeria head the list; under Dr. T. A. Lambo's leadership Nigerian psychiatry has blossomed. Special attention should be turned to Beiser's sophisticated studies among the Serer of Senegal (86), to the many French, psychoanalytically oriented studies, such as Parin et al.'s *Fear Thy Neighbor As Thyself: Psychoanalysis and*

Society Among the Anyi of West Africa (1114), to Wober's *Psychology in Africa* (1601), to Janzen's *The Quest for Therapy in Lower Zaire* (664), to excellent lengthy reviews by Corin (258, 259) and by Edgerton (352), and to Lee and DeVore's book on Kalahari hunter-gatherers (824).

Included in the *Europe* category are fourteen general references as well as references dealing with the following areas and peoples:

Albania (2)	Belorussian (1)
Alsatians (1)	Bocage (1)
Algeria (2)	Bosnian Muslim (1)
Andalusia (1)	Brittany (1)
Austria (6)	Bulgaria (1)
Balkan (1)	Corsica (1)
Basques (1)	Czechoslovakia (4)
Belgium (7)	Denmark (6)
Eastern Catholic (1)	Portugal (6)
Estonians (1)	Romania (2)
Finland (5)	Sardinia (1)
France (15)	Scandinavia (1)
Germany (17)	Scotch-Irish (1)
Great Britain (47)	Scotland (9)
Greece (24)	Serbia (2)
Hungary (3)	Shetland Islands (1)
Iceland (3)	Sicily (2)
Ireland (19)	Skanland (1)
Italy (19)	Slovak (1)
Lapp (2)	Slovene (1)
Latvia (1)	Spain (10)
Lithuania (1)	Sweden (17)
Luxembourg (1)	Switzerland (7)
Macedonian (1)	Turkey (17)
Malta (1)	Turkistani (1)
Manx (1)	Ukraine (1)
Middle Europeans (1)	USSR (24)
Netherlands (5)	Wales (3)
Norway (8)	Wends (1)
Poland (8)	Yugoslavia (8)

Many of the articles from Great Britain reflect the interests of cultural psychiatrists there who deal with immigrants, especially those in London, Manchester, and Birmingham. *Aliens and Alienists* (Penguin Books, 1982) by R. Littlewood and M. Lipsedge is a comprehensive and masterful study of ethnic minorities and psychiatry in London. Special mention should also be made of Scheper-Hughes's *Saints, Scholars, and Schizophrenics: Mental Illness in Rural Ireland* (1286). R. Giel's work reflects the expertise of cultural psychiatry in the Netherlands (495–500).

The category *Native North Americans* contains sixty-one general references as well as references to the following peoples:

Aleuts (2)	Cherokee (1)
Algonquin (3)	Cheyenne (1)
Apache (4)	Chippewa (2)
Arapahoe (2)	Choctaw (1)
Athabascan (3)	Coast Salish (7)
Carrier (1)	Cree (1)

Eskimo (22)
Forest Potawatomi (1)
Hopi (3)
Hupa (1)
Huron (1)
Inuit (2)
Iroquois (2)
Kaska (1)
Kiowa (1)
Kwakiutl (1)
Lumbee (1)
Micmac (1)

Mohave (1)
Naskapi (1)
Navajo (9)
Oglala Sioux (1)
Ojibway (5)
Papago (3)
Paite (1)
Plateau (1)
Pueblo (1)
Shoshone (2)
Tsimshin (1)
Zuni (2)

The literature on Native North Americans is not particularly joyous, with many references to alcoholism and suicide, for example, Hobfoll's study of an Anchorage skid row (615), Foulks's study of dissociative states, alcohol use, and suicide in Arctic populations (438), and Shore's article on suicide (1334). Westermeyer's description of the Apple Syndrome (1559)—a condition characterized by severe behavioral symptoms in Indian children who are reared by white foster parents and rejected during adolescence by their white peers—is a poignant example of the consequences of racial-ethnic discontinuity. The Jileks' studies of the Coast Salish Indians (669, 673) are especially sensitive, as is the Boyers' work·on the Apache Indians (139).

The category *Middle East* contains one general reference as well as references on the following areas and peoples:

Arab (13)
Armenia (1)
Baluch (1)
Bandari (1)
Black Hebrew (1)
Cyprus (3)
Egypt (12)
Iran (11)
Israel (36)
Jordan (1)

Kuwait (2)
Lebanon (3)
Libya (1)
Moroccan-Jew (3)
Palestinians (1)
Qashqa'i (1)
Qatar (2)
Saudi Arabia (3)
Yemen (1)

Israel, a country where psychiatry is highly developed, is the focus of many important studies dealing with such topics as the kibbutz movement and the integration of folk healing with modern psychiatry; see the studies of Moroccan-Jews (105, 106, 108) and Levau and Bilu's overview of Israeli psychiatry (843). Arab psychiatrists are beginning to publish the results of their research, for example, Zarroug's study of visual hallucinations among Saudi Arabian schizophrenics (1633) and El Sendiony's study relating culture change to the frequency of mental illness in Cairo (366).

The category *Latin and South America* contains references to the following areas and peoples:

Afro-Brazilian (2)
Afro-Cuban (1)
Afro-Curacaoan (1)
Andean Indian (1)
Argentina (4)
Aymara (1)
Aztec (2)

Bahamas (1)
Barbados (2)
Batuque (1)
Belize (1)
Bimini (1)
Black Caribe (1)
Bolivia (1)

Bororo (2)
Brazil (11)
Caribbean (General) (6)
Central America (General) (1)
Chipas (1)
Chile (7)
Chinese-Mexican (1)
Colombia (5)
Costa Rica (2)
Cuba (6)
Curacao (1)
Dominica (4)
Dominican Republic (3)
Ecuador (1)
Garifuna (1)
Guatemala (7)
Guyana (3)
Haiti (8)
Huichol (3)
Inca (1)
Jamaica (6)
Latin American (7)
Maka (1)

Maya (6)
Mazatec (1)
Mexico (45)
Mopan (1)
Nahua (2)
Oaxaca (1)
Paraguay (1)
Peru (9)
Quechua (1)
Quiche (1)
Rastafari (1)
Siriono (1)
South America (1)
St. Lucia (1)
Surinam (1)
Tarahumara (1)
Tarascan (2)
Trinidad (4)
Tukamo (1)
West Indian (13)
Yaqui (1)
Zapotuc (2)
Zinacanteco (1)

An increased interest in cultural psychiatry in this area was shown by the first Congreso Mundial De Medicina Folklorica, held in Peru in 1979 under the leadership of Dr. Fernando Cabieses of Peru and Dr. Carlos Sequin of Colombia. Of the many studies from Mexico perhaps the most sophisticated and significant are those by Horacio Fabrega.

Our last category, *Oceania,* contains references to the following areas and peoples:

Australia (10)
Admiralty Islands (2)
American Samoa (1)
Andaman Islands (1)
Anggor (1)
Australian Aborigine (23)
Australian-Greek (1)
Australian-Jew (1)
Baffin Islands (1)
Berawan (1)
Borneo (2)
Celebes Islands (1)
Cook Islands (3)
Easter Island (1)
East Indies (3)
Elema (1)
Enga (1)
Fiji (3)
Fore (3)
Gilbert Islands (1)
Gnau (1)
Guam (1)
Hua (1)
Huli (1)
Ibau (2)
Igorot (1)
Indonesia (7)

Java (5)
Kaiadilt (1)
Kaliali (1)
Kelantanese (1)
Kosrae Island (1)
Lardil (1)
Ma'anyan (1)
Malaysia (16)
Mambai (1)
Mandak (1)
Maori (4)
Maring (1)
Marquesas (1)
Melanesia (3)
Micronesia (6)
Molukkan Islands (1)
Mudang (1)
Namoluk Atoll (1)
Nekematigi (1)
New Britain (1)
New Caledonia (1)
New Zealand (10)
Oceania (General) (5)
Okinawa (2)
Pacific Islanders (1)
Pacific Rim (2)
Pakeha (1)

Papua New Guinea (23)	Timor (1)
Polynesia (5)	Tiwi (1)
Ponape (1)	Tokelanan (1)
Samoa (5)	Tonga (1)
Semai (or Senoi) (2)	Toradja (1)
Sepik (1)	Truk (2)
Singapore (4)	Walbiri (1)
Solomon Islands (1)	Yap (1)
South Pacific (1)	Yewan (1)
Sundanese (1)	Yolngu (3)

Although many of the islands of Oceania have a romantic aura, the plight of the Australian Aborigines is hardly romantic. Because they are one of the few remaining hunting and gathering groups, research among them can inform us of very ancient beliefs about illnesses and their treatment. As this group invariably comes more and more into contact with mainstream Australian culture, however, the old ways and beliefs may be lost. Many of the studies of Aborigines noted here may be among the last to reflect the old ways. The diverse cultural groups of Papua New Guinea have provided very important information to Western scientists. The saga of the transmission through cannibalism of a lethal show-virus among the Fore has become a classic of modern medical history (870). C. G. Burton-Bradley's many studies in Papua New Guinea are impressive (178–81), as are Virginia Abernethy's use of data from the area to develop an intriguing model relating population control to cultural processes (4), Davidson's study of aboriginal adolescent coping and culture conflict (285), and Howard's review article on Polynesia and Micronesia (630).

Specific Themes

The diversity and the special interests of cultural psychiatry from 1975 to 1980 are demonstrated not only by references to cultural areas and populations but also by references to specific themes. All the references for each specific theme are listed in the Subject Index of this book.

The concept of *culture-bound syndromes* continues to be problematic; W. P. Lebra's "Culture Bound Syndromes" (823) presents many examples. All are regarded as somewhat exotic, while some are strange in the extreme; *heva* (116) is a condition found only on Easter Island in which a person puts a rat in his mouth and runs around violently with a club! *Koro,* a condition most common in Southeast Asia, is characterized by the fear of death resulting from the belief that one's genitals are retracting into the abdomen (349, 672, 1418). Interestingly, it may occur as an epidemic. Hippler and Cawte's article on the *Malgri syndrome* in some Australian Aborigines provides a primitive paradigm for modern agoraphobia; the person afflicted with the syndrome experiences anxiety and fear upon moving into another lineage's or moiety's territory (608). Articles by Simons (1347) and by Kenny (724) on *latah,* by Carr (197) on *amok,* and by Freeman (447) on *Arctic hysteria* reveal the complex ways in which neurophysiological, experimental, and cultural variables interact to produce the social phenomenon called a culture-bound syndrome. While we find it easy to recognize the cultural factors in conditions such as *piblokto* and *amok,* we still are uncomfortable admitting that our "scientifically based" syndromes, such as schizophrenia and anxiety, have cultural components. Such an admission, however, need *not* undermine any biological validity, nor need it lead to the straitjacket of total cultural relativism. The following culture-bound syndromes are referenced in this volume:

Agali (1)
Amakiro (1)
Amok (6)
Arctic hysteria (3)
Ascetic syndrome (1)
Aslai (1)
Ataque de nervios (2)
Aumakua (1)
Bati-hot mouth complex (1)
Bon ba nsinga (1)
Brain fag (1)
Chiyoroso (1)
Chuvah (1)
Colerina (1)
Dhat syndrome (1)
Empache (2)
Espanto (1)
Evil spirit disease (1)
Falling out (4)
Ghost sickness (1)
Heva (1)

Ichaa (1)
Indisposition (2)
Koro (3)
Latah (3)
Malgri (1)
Matiruku (1)
Nit-ku-bon (1)
Phipop (1)
Piblokto (3)
Pobough Lang (1)
Shinkeshitu (1)
Spirit sickness (3)
Suchi Bai (1)
Susto (9)
Tawatl ye sni (1)
Thwasa (1)
Tsira (1)
Uzr illness (1)
Wacinko (1)
Windigo (1)
Wind illness (1)

The concept of *healing* is a theme of great importance to cultural psychiatry, and current studies and reviews, such as Prince's chapter (1171), are quite sophisticated in comparison with past ones. Harwood's *Spiritist As Needed* (575) is a brilliant study of Puerto Rican folk healing in New York City. Other examples of significant references include Jilek's review of American Indian folk healing (670), Ademuwagun et al.'s book on African therapeutic systems (10), Alegria's study of curanderismo (20), Chen's description of Kelantenese therapy (211), Comaroff's study of healing in Southern Africa (240), Corin's study of the Zebola ritual in Kinshasha (256), Figge's study of Brazilian umbanda healing (417), Horikoshi's report on the Sundanese of Java (628), Johanne's study of curing in Papua New Guinea (679), Kleinman's *Patients and Healers in the Context of Culture* (758), Landy's *Culture, Disease and Healing* (803) (a collection of classic papers), Luckert's presentation of the Navajo Coyoteway healing ceremony (894), Maloney's volume on the evil eye (928), Moerman's essay on symbolic healing (991), Morley and Wallis's *Culture and Curing* (1000), Ohnuki-Tierney's studies on Ainu illness and healing (1075), Sandoval's study of Afro-Cuban Santeria (1274), Sharon's study of Peruvian curanderismo (1324), Siikala's study of Siberian shamans (1339), and Young's study of Amhara magician-healers (1621). Contemporary Christian religious healing is represented by MacNutt's *The Power to Heal* (919) and by Hufford's study (634). Westermeyer has contributed an impressive series of reports on Laos demonstrating that folk healers have their fair share of therapeutic failures (1563, 1564; also see his article "Mental disorders in a peasant society: personal consequences" in *J Operational Psychiatry* 12:121–26, 1981).

The theme of *psychotherapy* is well represented by Spiegel's reexamination of transference and countertransference from a cultural perspective (1377), by Pedersen et al.'s *Counseling Across Cultures* (1132; the use of the word *counseling* in the title is somewhat of a misnomer), by Marcos's studies on bilingual patients (934, 935), by Lager and Zwerling's report on time orientation and psychotherapy in the ghetto (801), and by Tseng and McDermott's search for universal elements and cultural variations of psychotherapy (1472). Kinzie offers lessons from cross-cultural psychotherapy (742). Kleinman, Eisenberg, and Good present clinical findings from cross-cultural research (759); this paper (published in *Annals of Internal Medicine*) is a major statement on the relationship among culture, illness, and care. Reynolds's book *The Quiet Therapies* (1200) clearly delineates varieties of Japanese psychotherapy, such as Morita, Naikan, Shadan, Seiza, and Zen.

Psychoanalysis has gone through turbulent times recently. Although a number of significant works are referred to in this volume—including Kakar's study of childhood and society in India (697), Devereux's *Ethnopsychoanalysis* (307, 309), Holter's comments on field work (621), the Boyers' sensitive study of the Apache (139), and the French contributions from Africa (often reported in the journal *Psychopathologie Africaine*)—a great many articles deal with cultural concepts in a rather speculative manner. The *Journal of Psychological Anthropology* is devoted to a psychoanalytic perspective.

The theme of *social change* is often linked with epidemiological studies, such as Schwab et al.'s monumental *Social Order and Mental Health* (1300) and the Rosens' paper on the impact on mental health of industrialization and urbanization in the Shetland Islands (1225). *Culture change* is a more difficult topic to grasp since it does not lend itself to traditional, epidemiological methodology. Overviews of the topic are presented in papers by Barger (64), Berry (99), Favazza (404), and Taft (1529; his chapter on "Coping with Unfamiliar Cultures" can be found in Warren's *Studies In Cross-Cultural Psychology*, vol. 1). The notion of change is frequently linked with the themes of *acculturation* and *migration*. H. B. M. Murphy, perhaps the greatest scholar in the field, has written a succinct overview of "Migration, Culture, and Mental Health" (1020). A. W. Burke and his colleagues have contributed an important series of papers on immigrants to England (171–74). Kinzie, Bloom et al. present information on treatment approaches with Indochinese refugees (743); volume 4 (1977) of the European journal *Mental Health and Society* features articles on immigration. Keefe's study of urbanization, acculturation, and extended family ties among Mexican-Americans is a good example of current anthropological thinking (715). Padilla's edited *Acculturation: Theory, Models and Some New Findings* (1104) is the most up-to-date and comprehensive volume on that theme.

Aggression and *violence* have always been troublesome themes for psychiatry. Jolly West's plans to establish a center at UCLA were cancelled because of criticism of the center's proposed emphasis on the biological rather than the social and cultural causes of aggression. Some important references noted here include Eibl-Eibesfeldt's ethological treatise on war and peace (355), Vayda's book on wars in Oceania from an ecological perspective (1496), Montagu's work on the importance of cultural factors in aggression (996), Volkan's psychoanalytic study of war and adaption on Cyprus (1507), and Robarchek's study of the Semai, one of the most nonviolent cultural groups (1211).

The themes of *death and dying, grief,* and *bereavement* were revitalized following the publication of Elizabeth Kubler-Ross's books. Kalish's *Death and Dying: Views from Many Cultures* (698), Huntington and Metcalf's *Celebrations of Death* (636), and Rosenblatt et al.'s *Grief and Mourning in Cross-Cultural Perspective* (1128) present these themes from a cultural perspective that may enhance clinical understanding. Ahyi reports on an amazing therapeutic ritual (called *hoxosudide*) that is utilized by an African tribe in mourning the death of twins (15).

Suicide and culture is a theme of great importance. Beskow's study of suicide and mental disorder in Sweden (101) utilizes a socioepidemiological approach, while Fuse's (466–67) and Iga's studies (641–42) on Japanese suicide utilize an anthropological approach. Of special interest is seppuku, an institutionalized form of suicide in Japan. Also see M. Tousignant and B. L. Mishara's "Suicide and Culture: A Review of the Literature (1969–1980)" in *Transcultural Psychiatric Research Review* 18:5–32, 1981.

In keeping with the current psychiatric interest in *depression,* this theme is well represented in this volume by Marsella's cross-cultural approach (947, 948), by Mezzich and Raab's study of depressive symptomatology across the Americas (974), by Binitie's factor-analytical study of depression in Europe and in Africa, and by Brown and Harris's major study in Camberwell (109) and the Outer Hebrides on the *Social Origins of Depression* (160). Examples of references on *schizophrenia* include the World Health Organization's *Follow-up Study* (1610), Edgerton's perceptive comments on that study (352), and Scheper-Hughes's work in rural Ireland (1286). The theme of *anxiety* has lost some of its popularity; Spielberger and Diaz Guerrero's edited volume on *Cross-Cultural Anxiety* (1378) is the best book on the topic.

The *alcohol* literature is very extensive. Important references include Marshall's *Beliefs, Behaviors, and Alcoholic Beverages* (951), Hamer and Steinbring's *Alcohol and Native Peoples of the North* (557), Leland's *Firewater Myths* (834), Jilek-Aall's report on alcohol and the Indian-white relationship (677), Heath's sociocultural model of alcohol use (581), Ablon's study of cultural patterning in American ethnic families (5), Blaine's volume on *Alcoholism and the Jewish Community* (112), Singer's fascinating study of sobriety among black Hebrews (1351), Blumberg et al.'s book on *Skid Row as a Human Condition* (121), Dennis's study of the drunk role in a Mexican village (299), and reports by Gordon (521), by Paine (1105), and by Szapocynik on alcoholism among Hispanics (1420).

Books on *mind-altering drugs* other than alcohol include Schultes and Hofmann's graphically stunning *Plants of the Gods* (1298), du Toit's *Drugs, Rituals and Altered States of Consciousness* (338), de Rios's *The Wilderness of Mind: Sacred Plants in Cross-Cultural Perspective* (301), and Reichel-Dolmatoff's *The Shaman and the Jaguar* (1190). Qat use in Yemen is the focus of a brilliant study by Kennedy et al. (722).

The related themes of *spirits, spirit possession, exorcism,* and *religion* are found in a large number of references. Pattison and Wintrob's "Possession and Exorcism in Contemporary America" (*Journal of Operational Psychiatry* 12:13–20, 1981) offers the most successful categorization of trance and spirit possession. Other important references include Bourguignon's books *Possession* (134) and *Psychological Anthropology* (135), Davis's study of exorcistic religious sects in Japan (289), Claus's report utilizing Tulu oral traditions (220), and Pattison's psychosocial interpretations of exorcism (1123). Favazza and Faheem's case report "The Heavenly Vision of a Poor Woman" (405) and Spitzer et al.'s discussion (1382) provide an example of the difficulties of psychiatric diagnosis in a patient who claimed contact with the spirit world.

Although *ethnicity* is an essential theme both in anthropology and in cultural psychiatry, it is a difficult one to treat operationally. Examples of references in which ethnicity is the focus include the Giordanos' *The Ethno-cultural Factor in Mental Health* (506), Hraba's *American Ethnicity* (632), Lin et al.'s report on ethnicity and patterns of help-seeking (868), and the Jileks' study comparing Mennonites, Doukhobors, and Coast Salish Indians (678). Thernstrom's monumental *Harvard Encyclopedia of American Ethnic Groups* is the premier reference book on the topic (1441).

The themes of *family, marriage,* and *kinship* are well represented in this book. Important studies include that by Aschenbrenner on black families in Chicago (43), by Byrnes on communal families (the Zadruga) in the Balkans (184), by Degler on women and family life in America (297), by Doane on family interaction and communication deviance (323), by Fisher on the classification of families (422), by Lichtman and Challinor on *Kin and Communities* (859), by Mindel and Haberstein on *Ethnic Families in America* (986), by Schneider on *American Kinship* (1292), and by van den Berghe on human family systems from a sociobiological perspective (1490). Soliday's bibliography on the history of the family and kinship contains 6,200 entries (1371).

The themes of *social networks* and *support groups* are emerging as highly significant areas for both clinical and cultural psychiatry. The *Schizophrenia Bulletin* (vol. 4, no. 4, 1978) contains a series of articles (see Beels [83], Budson [165], and Garrison [477]) on the social networks of schizophrenics. The conceptual basis for the study of social networks in psychiatry has been reported by Mansell Pattison (1125) in the United States and by Scott Henderson (595–98) in Australia (especially see Pattison's chapter in Foulks et al.'s *Current Perspectives in Cultural Psychiatry* [440]). Caplan and Killilea's *Support Systems and Mental Health* is another important reference (190).

Child rearing is a theme that relates directly to many tenets of dynamic psychiatry. Current studies in child rearing are far more sophisticated than in the past (especially see the Whitings' *Children of Six Cultures* [1576] and Leiderman et al.'s *Culture and Infancy* [832]). Other important references include Bolman and Maretzki's book *Child Psychiatry in Asian Countries* (126), Robert Coles's sensitive series on *Children of Crisis* (234–35), de Vries and Super's report on uses of the Neonatal Behavioral Assessment Scale (311), Kaffman's studies of kibbutz children (692–95), Kett's historical review of adolescence and rites of passage (729), Korbin's *Child Abuse and Neglect: Cross-Cultural Perspectives* (776), Bronfenbrenner's *The Ecology of Human Development* (156), and Brazelton et al.'s studies of neonatal behavior in Zambia (150).

Old age, the other end of life's spectrum, has newly attracted the attention of scholars. Important books on the theme of *geriatrics* include those by Fry on *Aging in Culture and Society* (459), by Gelfand and Kutzik on *Ethnicity and Aging* (485), and by Myerhoff and Simi on cultural variations on growing old (1027). Among important articles are T. S. Lebra's report on aging among Japanese women (822) and the Bozzettis' reports on aging in Sweden (141–43).

Cross-cultural research is a major component of cultural psychiatry. Chapters by Barry (72) and by Brown and Sechrest (159) in the *Handbook of Cross-Cultural Psychology* deal with this theme, as do Adler's *Issues in Cross-Cultural Research* (12), Naroll et al.'s *Worldwide Theory Testing* (1037), and Dasen's volume on Piagetian psychology (280).

The *community mental health* literature provides many examples of the direct application of cultural understandings to clinical practice. Important references include Ruiz and Langrod's "The role of folk healers in community mental health services" (1248), Fritz's "Indian people and community psychiatry in Saskatchewan" (457), Giordano's "Community mental health in a pluralistic society" (505), and Wu and Windle's "Ethnic specificity in the relative minority use and staffing of community mental health centers" (1612).

Much of the literature on the provision of *mental health services in developing nations* stresses the importance of cultural factors (see Higginbotham's review of this topic [605]). Significant references include Binitie's "Mental health implications of economic growth in developing countries" (110), Chaudhry and Misza's "Rehabilitation of schizophrenics in a developing country" (210), and Minde's "Child psychiatry in developing countries" (983).

The theme of *women's issues* has exploded onto the psychiatric scene. Indeed, in our earlier bibliography covering 1925–1975 *women's issues* was not even listed in the index, but our current book includes 105 entries on this topic. In addition to general references about women (for example, those by Ardener [36], Blum [120], Caplan and Bujira [191], Donelson and Gullahorn [324], Heckerman [584], and Rohrlich-Leavitt [1221]) there are entire books devoted to such specific groups as lesbian women (385), Bengali women (1235), Mayan women (363), Yaqui women (720), Gusii women (840), Himalayan women (688), Muslim women (81), kibbutz women (1380), and alcoholic women (187). The theme of women's issues is frequently linked with the theme of *sex roles and sexuality,* as exemplified by Weitz's *Sex Roles* (1549) and Friedel's *Women and Men* (453).

Coda

H. B. M. Murphy wrote the following in the *Transcultural Psychiatry Newsletter* (vol. 2, no. 2, June 1981):

For Cultural Psychiatrists and Anthropologists, End of a Lonely Era

For years, persons seriously and consistently involved in transcultural psychiatry throughout the world could be numbered on one's fingers and toes. The chances of more than three or four of these persons meeting together were remote. Not long ago, very few psychiatrists took a direct interest in anthropology; anthropologists interested in practical psychiatry (as distinct from abstract psychiatric and psychoanalytic theory) were rare. A few months ago it was impressed on me how much the situation is changing. Early in April, the Transcultural Psychiatry Society (U.K.), meeting in Leeds, England, drew a substantial attendance from anthropologists as well as psychiatrists. Later that month I went to Dakar for the W.P.A. Regional Symposium on the theme, "Psychiatry and Culture." There I learned that the African Psychiatric Association had been reactivated. (Though the Association is concerned with many aspects of psychiatry and feels it should contribute to mainstream psychiatry rather than concentrating on distinctly African aspects, it fully realizes the importance of local cultural factors.) At this symposium I also learned that enough persons in the south of France are interested in transcultural psychiatry to make a regional organization a distinct possibility. At the end of April, the Society for Applied Anthropology, a largely American organization, met in Edinburgh. At least six psychiatrists attended. The meeting held great interest for any social psychiatrist; sessions were devoted to deinstitutionalization, substance abuse, social support networks, utilization of indigenous healers, and the comparison of outcomes of non-medical treatments. All included an awareness of the cultural dimension.

It seems evident that in many countries men and women can now meet and share their interest in transcultural psychiatry without traveling great distances. It is this sharing and meeting, this sense of support from colleagues, that can make interest become operational. Informal local meetings addressed to practical problems, rather than to doctrine, are a good starting point; social scientists are increasingly ready to be pulled into operational roles.

In 1975 to 1980 cultural psychiatry finally joined biological, psychological, and community psychiatry as a true foundation stone of psychiatry (see 407). During this period, as noted by Dr. Murphy, a worldwide network of psychiatrists sharing common cultural interests began to emerge. Entrance to the network can be achieved in differing ways, including through the Transcultural Psychiatry Section of the World Psychiatric Association, the Pacific Rim College of Psychiatrists, the Society for the Study of Culture and Psychiatry, the English transcultural psychiatry group, and the McGill University group (long the only real training center). The network can also be entered indirectly by familiarization with the books and articles noted in this bibliography and by reading current material in such journals as *Culture, Medicine and Psychiatry, Transcultural Psychiatric Research Review, The Journal of Operational Psychiatry, Social Science and Medicine,* and *Medical Anthropology.*

Just as culture is an integrative concept, so too cultural psychiatry can form interconnections among biological, psychological, and social forces that impinge on an individual. The research data base and theoretical underpinnings of cultural psychiatry have developed dramatically in the past five years. We have also witnessed the increase in mental health services to rapidly growing numbers of ethnic groups and refugees. These services will be successful only if the lessons of cultural psychiatry are heeded. The next steps for cultural psychiatry are (1) the development of training materials and curricula for use in general psychiatric residency and medical student programs (see Foulks's article [437] and Tseng and McDermott's excellent introductory textbook *Culture, Mind and Therapy* [Brunner/Mazel, 1981]); and (2) the demonstration of the importance of cultural factors for *all* patients and not merely those from certain ethnic groups.

Journals Cited in Annotations

Acta Psiquiatria y Psicologia de America Latina
Acta Psychiatrica Scandinavica
Africa
African Journal of Psychiatry
Alaska Medicine
American Anthropologist
American Ethnologist
American Journal of Mental Deficiency
American Journal of Orthopsychiatry
American Journal of Psychiatry
American Journal of Psychoanalysis
American Journal of Psychotherapy
Anthropological Quarterly
Archives of General Psychiatry
Archives of Sexual Behavior
Australian and New Zealand Journal of Psychiatry
Behavioral and Brain Sciences
British Journal of Medical Psychology
British Journal of Social and Clinical Psychology
Bulletin of the Menninger Clinic
Canadian Journal of Psychiatry (Canadian Psychiatric Association Journal)
Central African Medical Journal
Child Development
Colorado Medicine
Community Mental Health Journal
Comparative Medicine East and West
Comprehensive Psychiatry
Confina Psychiatrica
Confrontations Psychiatrique
Culture, Medicine and Psychiatry
Current Anthropology
Drug and Alcohol Dependence
Ethnicity
Ethnology
Ethnopsychiatrica
Ethos
Human Biology
Human Organization
Indian Journal of Psychiatry

Indonesia
International Journal of the Addictions
International Journal of Aging and Human Development
International Journal of Group Psychotherapy
International Journal of Mental Health
International Journal of Offender Therapy and Comparative Criminology
International Journal of Psychoanalysis
International Journal of Psychoanalytic Psychotherapy
International Journal of Social Psychiatry
Israel Annals of Psychiatry
Journal of Abnormal Psychology
Journal of the Addictions and Health
Journal of Adolescence
Journal of Alcohol and Drug Education
Journal of Alcoholism and Related Addictions
Journal of the American Academy of Child Psychiatry
Journal of the American Academy of Psychoanalysis
Journal of the American Medical Association
Journal of Child Psychology, Psychiatry and Allied Disciplines
Journal of Chronic Disease
Journal of Clinical Psychology
Journal of Consulting and Clinical Psychology
Journal of Cross-Cultural Psychology
Journal of the Korean Neuropsychiatric Association
Journal of Marriage and the Family
Journal of the National Medical Association
Journal of Nervous and Mental Disease
Journal of Operational Psychiatry
Journal of Psychological Anthropology
Journal of Psychosomatic Research
Journal of Studies on Alcohol
Lakartigningen
Mankind
Masyarakat Indonesia
Medical Journal of Australia
Mental Health and Society
Moana
Monographs of the Society for Research in Child Development
Papua New Guinea Medical Journal
Perspectives in Psychiatric Care
Phylon
Psyche
Psychiatric Annals
Psychiatric Journal of the University of Ottawa

Psychiatric Opinion
Psychiatric Quarterly
Psychiatrie, Neurologie, and Medizinische Psychologie
Psychiatry
Psychoanalytic Review
Psychoanalytic Study of the Child
Psychologia
Psychological Medicine
Psychological Reports
Psychopathologie Africaine
Psychosomatic Medicine
Psychotherapia
Psychotherapy: Theory, Research and Practice
Public Health Reports
Scandinavian Journal of Social Medicine
Schweizer Archiv fur Neurologie, Neurochirurgie und Psychiatrie
Seishin Igaku
Social Analysis: Journal of Cultural and Social Practice
Social Psychiatry
Social Science and Medicine
Transcultural Psychiatric Research Review
Transnational Mental Health Research Newsletter
Tropical and Geographical Medicine
Youth and Society

Annotations

1. Abad V, Boyce E: Issues in psychiatric evaluations of Puerto Ricans: a socio-cultural perspective. J Operational Psychiatry 10:28–39, 1979.

Language barriers and psychocultural distance present a disadvantage for Puerto Ricans competing with Anglos for mental health care. Critical issues in the psychiatric evaluation of Puerto Ricans include consideration of fear of loss of control, ataques, hallucinatory experiences, somatization, spiritismo beliefs, and spirit possession.

2. Abell T, Lyon L: Do the differences make a difference? An empirical evaluation of the culture of poverty in the United States. Amer Ethnologist 6:602–19, 1979.

The analysis of the culture of poverty in the United States produces several findings specific to Lewis's "perpetuation of poverty" hypothesis. All the variables predictive of educational, occupational, and financial achievement also differentiate the lower and middle classes. Two-thirds of the income gap between the descendants of the poor and those of the middle class is determined by structural factors beyond individual control.

3. Abernethy V: Cultural perspectives on the impact of women's changing roles on psychiatry. Amer J Psychiatry 133:657–61, 1976.

Sex role stereotypes and their impact on the self-concept of women in the United States are examined. The increasing flexibility in gender role will have a positive effect on the treatment of women by therapists.

4. Abernethy V: Population Pressure and Cultural Adjustment. New York, Human Sciences, 1979.

Population pressure triggers or results in the elaboration of cultural mechanisms that restrain further population growth. Evidence for this finding comes especially from study of the Enga, Fore, Yapese, and Eskimo.

5. Ablon J: The significance of cultural patterning for the "alcoholic family." Family Process 19:127–44, 1980.

To understand alcohol usage in a population of middle-class Catholic families of primarily Irish, German, and Italian heritage, a knowledge of the historical and cultural roles of drinking in the relevant ethnic or national groups and a holistic view of contemporary family life are essential.

6. Acosta FX: Self-described reasons for premature termination of psychotherapy by Mexican American, Black American, and Anglo-American patients. Psychological Reports 47:435–43, 1980.

Mexican-American, Black-American, and Anglo-American patients who prematurely terminate psychotherapy usually have negative attitudes toward therapists and perceive therapy as of no benefit. Mexican-Americans have the least negative attitude toward their therapists.

7. Acosta FX, Sheehan JG: Preferences toward Mexican-American and Anglo-American psychotherapists. J Consulting Clin Psychology 44: 272–79, 1976.

Both Mexican-Americans and Anglo-Americans attribute more skill, understanding, trustworthiness, and liking to therapists who are identified as either Anglo-American or as Mexican-American nonprofessionals.

8. Adebimpe VR, Gigandet J, Harris E: MMPI diagnosis of black psychiatric patients. Amer J Psychiatry 136:85–87, 1979.

The MMPI should be used with caution in the diagnosis of psychiatric illness in black Americans. There are spuriously elevated scales producing a false pathological picture.

9. Adejumo D: Conceptual tempo and visual perceptual ability of some Nigerian children. Psychological Reports 45:911–16, 1979.

The significant correlation between the subjects' conceptual tempo and performance in visual perceptual ability underscores the assertion that the tendency to respond quickly or slowly with varying degrees of accuracy in response is manifested across virtually all tasks that have the property of response uncertainty.

10. Ademuwagun ZA, Ayoade JAA, Harrison DE, Warren DM (eds): The African Therapeutic Systems. Waltham, Mass., Crossroads, 1979.

Many African tribes believe in a spiritual etiology of both physical and psychological illness. Traditional healing approaches of the Yoruba, Amhara, Wolof, Lebou, Bayanda, Hebe, Zulu, Liberians, and Ghanians are discussed. The coexistence of Western and traditional African medical systems poses problems both for patients and for practitioners.

11. Adler F: Sisters in Crime: The Rise of the New Female Criminal. New York, McGraw-Hill, 1975.

As women become increasingly liberated they can be expected to follow the same criminal careers as men.

12. Adler LL (ed): Issues in Cross-Cultural Research. NY Academy of Science Annals, 285, 1977.
Sixty articles discuss cross-cultural research, including sections on psychopathology, ethnopsychiatry, and psychotherapy.

13. Ahmed AH: Consanguinity and schizophrenia in Sudan. Brit J Psychiatry 134:635–36, 1979.
Schizophrenia is not significantly associated with first-cousin marriage in Sudan.

14. Ahmed SH: Cultural influence on delusion. Psychiatria Clinica 11:1–9, 1978.
Delusions of persecution, religion, and magic were the most common found in Pakistani schizophrenics, who often felt that their persecutors used spells, evil spirits, amulets, and influence with verses to torture them.

15. Ahyi RG: Victory over death: reflections on therapy for grief through "Hoxosudide." Psychopathologie Africaine 15:141–57, 1979.
Hoxosudide is a ritual to aid the mourning process following the death of twins among the Fon. A statue of the dead twins is made, and the twins' spirits promise to protect their parents provided that their parents live in peace without dispute or divorce, that their mother does not prepare a meal without inviting their father, and that their father does not become agitated. The statues then go through a period of "gestation," and the rebirth of the twins is celebrated.

16. Akhtar S: Obsessional neurosis, marriage, sex and fertility: some transcultural comparisons. Intl J Social Psychiatry 24:164–66, 1978.
Indian obsessives, unlike their counterparts in other countries, do not display a higher-than-expected rate of celibacy, bachelorhood, and low fertility.

17. Akins C, Beschner G (eds): Ethnography. Rockville, Md., Natl. Inst. Drug Abuse, 1980.
Attention to ethnographic studies and reports can be a research tool for policymakers in the drug and alcohol fields.

18. Albaugh B, Albaugh P: Alcoholism and substance sniffing among the Cheyenne and Arapaho Indians of Oklahoma. Intl J Addictions 14:1001–7, 1979.
Confusing family interpersonal relationships, alcoholism in the immediate family, and severe parent-child emotional deprivation predispose these groups to alcoholism.

19. Albert S, Amgatt T, Krakow M, Marcus H: Children's bedtime rituals as a prototype rite of safe passage. J Psychol Anthropology 2:85–105, 1979.
The rite of safe passage, as the protector and maintainer of identity during a period of undesired change, is illustrated in the rituals of a child's going to sleep and reawakening.

20. Alegria D, Guerra E, Martinez C Jr, Meyer GG: El hospital invisible: a study of curanderismo. Arch Gen Psychiatry 34:1354–57, 1977.
Practitioners and their clients simultaneously utilize the folk medical system and the scientific medical system. Curanderos and curanderas (folk healers) provide valuable services to the people whom they treat.

21. Alexander J: The culture of race in middle-class Kingston, Jamaica. Amer Ethnologist 4(3):413–35, 1977.
To suppose that the idea of race refers simply to physical characteristics or to an inherent physical hierarchy is wrong. Understanding of race as a cultural phenomenon in the Caribbean shows that race symbolizes mythological time and thereby anchors in the past a belief in the fragmented nature of society.

22. Alexander J: The cultural domain of marriage. Amer Ethnologist 5(1):5–14, 1978.
Conjugal love and marriage involve a conscious and voluntary aspect of the personality as well as an unconscious involuntary element.

23. Al-Issa I: Sociocultural factors in hallucinations. Intl J Social Psychiatry 24:167–76, 1978.
One of the most basic differences between the organic and the sociocultural approaches to hallucinations is whether they indicate an underlying disease process such as schizophrenia or whether they are subjective experiences with true individual and social significance.

24. Al-Issa I: The Psychopathology of Women. Englewood Cliffs, N.J., Prentice-Hall, 1980.
Cultural and social factors influence the prevalence and diagnosis of mental illness in women.

25. Alissi AS: Boys in Little Italy. San Francisco, R & E Research Assoc., 1978.
A study conducted in a small Italian-American neighborhood in Cleveland supports the following hypotheses: the traditional subsystem is made up of boys with existing value orientations

who come from expanded families and belong to corner-boy groups; the mobile subsystem is made up of boys with achieving value orientations who come from nuclear families and belong to college-boy groups; and the deviant subsystem is made up of boys with conflicting value orientations who come from mixed families and belong to deviant-boy groups.

26. Allen IM, Brown JL, Jackson J, Lewis R: Psychological stress of young black children as a result of school desegregation. J Amer Acad Child Psychiatry 16:739–47, 1977.

Two black children, undergoing the stress of the Boston school desegregation program, experienced reactions suggesting that the maintenance of self-identity was severely threatened. While both were especially vulnerable due to their early family losses, most children, particularly of latency age, subjected to similar stresses would manifest negative reactions.

27. Allodi J, Dukszta J: Psychiatric services in China. Canadian Psychiatric Assn J 23:361–71, 1978.

Psychiatric services in China are concerned primarily with cases of psychosis and severe neurosis. Neurosis is viewed as a general health problem, and personality and behavior disorders are considered social or community matters.

28. Al-Najjar SY: Suicide and Islamic law. Mental Health Society 3:137–41, 1976.

Islamic law considers the act of abandoning life by destroying it as equal to wrecking of an edifice constructed by God. Martyrdom and self-sacrifice are rewarded by everlasting life in paradise, while suicide is punished by eternal fire. For those in a hopeless impasse, suicide is forgiven.

29. Altman I, Chemers MM: Cultural aspects of environmental-behavior relationships. In Handbook of Cross-Cultural Psychology, edited by HC Triandis and RW Brislin, 5:335–93. Boston, Allyn and Bacon, 1980.

Cultural and environmental phenomena are best viewed from a "systems" perspective and involve interdependency and multicausal relationships, with environment and culture operating on one another in a reciprocal fashion.

30. Amarasingham LR: Movement among healers in Sri Lanka: a case study of a Sinhalese patient. Culture Medicine Psychiatry 4:71–92, 1980.

Movement of the patient among a variety of treatment systems (Ayurvedic, Western, ritual practitioners) in Sri Lanka allows a fluidity of diagnosis that prevents any one explanatory system from dominating the patient's perception of mental illness. Treatments are linked by an underlying continuity of process in which the personal antecedents of the illness are reinterpreted in terms of public representations of affliction and in which all treatments focus on illness most basically in terms of excess and imbalance.

31. Amarasingham LR: Social and cultural perspectives on medication refusal. Amer J Psychiatry 137:353–57, 1980.

A complex interplay of social and cultural factors affects drug refusal. In prescribing medications, culturally shaped expectations and the meaning of the act of taking drugs should be explored to improve compliance.

32. Ananth J: Psychopathology in Indian females. Social Science and Medicine 12(3B):177–78, 1978.

The position of women in India is one of considerable stress, but the psychopathology they exhibit is not what one would find in Western women under similar conditions. Indian women manifest depression less frequently in spite of social pressures, and this is more so in rural settings than in urban. They do not aspire to change unfortunate circumstances.

33. Ananth J: The problems of Indian psychiatrists in an alien culture. Indian J Psychiatry 22:32–38, 1980.

Coming from a society that stresses family strength and discourages initiative and competitiveness, the Indian psychiatrist may have trouble adjusting to North American culture. The Indian psychiatrist can make a contribution to North American culture through the understanding brought about by his own struggles in the new country, through his cultural values of respect for the family and the aged, through an understanding of the principles of yoga and relaxation, and through a positive utilization of the dependency needs of some patients.

34. Anderson T: Ill health in two contrasting societies, particularly nonpsychiatric morbidity among those with a psychiatric diagnosis. Psychotherapy Psychosomatics 32:249–56, 1979.

A study of two culturally contrasting northern Norwegian societies—a coastal group and a Lapp group—indicates that those with psychiatric diagnoses are more prone to nonpsychiatric illnesses than those without psychiatric diagnoses. The nonpsychiatric illnesses began before the onset of the psychiatric conditions.

35. Andress VR, Corey DM: Regional suicide rates as a function of national political change. Psychological Reports 39:955–58, 1976.

Although the American presidential elective process is considered to be an orderly process of change representing stability in the international arena, some individuals may interpret the transitional uncertainties as a chaotic and stressful period that they cannot endure.

36. Angrosino MV: Applied anthropology and the concept of the underdog: implications for community mental health planning and evaluation. Comm Ment Health Journal 14:291–99, 1978.

Assessing the reasons for the success or failure of a program should not be an end in itself, but should instead be a process that generates guidelines for the development of similar programs elsewhere.

37. Ardener S (ed): Perceiving Women. New York, Halsted, 1975.

Women, as demonstrated by accounts of nuns, African militants, and gypsies, possess a hidden, muted structure from which they can detach themselves from men's designations and describe the deepest sense of their femininity.

38. Ardener S (ed): Defining Females. New York, Halsted, 1978.

The nature of women in society is studied by examining cultural conceptions of virginity, motherhood, and childbirth, socially imposed constraints on female behavior in Greece and Mongolia, and sociobiology.

39. Argyle M: Bodily Communication. New York, Intl. Universities Press, 1975.

Cultural differences, as demonstrated by case studies from Japan and the Arab world, greatly affect bodily communication.

40. Arieti S, Chrzanowski G (eds): New Dimensions in Psychiatry, Vol. 2. New York, Wiley-Interscience, 1977.

Topics discussed include sociogenic brain damage, folklore therapy in Japan, residential and day-care treatment in Czechoslovakia, a cross-cultural consideration of dependence, and various psychiatric issues in Sardinia, India, Spain, and Nigeria.

41. Armstrong H, Patterson P: Seizures in Canadian Indian children: individual, family and community approaches. Canadian Psychiatric Assn J 20:247–55, 1975.

Seizures in Canadian Indian children have a hysterical flavor and resemble the Eskimo culture-bound syndrome, piblokto.

42. Arthur GK, Brooks R, Long ML: A language-cultural course for foreign psychiatric residents. Amer J Psychiatry 136:1064–67, 1979.

Tailoring a course of study to the particular needs of foreign medical graduates in psychiatry is productive and gratifying. Such a course should focus on the intrapersonal, interpersonal, and social adjustment problems of foreign-trained physicians through the educational vehicles of communication and language.

43. Aschenbrenner J: Lifelines: Black Families in Chicago. New York, Holt, Rinehart & Winston, 1975.

Values attributed to blacks include (1) a high value on children, (2) approval of strong, protective mothers, (3) emphasis on strict discipline and respect for elders, (4) the strength of family bonds, and (5) the ideal of an independent spirit.

44. Ashcraft N, Scheflen A: People Space. Garden City, N.Y., Anchor, 1976.

Each person lives in psychological and physical space that has defined boundaries.

45. Asuni T: The dilemma of traditional healing with special reference to Nigeria. Social Science Medicine 13B(1):33–39, 1979.

Although herbalists in Nigeria find dramatic success with some of their potent medicines, they lack an adequate knowledge of the effects these potions may have on the patient.

46. Aurelius G: Adjustment and behavior of Finnish and southern European immigrant children in Stockholm: the teacher's assessment. Scand J Soc Medicine 7:105–13, 1979.

Immigrants as a whole have adjustment difficulties more often than the controls. Compared with controls (Swedish children who have lived in the country for more than four years), immigrant children show a higher frequency of symptoms relating to a disordered self-esteem, have a lower status, and are less trustworthy. Schooling of immigrant children demands serious attention in order to prevent discrimination and to promote a feeling of personal worth among them.

47. Aurelius G: Adjustment and behavior of Finnish immigrant children in Stockholm: the parent's assessment. Scand J Soc Medicine 8:43–48, 1980.

Behavior disorders are found in immigrant children more often soon after immigration than prior to it or three years after. Children from homes where there are relationship disturbances, alcoholism, or depression are more often maladjusted and have greater difficulty in being accepted at school.

48. Aurelius G: Oka vardpersonalens sprak—och kulturkompeten Beakta minoritetemas krav i planeringin. Lakartidningen 77:432–34, 1980.

With an increase in the number of immigrants in Sweden there is a greater need for bilingual interpreters to instruct health professionals on immigrant problems, and to extend cooperation between immigrant organizations and social welfare services.

49. Ausubel DP: The role of race and social class in the psychiatric disorders of treated narcotic addicts. Intl J Addictions 15:303–7, 1980.

Lower-class black narcotic addicts from a ghetto "welfare" setting primarily manifest reactive schizophrenia when they become mentally ill, whereas white lower-middle or working-class addicts primarily manifest reactive depression when they become mentally ill.

50. Avgar A, Bronfenbrenner U, Henderson CR: Socialization practices of parents, teachers, and peers in Israel: kibbutz, moshav, and city. Child Development 48:1219–27, 1977.

The cooperative organization of the larger society exerting a stronger effect than a traditional family structure is reflected by the moshav falling closer to the kibbutz than the city on a continuum of child-rearing patterns.

51. Aviram A, Milgram RM: Dogmatism, locus of control and creativity in children educated in the Soviet Union, the United States and Israel. Psychological Reports 4:27–34, 1977.

American and Israeli children are more open-minded, more internal in feelings of locus of control, and more creative in their thinking than Soviet children.

52. Awonigi TA: The dilemma of traditional childhood education in Africa, south of the Sahara. Mental Health Society 4:9–25, 1977.

Social, religious, economic, and political contacts with Europeans and Arabs have radically altered the African community's view of childhood and child-rearing practices. Africans are faced with the dilemma of how to advance with the rest of the world economically, politically, educationally, and socially and at the same time maintain their traditional value systems with minimum maladjustment to their mental health.

53. Ayonrinde A, Erinosho A: The development of a community psychiatric program at Igbo-Ora, Nigeria. Intl J Social Psychiatry 26:190–95, 1980.

Mental health education conducted in an atmosphere of equality and respect for the belief system of others helps in removing resistance and in developing enough trust for cooperation between Western therapeutic approaches and traditional healing practices.

54. Azayem GMA: The Islamic psycho-social approach to alcoholism. Comp Med East West 6:237–40, 1978.

Alcoholism in Islamic countries has such a low incidence that it is not yet considered a serious public-health problem of the Moslem states. The reason is that the precepts of Islam succeeded in reducing alcoholic dependence and offer a unique example in prohibiting this social evil.

55. Baasher TA: Mental health services for children in the Eastern Mediterranean region. Intl J Mental Health 7:49–64, 1978.

In most countries of the Eastern Mediterranean, the services for children are disjointed and isolated. Therefore, close coordination among medical, social, educational, judicial, and vocational services is needed to pool the resources and provide better, more comprehensive care and a more effective organizational framework to deal with the complexities of child mental health.

56. Babiker IE, Cox JL, Miller PM: The measurement of cultural distance and its relationship to medical consultations, symptomatology and examination performance of overseas students at Edinburgh University. Social Psychiatry 15:109–16, 1980.

Cultural distance per se is no handicap to overseas students.

57. Bachtold LM, Eckvall KL: Current value orientations of American Indians in northern California: the Hupa. J Cross-Cultural Psychology 9:367–75, 1978.

Maintenance of dual identity systems depends on a continuing commitment of the Hupa to a collateral orientation.

58. Bainbridge W: Satan's Power. Berkeley, U. of California Press, 1978.

The rise and fall of a strange, modern religious cult in Boston are recounted.

59. Bakan D: And They Took Themselves Wives: The Emergence of Patriarchy in Western Civilization. New York, Harper & Row, 1979.

As seen through Biblical studies, the ancient Semitic matriarchal society developed into a patriarchy with consequent stability of family life and unification of dispersed tribes. Christianity is the natural sociologic outgrowth of patrilineality and extends brotherhood to exist through faith.

60. Bakos M, Bozic R, Chapin D, Neuman S: Effects of environmental changes on elderly residents' behavior. Hosp Community Psychiatry 31:677–82, 1980.

Measurable, positive changes in residents' behavior occur among those who take part in decisionmaking about the environmental changes.

61. Baldanf RB, Ayabe HI: Acculturation and educational achievement in American Samoan adolescents. J Cross-Cultural Psychology 8:241–56, 1977.

Although several alternative approaches are operative, the modern-man approach to acculturation is clearly dominant when dealing with adolescents, regardless of sex.

62. Balkwell C, Balswick J, Balkwell JW: On black and white family patterns in America: their impact on the expressive aspect of sex-role socialization. J Marriage Family 40:743–48, 1978.

Black students tend to have lower levels of expressiveness of each of four emotions (fondness, sadness, pleasure, and antipathy) than white students. Black males are more expressive of antipathy, while females are more expressive of fondness, pleasure, and sadness. There is less sexual dimorphism among blacks than among whites in the expressiveness of pleasure.

63. Barash DP: Sociobiology and Behavior. New York, Elsevier, 1977.

When any behavior under study reflects some component of genotype, then animals should behave so as to maximize their inclusive fitness. The relationship between ecology and social organization is a correlation that does not necessarily imply causation.

64. Barger WK: Culture change and psychosocial adjustment. Amer Ethnologist 4(3):471–95, 1977.

Three general positions can be identified in the literature dealing with culture change and psychosocial adjustment: (1) change has a negative impact on adjustment, (2) adjustment hinges on the context of change, and (3) no universal relationship exists between change and adjustment. Any association between change and adjustment is case-specific rather than a universal phenomenon and is dependent upon the context in which change takes place.

65. Barkow JH: Culture and sociobiology. Amer Anthropologist 80:5–20, 1978.

Because biological and cultural evolution are two linked but conceptually distinct processes, sociobiology is more readily applied to the evolution of cultural capacity than to contemporary cultural behavior.

66. Barlett PG, Low SM: Nervios in rural Costa Rica. Medical Anthropology 4:523–59, 1980.

Nervios, a neurotic condition found more in women than in men, typically occurs during the early parenting years and when children have grown up and left home. Symptoms include anxiety, depression, and somatic complaints. Rural Costa Ricans perceive nervios to be caused by forces such as heredity. Since it results from unchangeable psychosocial stresses, the condition absolves the individual from responsibility for the situation.

67. Barnes FF: A psychiatric unit serving as an international community. Hosp Community Psychiatry 31:756–58, 1980.

Travel and a transcultural milieu may impart a special quality to mental illness and pose special difficulties in its management and treatment.

68. Barnlund DC: Public and Private Self in Japan and the United States. Tokyo, Simul, 1975.

Japanese and Americans have differing communication styles. The Japanese have a smaller "public self" and a larger "private self" than do Americans.

69. Barocas HA: Children of purgatory: reflections on the concentration camp survival syndrome. Intl J Social Psychiatry 21:87–92, 1975.

Children of concentration camp survivors may become the transferential recipients of parental unconscious and unexpressed rage. The survivors, being terrified of their own aggression and unable to express it, may broadcast explicit or implicit cues for their children to act it out, and vicariously gratify the wishes of the parents.

70. Barrera M Jr: Mexican-American mental health service utilization: a critical examination of some proposed variables. Comm Ment Health Journal 14:35–45, 1978.

Mexican-Americans are primarily underrepresented in the prevalence figures of public mental health facilities.

71. Barrett CJ, James-Cairns D: The social network in marijuana-using groups. Intl J Addictions 15:677–88, 1980.

Despite high levels of drug use, the most frequent reason for group participation is friendship. Popularity is related to frequency of group participation, but not to the extent of drug use.

72. Barry H: Description and uses of the Human Relations Area Files. In Handbook of Cross-Cultural Psychology, edited by HC Triandis and JW Berry, 2:445–78. Boston, Allyn and Bacon, 1980.

The Human Relations Area Files contain ethnographic source materials on more than 300 cultural units throughout the world. The extensive compilations of cultural information are powerful and widely available tools with applications to a wide variety of cross-cultural studies.

73. Bartollas C, Miller SJ, Dinitz S: Juvenile Victimization. New York, Sage, 1976.

The social structure of juvenile institutions includes a subculture of exploitation in which both staff and inmates participate.

74. Bartz KW, Levine ES: Childrearing by black parents: a description and comparison to Anglo and Chicano parents. J Marriage Family 40:709–19, 1978.

Black parents differ from Anglo and Chicano parents on several dimensions of childrearing. Black parents expect early autonomy, do not allow wasted time, are highly supportive and controlling, value strictness, and encourage equalitarian family roles.

75. Battegay R, Ladewig D, Muhlemann R, Weidmann M: The culture of youth and drug abuse in some European countries. Intl J Addictions 2:245–61, 1976.

Three general factors are responsible for drug use among Swiss juveniles: the family situation of childhood, the conflicts of norms of the society in which they are involved, and the milieu provocation. The replacement of old patterns of education by different ideological norms of the various groups composing modern society in some European countries has created a feeling of insecurity among the youth. Drug abuse primarily represents an attempt to get over this insecurity.

76. Beaglehole R: Blood pressure and social interaction in Tokelauan migrants in New Zealand. J Chronic Disease 30:803–12, 1977.

A study of 635 adult Tokelauans in New Zealand showed a significant positive association between blood pressure and social interaction, with persons who interact more with society having higher levels of blood pressure than those who have less interaction. The interaction of Tokelauans with the mainly white New Zealanders is found to be a risk factor for hypertension.

77. Bean P: Psychiatrists' assessments of mental illness: a comparison of some aspects of Thomas Scheff's approach to labelling theory. Brit J Psychiatry 135:122–28, 1979.

Labelling theory as formulated by Thomas Scheff is not supported by British psychiatrists.

78. Beardslee WR: The Way Out Must Lead In. Atlanta, Ga., Emory U. Center for Research in Social Change, 1977.

Eleven life histories of leaders in the American civil rights movement are presented.

79. Beck E, Daniel P: Kuru. Psychological Medicine 6:343–45, 1976.

Creutzfelot-Jakob disease, found primarily among the Fore of Eastern New Guinea, may be transmissible to mice, and it is hoped that progress in elucidating the basic causes of these degenerative diseases of the brain will advance more rapidly than it has done in the past, when the only animal available for experimental work was the rare and expensive primate.

80. Beck JC: To Windward of Land: The Occult World of Alexander Charles. Bloomington, Indiana U. Press, 1979.

Obeah is practiced on the Caribbean islands of St. Lucia and Dominica.

81. Beck L, Keddie N (eds): Women in the Muslim World. Cambridge, Mass., Harvard U. Press, 1978.

Muslim women are devalued, subjugated, and exploited by male-dominated society, and male-female relations are of an adversary nature.

82. Becker T: Other voices, self, and social responsibility: a comparative view of American and Israeli youth. Amer J Psychoanalysis 36:155–62, 1976.

Compared with young Israelis, young Americans are much more committed to the ideal of early independence and self-reliance, are more resentful of being encumbered by any social obligations, display a greater sense of detachment from other individuals and the collective, and exhibit a lower level of trust of others. Israelis tend to view their society as an extension of their own family and acknowledge their obligation to both; in the Americans' view, the family alone is to be trusted and rivals all other social entities that oblige the individual in any way.

83. Beels CC: Social networks, the family, and the schizophrenic patient: introduction to the issue. Schizophrenia Bull 4:512–21, 1978.

Ideology, morale, structure, and the larger social context are aspects of the social network of the schizophrenic patient that need to be examined in future research. Consumer organizations of schizophrenics and their families need to cooperate with organized psychiatry for social network formation.

84. Beels CC: Social networks and schizophrenia. Psychiatric Quarterly 51:209–15, 1979.

Schizophrenics are acutely sensitive to the influence of current social supports. Feeling they have nothing to offer in a social exchange, they often sever the relationships they were in before the schizophrenic episode, and establish a social network consisting of fellow patients, their relatives, and friends.

85. Begler EB: Sex, states, and authority in egalitarian society. Amer Anthropologist 80:571–88, 1978.

Examination of hunting and gathering societies reveals that in some (Australian Aborigine) men have great authority over women, while in others (Mbuti Pygmies) the relationship between the sexes operates in an egalitarian mode.

86. Beiser M: Coping with past and future: a study of adaptation to social change in West Africa. J Operational Psychiatry 11:140–55, 1980.

The effect of social change on the city of Dakar and traditional villages in Senegal challenges the assumption that social change is bad for mental health. The openness of society to satisfy aspirations is a critical variable affecting mental health.

87. Beit-Hallahmi B: Encountering orthodox religion in psychotherapy. Psychotherapy: Theory, Research, Practice 12:357–59, 1975.

The issue of the religious gap in the therapist-client relationship is best handled openly and directly, facilitating a smoother working alliance between the therapist and the client. The problem is one of encouraging differentiation without creating too much tension. Therapist-client differences have to be recognized, and the separation process in this instance can be used to encourage the client's individuality in the face of the therapist's obvious authority.

88. Beit-Hallahmi B, Argyle M: Religious ideas and psychiatric disorders. Intl J Social Psychiatry 23:26–30, 1977.

Occurrence of religious ideas as part of the content of individual delusional systems in psychiatric patients can be explained on the basis of exposure to religious ideas through the social environment.

89. Bell C: The Navajo patient. Colorado Medicine 77:127–30, 1980.

Though their religious/medical views have changed only slightly, a rise of confidence for the non-Navajo medicine is evidenced by the ability of non-Navajo doctors and medicine men to work together.

90. Beltrane T, McQueen DV: Urban and rural Indian drinking patterns: the special case of the Lumbee. Intl J Addictions 14:533–48, 1979.

The urban Lumbee have a drinking pattern that is heavier than that of the rural group. Low achievement and low satisfaction usually result in excessive drinking patterns.

91. Berger MM: Beyond the Double Bind. New York, Brunner/Mazel, 1978.

The concept of the double bind is discussed as it relates to communication, family systems, theories, and techniques with schizophrenics.

92. Bergin AE: Psychotherapy and religious values. J Consulting Clin Psychology 48:95–105, 1980.

Until the theistic belief systems of a large percentage of the population are sincerely considered and conceptually integrated into clinical psychology, psychotherapists are unlikely to be fully effective professionals.

93. Berglund AI: Zulu Thought Patterns and Symbolism. New York, Africana, 1976.

Zulu thought patterns and symbols include divinities and shades (living and dead senior relatives) that are associated with sacrifice, initiation, healing, and witchcraft.

94. Berlin IN: Anglo adoptions of Native Americans: repercussions in adolescence. J Amer Acad Child Psychiatry 17:387–88, 1978.

Native Americans placed in white foster homes suffer an estrangement from both cultures during their adolescence as the foster care is ended. Both long-term developmental needs and preservation of cultural ties need to be considered in the case of Native-American and other minority children placed in foster homes.

95. Berman J: Individual versus societal focus: problem disgnoses of black and white male and female counselors. J Cross-Cultural Psychology 10:497–507, 1979.

Black males and females tend to use a societal focus more frequently than do white males and females.

96. Bernard J: Women, Wives, Mothers. Hawthorne, N.Y., Aldine, 1975.

Research should focus on individual differences between men and women and should not assume a position of moral superiority on the part of women. New societal forms should be developed to help women integrate their roles as mothers and as labor-force participants.

97. Berndt RM (ed): Aborigines and Change: Australia in the '70's. Atlantic Highlands, N.J., Humanities, 1978.

Aborigines can go to outstations to avoid the pressure of assimilation. Those in urban areas are developing a new political consciousness.

98. Berry JW: Human Ecology and Cognitive Styles. New York, Sage, 1976.

Members of preliterate, nomadic, loose cultural groups tend to be field independent, while members of tight, sedentary, agricultural groups tend to be field dependent in their cognitive styles.

99. Berry JW: Social and cultural change. In Handbook of Cross-Cultural Psychology, edited by HC Triandis and RW Brislin, 5:211–79. Boston, Allyn and Bacon, 1980.

A developing role for psychology is being recognized in the study of social and cultural change. A schematic model is proposed that makes a number of distinctions, such as the differences between sociocultural and individual focus of change and between psychological antecedents and psychological consequents of change. Representative studies of psychological antecedents to change and psychological consequents of change are considered. Suggestions are made for reorienting the field of inquiry and for pursuing urgent research questions.

100. Berstein M: Causes and effects of marginality, a Latin American view of the mental health aspects. Intl J Mental Health 5:80–95, 1976.

Socioeconomic and cultural factors and criteria of health and illness create situations that give rise to discrimination against certain groups and cause them to become marginal to the general society. This condition of marginality produces certain mental disorders.

101. Beskow J: Suicide and mental disorder in Swedish men. Acta Psychiatrica Scandinavica, supplement 277:132, 1979.

The male suicide rate in Sweden is increasing slowly, due to an increase in the number of people below the age of 45. The major difference between urban suicides and rural suicides is the high proportion of drug abusers in the urban area.

102. Best DL, Williams JE, Cloud JM, Davis SW, Robertson LS, Edwards JR, Giles H, Fowles J: Development of sex-trait stereotypes among young children in the United States, England and Ireland. Child Development 48:1375–84, 1977.

The nature of sex stereotypes being learned by children in the three countries is very similar, with Irish children learning them slower than the others. There is a clear progression in sex-stereotype learning from age five to age eight.

103. Bhaskaran K: Psychiatry in India. Psychiatric Opinion 12:24–26, 1975.

The problem of mental health services in India is one of bridging the wide gap between community needs and meager resources in terms of professional personnel and funds.

104. Billig O, Burton-Bradley BG: The Painted Message. Cambridge, Mass., Schenkman, 1978.

Schizophrenic art in Western culture and in Papua New Guinea is examined. Commonalities in such art point to the universality of the basic psychopathology of schizophrenia.

105. Bilu Y: General characteristics of referrals to traditional healers in Israel. Israel Ann Psychiatry 15:245–52, 1977.

The majority of Moroccan-born Jews who seek help from traditional healers do so for a mixture of mental and somatic symptoms assumed to be caused by demons. Meetings with healers outside the patient's home community become a broad social-familial event in which family support is demonstrated.

106. Bilu Y: Demonic explanations among Moroccan Jews in Israel. Culture Medicine Psychiatry 3:363–80, 1979.

Demonic explanations of disease among Moroccan Jews living in Israel can be construed as a two-level ordered sequence of steps including elements from both ordinary reality and the demonic world. Traditional patients are usually more aware of the manifest chain of precipitating events centering around emotional consequences of real trauma. Their rabbi-healers, however, are predisposed toward molding these events into a covert demonic pattern, the core of which involves a human injuring a jinn and the latter's retaliation. Reasons for the hitherto tenacious preservation of the demonic component among traditional segments of Israel can be explained by comparing the explanatory status of demons and psychoanalytic concepts.

107. Bilu Y: Sigmund Freud and Rabbi Yehudah: on a Jewish mystical tradition of "psychoanalytic" dream interpretation. J Psychol Anthropology 2:443–63, 1979.

Kabbalists, modern religious scholars of Jewish mysticism, share the ideas and principles of psychoanalytic conceptions that Freud borrowed from Jewish tradition. Two Jewish dream interpreters differ from Freud in that they view dreams as expressions not of wish-fulfillment but of wishes fulfilled.

108. Bilu Y: The Moroccan demon in Israel: the case of the "evil spirit disease." Ethos 8:24–39, 1980.

Moroccan Jews in Israel may experience a possession syndrome characterized by immobility and muteness followed by disorganized and uncontrollably agitated behavior, including indiscriminate verbal and physical violence. Exorcism is the preferred method of treatment. Belief in demons is decreasing in this group because of contact with modern Israeli culture.

109. Binitie A: A factor-analytical study of depression across cultures (African and European). British J Psychiatry 127:559–63, 1975.

Depression in African cultures presents principally as depressed mood, somatic symptoms, and motor retardation. In European cultures depression presents as depressed mood, guilt, suicidal ideas, motor retardation, and anxiety. Guilt and suicidal ideas and acts are common in the African sample and appear to be culturally determined.

110. Binitie A: Mental health implications of economic growth in developing countries. Mental Health Society 3:272–85, 1976.

Developing countries are able as yet to manage neither poverty nor wealth, and this failure has a deleterious effect on physical and mental health. The problems of rural poverty, unplanned urban growth, and a rapid rise in population have to be tackled if the emotional and physical health problems of developing nations are to be adequately treated.

111. Binitie A: The psychological basis of certain culturally held beliefs. Intl J Social Psychiatry 23: 204–8, 1977.

Although belief in witchcraft, the spirit world, and the evil machinations of one's enemies is common in Nigeria, only a portion of people seem to utilize this cultural mechanism for the explanation of psychopathology.

112. Blaine A (ed): Alcoholism and the Jewish Community. NY Commission on Synagogue Relations, 1980.

With the increased secularization of the Jewish community in America, the same problems that face the general community now face the Jewish community. Alcohol abuse is concomitant with the weakening and destabilization of the Jewish family and with the erosion of traditional Jewish ideas and values.

113. Blane HT: Acculturation and drinking in an Italian-American community. J Stud Alcohol 38(7):1324–46, 1977.

Drinking practices among Italian-Americans involve aspects from both parent and host cultures that are selected and blended to form an amalgam that is unique to both societies. Italian men, who are more exposed to new patterns of behavior, adopt new ways and relinquish old ways more rapidly than women.

114. Blank RJ, Silk KR: Racism as a response to change: the introduction of residents onto a psychiatry ward. J Nerv Ment Disease 167(7): 416–21, 1979.

Covert staff disagreement can result in the scapegoating of black patients on a psychiatric ward. The scapegoating can be avoided by a process of reeducation of ward staff.

115. Blaxter M: Diagnosis as category and process: the case of alcoholism. Social Science Medicine 12(A):9–17, 1978.

Diagnostic activity is essentially a prescriptive one, and even though a condition may have been clearly accepted into the medical gallery, doctors may be reluctant to use it as a classification if it is one for which no clear medical treatment exists.

116. Blixin O: El heva de los antiguos Pascuenses. Moana 1:1–13, 1977.

Heva is a condition found on Easter Island in which a person puts a rat in his mouth and runs around violently with a club. Upon being told that a relative has been murdered, he then seeks vengeance on the killer. The condition, similar to amok, occurs when a person is worried about a missing relative, and it induces others to talk with him about the relative.

117. Block S, Reddaway P: Psychiatric Terror. New York, Basic Books, 1977.

Psychiatry is misused in the Soviet Union for political purposes.

118. Bloom JD, Bloom JL: Psychiatric participation in the Hootch Case: effects on Alaska native education. Amer J Psychiatry 137:959–62, 1980.

Psychiatric participation in cases involving important social issues helps with primary prevention and decreases psychiatric morbidity.

119. Bloomingdale LW: Chinese psychiatry after Mao Zedong. Psychiatric Annals 10(6):7–24, 1980.

Psychotherapy in China consists of telling the patient in what way his thoughts are abnormal. "Face" is very important, so shame over nonconformity is a powerful motivating force for improvement.

120. Blum H (ed): Female Psychology. New York, Intl. Universities Press, 1977.

Contemporary psychoanalytic views of female psychology are presented, as are discussions of the influence of social attitudes.

121. Blumberg LV, Shipley TE, Barsky SF: Liquor and Poverty: Skid Row as a Human Condition. New Brunswick, N.J., Rutgers Center of Alcohol Studies, 1978.

Skid row is not a specific geographic area; rather, skid row people are found whenever there is poverty, in slum neighborhoods, the low-income ethnic enclaves, even in the suburbs. Poverty and addiction lead to disaffiliation and the skid row condition. Only through urban planning and renewal can future skid rows be prevented.

122. Bochner S: Unobtrusive methods in cross-cultural experimentations. In Handbook of Cross-Cultural Psychology, edited by HC Triandis and JW Berry, 2:319–87. Boston, Allyn and Bacon, 1980.

The major contribution of the unobtrusive method will be to foster the development of a cross-cultural psychology of social behavior. The current emphasis in psychology is to select for research those phenomena suited to existing methods. The unobtrusive approach reverses this trend by shaping and developing experimental procedures to fit phenomena; that is why the unobtrusive method will continue to be used in studies that address real-life problems.

123. Bodley JH: Victims of Progress. Menlo Park, Calif., Cummings, 1975.

Government policies and attitudes, often under the guise of "progress" or "raising standards of living," have undermined and destroyed tribal cultures throughout the world. The price of progress, as exemplified especially by Australian Aborigines and Native Americans, has been poverty, disease, mental illness, and discrimination.

124. Boissevain J: Network analysis: a reappraisal. Current Anthropology 20:392–94, 1979.

Network analysis is a research instrument which can help resolve certain social and theoretical problems. It must not become an esoteric area where practitioners can communicate only with each other about scientific puzzles of interest only to themselves.

125. Boles J, Tatro C: The new male role. Amer J Psychoanalysis 40:227–37, 1980.

In the future, men will continue to ideologically support the traditional male stereotype though they may incorporate some feminine attributes. Men will continue to experience role conflict as they are forced to accommodate to the structure of modern society and the limits that it puts on male activity.

126. Bolman W, Maretzki T: Child Psychiatry in Asian Countries: A Book of Readings. Quezon City, Philippines, New Day, 1979.

Indonesia, Malaysia, the Philippines, Singapore, and Thailand are nations with a large population of children but very few child psychiatrists. Child-rearing patterns in these countries often differ greatly from Western patterns. Community family life centers and community information centers may assist persons caught in the shift from peasant-rural to industrial life.

127. Bolton R: Andean coca chewing. Amer Anthropologist 78:630–34, 1976.

Coca chewing may be critical for the adaptation and survival of Andean Indians under high altitude conditions since it has metabolic functions that enhance glucose homeostasis.

128. Bond TC: The why of fragging. Amer J Psychiatry 133:1328–31, 1976.

The men convicted of using explosives in assaults on superior officers during the Vietnam War shared several characteristics, including deprived and/or brutal family backgrounds, poor self-image, externalization, insecurity and vulnerability, and lack of critical self-observation. Drug use and the situation these men found in Vietnam combined with their personal characteristics led to the assault of a figure perceived as powerful and threatening.

129. Bonfiglio G, Falli S, Pacini A: Alcoholism in Italy. Intl J Mental Health 5:52–62, 1976.

In Italy, alcoholism is the concern of isolated physicians (chiefly psychiatrists) and social workers, but has not yet received recognition by government agencies as a national medical and social problem. Currently, there are no provisions for treating the underlying psychological and social components of the disorder.

130. Boroffka A, Olatawura MO: Community psychiatry in Nigeria—the current status. Intl J Social Psychiatry 23:275–81, 1977.

Patients treated in a village hospital under no pressure to be discharged have fewer symptoms on discharge than those patients treated in a university hospital where there is great pressure to be discharged.

131. Boroffka A, Pfeiffer WM (eds): Fragen der Transkulturell-Vergleickenden Psychiatrie in Europa. Meunster, Germany, Westfalische Wilhelms-Universitat, 1977.

Topics discussed include intelligence tests and culture, and psychiatric profiles of immigrants, especially foreign workers in Germany.

132. Borunda P, Shore JH: Neglected minority urban Indians and mental health. Intl J Social Psychiatry 24:220–24, 1978.

Effective health services for a clearly neglected population can be obtained by sensitive treatment of issues such as tribal diversity, traditional values, and positive cultural reinforcements.

133. Boton R: Child-holding patterns. Current Anthropology 19:134–35, 1979.

There is a universal tendency for women to hold their infants on the left side.

134. Bourguignon E: Possession. San Francisco, Chandler and Sharp, 1976.

Possession beliefs can be divided into trance behavior and nontrance behavior. The former may be associated with spirit impersonation and the latter with illness and witchcraft. Trance is an experience while possession trance is a performance.

135. Bourguignon E: Psychological Anthropology. New York, Holt, Rinehart & Winston, 1979.

Psychological anthropology is distinguished by an explicit concern for psychological and psychodynamic elements in human behavior and a focus on the study of socialization and child development.

136. Bourne P: The Chinese student—acculturation and mental illness. Psychiatry 38:269–77, 1975.

Demands are mixed and conflicting on Chinese students, and too often these students are ill equipped in dealing with the Caucasian campus population. A better appreciation of the problems of assimilation will not only ease the process for the Chinese students but will benefit the whole society.

137. Bowen WT, Twemlow SW, Boquet RE: Assessing community attitudes toward mental illness. Hosp Community Psychiatry 29:251–53, 1978.

Respondents believe that mental illness is caused by a lack either of physical health or of proper nurturing, rather than seeing it as punishment for sins. Respondents with no children at home are more receptive to the idea of accepting a family-care patient, while those with children at home are highly ambivalent.

138. Boyer LB: On aspects of the mutual influences of anthropology and psychoanalysis. J Psychol Anthropology 1:265–96, 1978.

Psychoanalytic ideas about mental functioning and personality development have been useful to those anthropologists interested in the study of the mutual influences of personality and culture, and in expressive culture. Similarly, psychoanalysts are using anthropological data to validate and modify some of their ethnocentric ideas.

139. Boyer LB: Childhood and Folklore. New York, Library of Psychological Anthropology, 1979.

Apache personality development, socialization, and behavior disorders can be understood from a psychoanalytic viewpoint.

140. Boyer LB, Devos G, Borders O, Tani-Borders A: The "burnt child reaction" among the Yukon Eskimos. J Psychol Anthropology 1:7–56, 1978.

The burnt child reaction, a Rorschach response constellation that indicates an intense early emotional gratification followed by severe early emotional traumatization, is found in a high proportion of Eskimos. The physical contact between Eskimo mother and child provides both gratification and frustration. With the birth of the next sibling, the displaced child loses his previous intimacy with his mother and is further frustrated.

141. Bozzetti IL, Bozzetti LP: The aged in Sweden: samaritans and the marginal elderly. Psychiatric Annals 7(3):87–91, 1977.

The home-help or "samaritan" program in Sweden seeks to reduce the decrements in function brought about by secondary aging, which reflects the effects of environment on aging. By allowing the aged to function at a level they consider optimal and by allowing them to rely upon themselves, the program helps to slow down the passivity and emotional withdrawal brought on by debilitating illness.

142. Bozzetti LP: The aged in Sweden: a systems approach—the Swedish model. Psychiatric Annals 7(3):63–81, 1977.

To avoid the despair that older Swedes face as they approach retirement, the government has encouraged the idea of a "preretirement period" to allow them to gradually relinquish their roles as workers and accept retirement. Various social supports, in the areas of housing and health care, allow the elderly to maintain their independence.

143. Bozzetti LP, Sherman S: The aged in Sweden: the country, its people and institutions. Psychiatric Annals 7(3):46–62, 1977.

Within the Swedish health-care system the specialty of long-term care sets ambitious goals for patients. Each person who is handicapped by age or illness should have a reasonable chance to improve through facilities that provide a pleasant environment, excellent medical services, a strong rehabilitation program, and a full range of activities while hospitalized.

144. Bradley S, Sloman L: Elective mutism in immigrant families. J Amer Acad Child Psychiatry 14:510–14, 1975.

Elective mutism is more likely among children whose mothers, often unwilling immigrants, demonstrate fear and hostility to their new surroundings. By refusing to speak in class, the child reinforces the mother's dream of returning home, as the parents often threaten to send the child back to their native land.

145. Bradshaw WH: Training psychiatrists for working with blacks in basic residency programs. Amer J Psychiatry 135:1520–24, 1978.

Psychiatrists are lacking in critical knowledge of black people, the systems that impinge on them, pertinent growth and development data, and the understanding of the psychodynamics of racial relationships in the United States. Specific training for working with black patients, psychotherapeutic issues, and problems encountered in biracial and/or transcultural therapy should be integrated in the traditional residency programs.

146. Brain JL: Sex, incest, and death: initiation rites reconsidered. Current Anthropology 18:191–208, 1977.

Cause and effect in initiation rites are intertwined. The causes of rites are only to be sought in unconscious psychological processes of thought, which have a feedback effect through the immensely complex medium of human language and response to symbols.

147. Brandes S: Metaphors of Masculinity: Sex and Status in Andalusian Folklore. Philadelphia, U. of Pennsylvania Press, 1980.

The maintenance of masculinity and man's place in the social hierarchy are concerns of the Andalusian (Spain) man.

148. Brautigam W, Osei Y: Psychosomatic illness, concept and psychotherapy among the Akan of Ghana. Canadian J Psychiatry 24:451–57, 1979.

Western medicine has no psychotherapeutic alternative to offer for a "developing country" like Ghana. The traditional healing methods existing in such countries must be preserved and researched in order to maintain them at least at their present standard.

149. Braxton ET: Structuring the black family for survival and growth. Perspectives Psychiatric Care 14:165–73, 1976.

The black family, as the primary unit of socialization for the black community, must maximize the survival and facilitate the growth of its members. Blacks are still an oppressed group in this country, not only economically but, more significantly, psychologically, and the condition of oppression, with its racist components, is a determinant in conceptualizing the black family system.

150. Brazelton TB, Koslowski B, Tronick E: Neonatal behavior among urban Zambians and

Americans. J Amer Acad Child Psychiatry 15:97–107, 1976.

The Zambian infant recovers rapidly from his inadequate intrauterine environment due to his genetic abilities, supportive child-rearing practices, and cultural expectations of precocious development. The American child, with a more favorable intrauterine environment, is expected to have a prolonged infancy, and child-rearing practices are more protective and relatively nonstimulating.

151. Brenneis CB, Roll S: Ego modalities in the manifest dreams of male and female Chicanos. Psychiatry 38:172–85, 1975.

When the manifest dreams of young adult male and female Chicanos are examined, striking differences are found in the areas of setting, characters, interaction, self, instinctual modalities, and realism.

152. Brenneis CB, Roll S: Dream patterns in Anglo and Chicano young adults. Psychiatry 39:280–90, 1976.

Polarization of dreamers' preferred modes of activation (preferred ego modalities) for males and females in the Chicano subculture is not carried through to the same extreme for male and female Anglos. Cultural differences also exist in the perception and interpretation of dreams among the Chicanos and Anglos.

153. Brislin RW: Translation and content analysis of oral and written material. In Handbook of Cross-Cultural Psychology, edited by HC Triandis and JW Berry, 2:389–444. Boston, Allyn and Bacon, 1980.

The future of cross-cultural research will depend on its contribution to theory in general psychology. Methods will be only a means to the major goal of discovering important, central facts about human behavior. Every cross-cultural researcher, at one time or another, will deal with oral and written materials in the form of instructions to subjects, response protocols obtained from subjects, and content analysis of existing materials. Hence some knowledge concerning the processing of such materials is mandatory.

154. Brody EB, Ottey F, Lagranade J: Early sex education in relationship to later coital and reproductive behavior: evidence from Jamaican women. Amer J Psychiatry 133:969–72, 1976.

Lack of special information from the mothers of a group of Jamaican women coupled with chronic resentment was associated with multi-ple sexual partners and more pregnancies. Age at first pregnancy did not relate to early availability of sexual information, and was less significantly correlated with overall education, in contrast to age at first coitus.

155. Bromberg W: From Shaman to Psychotherapist. Chicago, Henry Regnery, 1975.

The history of the treatment of mental illness is recorded from ancient times to the present.

156. Bronfenbrenner U: The Ecology of Human Development. Cambridge, Mass., Harvard U. Press, 1979.

Human development is a process of a mutual accommodation between an active, growing human being and the changing properties of the immediate settings in which the developing person lives. The process is affected by relations between these settings and by the larger contexts in which the settings are embedded.

157. Broude GJ, Greene SJ: Cross-cultural codes on twenty sexual attitudes and practices. Ethnology 15:409–29, 1976.

Codes may be developed for a long-range study on styles of male-female attachment. Such a study would examine the patterning of opposite-sex relationships in cross-cultural perspective and isolate any social, structural, or psychological antecedents that might help to explain variations in heterosexual relationships from one culture to the next.

158. Browman DL, Schwarz R (eds): Spirits, Shamans, and Stars: Perspectives from South America. The Hague, Mouton, 1979.

Topics discussed include innovative mental health therapists' approaches in Guyana and a Peruvian curer's seance.

159. Brown ED, Sechrest L: Experiments in cross-cultural research. In Handbook of Cross-Cultural Psychology, edited by HC Triandis and JW Berry, 2:297–318. Boston, Allyn and Bacon, 1980.

Cross-cultural research can fulfill a necessary and valuable role in the advancement of theoretical knowledge, particularly in those areas of study where answers cannot be found within an individual culture, or where there are too many natural sources of confounding in a culture to allow valid conclusions to be made.

160. Brown GW, Harris T: Social Origins of Depression. New York, Free Press, 1978.

A study of women in Camberwell (London)

and the Outer Hebrides (Scotland) points to social factors that lead to increased risk of depression in women and explores links among social, economic, and cultural systems and their impact on the individual.

161. Brown LC, Itzkowitz N: Psychological Dimensions of Near Eastern Studies. Princeton, N.J., Darwin, 1977.

Topics discussed include culture, psychopathology, and psychiatry in the Arab East, mother-child and other human relations in Islam, psychiatry in Turkey, and Iranian national character.

162. Bruhn JG, Fuentes RG Jr: Cultural factors affecting utilization of services by Mexican-Americans. Psychiatric Annals 7(12):20–29, 1977.

Mexican-Americans believe illness to be God's will, and that such illnesses as susto (shock) and mal ojo (evil eye) are supernaturally caused and can be treated only by curanderos and other folk healers. Folk healers openly deal with the interpersonal relationships of their patients, and most physicians and nurses fail to achieve the close patient relationship that the folk healer achieves.

163. Brummit H: Impressions of a black psychiatrist in a college dealing with black and other minority students. Amer J Psychoanalysis 37:13–21, 1977.

Minority students on predominantly white, middle-class college campuses have various psychosocial problems including educational and psychiatric handicaps mainly due to deprivations in economic, educational, and other environmental factors. A black psychiatrist acting as a consultant can help as a facilitating bridge to the black students who do not want to communicate with white professionals.

164. Bruni P, Eysenck HJ: Structure of attitudes: an Italian sample. Psychological Reports 38:956–58, 1976.

Italians show a patterning of attitudes very similar to that of people in other industrialized nations.

165. Budson RD, Jolley RE: A crucial factor in community program success: the extended psychosocial kinship system. Schizophrenia Bull 4:609–21, 1978.

A crucial factor in community program success is the program's capacity to foster and strengthen an extended psychosocial network of neighbors, friends, and associates at work or school, as well as the extended kinship system. The chronically hospitalized patient and the young, isolated, acutely psychotic adult are both in need of an enhanced psychosocial system when entering a community program.

166. Bulka R (ed): Mystics and Medics. New York, Human Sciences, 1979.

There are many similarities between mystical experiences and psychotherapeutic encounters.

167. Burch EA, Powell CH: The psychiatric assessment of a Vietnamese refugee through art. Amer J Psychiatry 137:236–37, 1980.

Patients with cross-cultural language difficulties can be helped using art therapy to assess their mental status and progress.

168. Burgoyne RW: Effect of drug ritual changes in schizophrenic patients. Amer J Psychiatry 133:284–89, 1976.

Evaluation of chronic schizophrenics to determine the effect of changes in long-term medication regimens revealed no significant differences between group attendance and change or no change in medication routine.

169. Burgoyne RW, Burgoyne RH: Conflicts secondary to overt paradoxes in belief systems —the Mormon women example. J Operational Psychiatry 8(2):39–45, 1977.

The problems of religious women seen in psychiatric treatment have a partial basis in the institutionalized paradoxes inherent in their role in modern society. By attacking these reality-based conflicts and assaulting the patient's belief system, the trust needed for a therapeutic relationship is not achieved and results of psychotherapy are poor. To successfully treat these women, one must have an understanding of the depth of their traditions and commitment to their church.

170. Buriel R: Cognitive styles among three generations of Mexican American children. J Cross-Cultural Psychology 6:417–29, 1975.

Anglo-American children are the most field dependent and show the smallest sex difference, followed respectively by second, first, and third generation Mexican-American children.

171. Burke AW: Attempted suicide among Asian immigrants in Birmingham. Brit J Psychiatry 128:528–33, 1976.

The immigrant group is underrepresented among attempted suicide admissions to Birmingham (England) hospitals. The attempted suicide rates in immigrants (South Asian) are lower than the rates found among natives in Britain, but the female immigrant rate is higher than that found in India. Asian patients who attempt suicide are younger than forty-five, rarely abuse drugs and alcohol, and make repeated attempts infrequently.

172. Burke AW: Attempted suicide among the Irish-born population in Birmingham. Brit J Psychiatry 128:534–37, 1976.
The average annual rate of admission for attempted suicide among the Irish-born population in Birmingham (England) is higher than the rates in Ireland. Fewer Irish than British admissions give a history of previous attempted suicide or repeat their attempt.

173. Burke AW: Socio-cultural determinants of attempted suicide among West Indians in Birmingham: ethnic origin and immigrant status. Brit J Psychiatry 129:261–66, 1976.
Self-poisoning among West Indian immigrants in Birmingham (England) is less prevalent than among natives there, but more prevalent than in the West Indies. Attempted suicide among immigrants is often relatively benign; few abuse alcohol or drugs or make repeated suicide attempts.

174. Burke AW: Attempted suicide among Commonwealth immigrants in Birmingham. Intl J Social Psychiatry 24:7–11, 1978.
Attempted suicide among immigrants in Birmingham (England) is benign in comparison with that among the natives there.

175. Burke AW: Social attempted suicide: young women in two contrasting areas. Intl J Social Psychiatry 25:198–202, 1979.
In the inner zones of the industrial city where migrants live in poor social conditions, the suicide rates are significantly higher than those found in West Indian island societies where, despite the lower living standards, the sociocultural environment may be more supportive.

176. Burke AW: Trends in social psychiatry in the Caribbean. Intl J Social Psychiatry 25:110–17, 1979.
Two recent trends in social psychiatry in the Caribbean are (1) the minority status of the Western-trained psychiatrists and their inability to make contact with traditional therapists, and (2) the pervasive and impossible task of unravelling social psychiatric pathology in an area disrupted by internal and external migration and remigration and disorganized by social change and a population deprived of adequate living standards.

177. Burke AW: A cross cultural study of delinquency among West Indian boys. Intl J Social Psychiatry 26:81–87, 1980.
One-third of West Indian school boys have a neurotic disorder that can be treated by psychotherapy. Delinquency is associated with personal aggression rather than with property offenses. Evidence of parental deviance is infrequently found.

178. Burton-Bradley BG: Stone Age Crisis. Nashville, Tenn., Vanderbilt U. Press, 1975.
Mental illness and psychiatric practice in Papua New Guinea are described. Cargo cult leaders are usually psychotic. Popular modes of suicide include poisoning by derris root and by running amok. Amok is a psychogenic disorder that is seriously influenced by group expectations.

179. Burton-Bradley BG: Single case study: cannibalism for cargo. J Nerv Ment Disease 163(6):428–31, 1976.
Cannibalism is not confined to exotic people but is part of the human condition. It occurs as a preferred form of protein consumption or as the result of extreme necessity, to absorb the virtues of others, to facilitate conception, for magicoreligious reasons, in warfare, famine, revenge, filial piety, and justice.

180. Burton-Bradley BG: Kung fu for cargo. J Nerv Ment Disease 166(2):885–89, 1978.
A patient who suffered a grandiose paranoia following head injury used kung fu in his attempts toward acquisition of both material and spiritual cargo in a Melanesian cargo cult.

181. Burton-Bradley BG: Arecaidinism: betel chewing in transcultural perspective. Canadian J Psychiatry 24:481–88, 1979.
Arecaidinism, or betel-nut habituation, has existed since earliest recorded times in Australia and is inextricably interwoven with the overall patterning of psychological, social, cultural, and economic behavior. Betel nut is a fairly harmless stimulant and addictive agent. Arguments against its use are scientifically unsupported.

182. Butcher JN, Panchari P: A Handbook of Cross-National MMPI Research. Minneapolis, U. of Minnesota Press, 1976.

Although there are some problems, the MMPI can be used worldwide.

183. Butler RM: Why Survive? Being Old in America. New York, Harper and Row, 1975.

Many elderly Americans live in substandard housing and are financially impoverished. Depression and hypochondriasis commonly accompany the many physical ailments of old age. Simply extending the human life span for more years is inhumane without an improvement in the quality of late life. In regard to the elderly, American society must adopt new attitudes and reform its institutions and social programs.

184. Byrnes RF (ed): Communal Families in the Balkans: The Zadruga. Notre Dame, Ind., U. of Notre Dame Press, 1976.

The Zadruga, a communal family organization, is disappearing in the Balkans.

185. Cairns E, Hunter D, Herring L: Young children's awareness of violence in Northern Ireland: the influence of Northern Irish television in Scotland and Northern Ireland. Brit J Social Clinical Psychology 19:3–6, 1980.

Severe pathological reactions to stress in children have been the exception rather than the rule. Television news can distort perceptions of reality.

186. Caldwell BM: Social changes and patterns of child care in the United States. Intl J Mental Health 6:32–48, 1977.

Many of the social changes that have alarmed those concerned about child welfare express the needs of adults, not children.

187. Camberwell Council on Alcoholism: Women and Alcohol. New York, Tavistock, 1980.

The broad sociological and psychological factors underlying the causes, patterns, and consequences of drinking problems and alcoholism are noted.

188. Campbell J: The Mythic Image. Princeton, N.J., Princeton U. Press, 1975.

The major civilizations of the world share many mythological motifs that originate in the remains of the primal physical and fantastic experience, the immediate interpersonal environment, and the perceived mathematical order of the earth and of the heavens.

189. Campbell JD: Illness is a point of view: the development of children's concepts of illness. Child Development 46:92–100, 1975.

In the domain of illness concepts, children pro-

fit from experiences, but the extent to which they do so may be contingent on their level of development.

190. Caplan G, Killilea M (eds): Support Systems and Mutual Help. New York, Grune and Stratton, 1976.

Support systems—such as the family, self and mutual help groups, and religious groups—help individuals with acute crises and long-term stresses by promoting emotional mastery, offering guidance in dealing with problems, and by providing feedback about a person's behavior.

191. Caplan P, Bujira J (eds): Women United, Women Divided. Bloomington, Indiana U. Press, 1979.

Women in various cultures (China, Kenya, India, England, Sierra Leone, Australia, Sudan, Caribbean) express both solidarity and antagonism to class structure.

192. Cappanari SC: Voodoo in the general hospital. JAMA 232:938–40, 1975.

The case of a young black woman who believed herself hexed emphasizes the interplay between modern medicine and the influence of a voodoo subculture. The patient was able to use the hex to adequately explain her stillborn child, her husband's desertion, and the development of regional enteritis. The ambivalence of the patient toward the acceptance of either modern medicine or voodoo probably allowed her to avoid her predicted death.

193. Cappon J: Masochism: a trait in the Mexican national character. Psychoanalytic Review 64:163–71, 1977.

The conquest of Mexico by Cortez influenced Mexican national character traits, especially instituting masochism into the Mexican social character.

194. Carleton JL, Stentz KT: Socio-cultural modalities in population control. Mental Health Society 3:197–204, 1976.

All efforts to achieve world population control will be ineffective unless the insights of the holistically oriented science of social psychiatry are refined into principles and rules that direct population control endeavors. Effective population control is possible if the actions of world leaders are directed toward efforts to achieve satisfaction of the basic needs of all individuals and groups for physical survival, socialization, and transcendence.

195. Carpenter L, Brockington IF: A study of mental illness in Asians, West Indians and Africans living in Manchester. Brit J Psychiatry 137:201–5, 1980.

Migrant populations have a higher rate of psychiatric morbidity than nonmigrants in Manchester (England). Asians and women have the highest rate of psychiatric disorders. Most of the immigrants suffer from paranoid psychosis, not schizophrenia.

196. Carr JE: Ethno-behaviorism and the culture-bound syndromes: the case of amok. Culture Medicine Psychiatry 2:269–93, 1978.

The ethno-behavioral model postulates that culture-bound syndromes consist of culturally specific behavioral repertoires legitimated by culturally sanctioned norms and concepts but with both behavior and norms acquired in accordance with basic principles of human learning universal to all cultures. Amok is a common behavioral pathway for multiple participants but with a distinct form and conceptualization that can be traced to the social-learning practices and beliefs of the Malay.

197. Carr JE, Tan EK: In search of the true amok: amok as viewed within the Malay culture. Am J Psychiatry 133:1295–99, 1976.

Twenty-one Malaysian amoks are interviewed to discover how the phenomenon of amok is viewed within its indigenous culture. Both the subjects and their culture view amok, a violent homicidal assault, as psychopathological.

198. Carrier JM: Cultural factors affecting urban Mexican male homosexual behavior. Arch Sex Behavior 5:103–24, 1976.

Effeminate Mexican men are characterized as homosexuals by the macho culture and may act out a self-fulfilling prophecy.

199. Carstairs GM: Revolutions and the rights of man. Amer J Psychiatry 134:979–83, 1977.

There is an ongoing struggle in psychiatric treatment between those who advocate maximum liberty in management of the mentally disordered and those who believe such patients will benefit more from firm guidance and discipline. Two current challenges to psychiatry worldwide are the unconstructive hostility of the various schools of antipsychiatry and the political abuse of psychiatric diagnosis and treatment, particularly in the Soviet Union.

200. Carstairs GM, Kapur RL: The Great Universe of Kota: Stress, Change, and Mental Disorder in an Indian Village. Berkeley, U. of California Press, 1976.

The Brahmins, Bants, and Mogers who live in the small village of Kota (southwest India) usually go to healers known as vaids, mantarwadis, and patris as well as to modern medical doctors. Complaints of spirit possession and of psychiatric symptoms are common.

201. Cassell EJ: The Healer's Art. New York, J. B. Lippincott, 1976.

By distinguishing between illness and disease, and by not acting as technicians, physicians may restore the art of healing to medicine.

202. Cawte J: Psychosexual and cultural determinants of fertility choice behavior. Amer J Psychiatry 132:750–53, 1975.

The fertility-choice behavior of traditional societies in Oceania, while directed toward spirits and magic, has an empirical basis. The alternatives to population control sometimes used—murder and starvation—should be replaced by more modern methods.

203. Cawte J: Mockery for the ancestors: the dynamics of disrespect in aboriginal society. J Psychol Anthropology 1:211–20, 1978.

The dynamics of mockery, the disrespect that it entails, and the psychodynamic elements underlying it are illustrated by the Yolngu aborigines of Australia.

204. Chakraborty A: Rejoinder to Estroff's "The anthropology-psychiatry fantasy." Transcult Psych Res Review 16:109–11, 1979.

It is feasible for psychiatrists to learn a little anthropology, but it is futile and dangerous for anthropologists to acquire only a little psychiatry.

205. Chandler CR: Traditionalism in a modern setting: a comparison of Anglo- and Mexican-American value orientations. Human Organization 38:153–59, 1979.

Traditionalism among Mexican-Americans makes their adjustment to urban life more difficult than it otherwise would be.

206. Chandrasena R, Rodrigo A: Schneider's first rank symptoms: their prevalence and diagnostic implications in an Asian population. Brit J Psychiatry 135:348–51, 1979.

In Sri Lanka Schneider's first rank symptoms are present in only those receiving a diagnosis of schizophrenia. Low prevalence of first rank symptoms is culturally related. Those patients with first rank symptoms in the first episode develop more symptoms during subsequent episodes.

207. Charles C: Brief comments on the occurrence of etiology and treatment of indisposition. Social Science Medicine 13B(2):135–36, 1979.

Haitians in general experience indisposition on occasions of great grief following the loss of someone dear. It is commonly acknowledged to occur among children when there are such problems as intestinal worms.

208. Chatel J, Joe B: Psychiatry in Spain: past and present. Amer J Psychiatry 132:1182–86, 1975.

The history of Spanish psychiatry includes pioneering efforts in establishing mental institutions and a strong alliance between psychiatry and literature. Modern Spanish psychiatrists are less innovative than their foreign contemporaries, emphasizing the historical and cultural context of psychiatry and the importance of family and other sociocultural factors.

209. Chaudhry MR: First experience of a rehabilitation centre for schizophrenics in a developing country. Comp Med East West 6:103–8, 1978.

Mental health services in Pakistan are still at the elementary level. Discharged patients from the mental hospitals find great difficulty in rehabilitating themselves in the community, particularly when the period of hospitalization has been long.

210. Chaudhry MR, Misza L: Rehabilitation of schizophrenics in a developing country. Mental Health Society 4:301–7, 1977.

Results from a four-year follow-up study of a rehabilitation center for the mentally ill in Labore, Pakistan, having collaborative ties with the Fountain House Rehabilitation Center in New York City show that programs and ideas developed in one country can be profitably utilized in another country.

211. Chen PCY: Main puteri: an indigenous Kelantanese form of psychotherapy. Intl J Social Psychiatry 25:167–75, 1979.

The *main puteri* is the most elaborate of all the traditional healing ceremonies available to the Kelantanese and is only resorted to after the family of the sick individual has exhausted the more mundane healing ceremonies. The involvement of family, relatives, and friends tends to enhance group solidarity and reintegrate the sick individual into his immediate social group.

212. Chen RM: The education and training of Asian foreign medical graduates in the United States. Amer J Psychiatry 135:451–53, 1978.

Asian physicians are a growing majority among foreign medical graduates practicing psychiatry in the United States. Particular attention should be given to curriculum enrichment programs, the acculturation process, and role models and supervision in the training of Asian physicians.

213. Chess S, Thomas A, Cameron M: Sexual attitudes and behavior patterns in a middle-class adolescent population. Amer J Orthopsychiatry 46:689–701, 1976.

Present generation adolescents evince a more matter-of-fact, less fearful attitude toward sex than previous generations, but are not more prone to casual sexual encounters. Sexual conflicts occur only in relation to overall psychological conflict.

214. Chimbos PD: Marital Violence: A Study of Interspouse Homicide. San Francisco, R & E Research Associates, 1978.

Social conditions and processes under which interspouse homicide is likely to occur are examined in the Canadian cultural setting. Early life experiences predispose individuals to violent behavior in their adult marriages, and there are major difficulties with the marital relationships and with conflicts that "build up to" the commission of the final act or crime. The factor that triggers the homicide in most cases is a perception of identity threat by the slayer. The role of alcohol, lack of impulse control, absence of persons with intervening capability (such as police), and other factors are examined. Preventive programs for the interspouse homicide are discussed.

215. Christensen HF, Johnson LB: Premarital coitus and the southern black: a comparative view. J Marriage Family 40:721–32, 1978.

Blacks have higher premarital coital rates than their white counterparts and are less deterred by religiosity. Black males incline more toward the permissive Scandinavian model while black females resemble the more conservative American model. Trends are generally in the direction of increased coital incidence coupled with decreased relationship commitment and decreased negative feelings following first coitus.

216. Ciborowski T: The role of context, skill, and transfer in cross-cultural experimentation. In

Handbook of Cross-Cultural Psychology, edited by HC Triandis and JW Berry, 2:279–95. Boston, Allyn and Bacon, 1980.

The importance of such variables as experimental context and transfer of cognitive skills needs to be strongly reemphasized in cross-cultural research methodology.

217. Clark RA: Religious delusions among Jews. Amer J Psychotherapy 34:62–71, 1980.

Religious delusions among Jews may have either Old Testament or Christian contents. One delusion relates to Sabbatai Sevi and the individual and social conditions that led to the Messianic idea.

218. Clarke J, Haughton H: A study of intellectual impairment and recovery rates in heavy drinkers in Ireland. Brit J Psychiatry 126:178–84, 1975.

In an Irish population, heavy drinkers perform significantly poorer on tests of visual/spatial and visual/motor coordination, visual reproduction, and abstract reasoning compared with a matched control group, even when they have not been drinking for ten weeks.

219. Claus PJ: The Siri myth and ritual: a mass possession cult of South India. Ethnology 14:47–58, 1975.

The legend of Siri charters the establishment of a kinship institution, matrilineality, among the dominant Indian caste, the Bants. Siri is unique in lacking the fearful characteristics associated with other *Bhūtas;* ritual possession by Siri is always considered beneficial, never malicious. The significance of the Siri *Paddana* lies in its ability to gather and organize into a perpetual group the many women afflicted with the problems of matrilineal kinship organization.

220. Claus PJ: Spirit possession and spirit mediumship from the perspective of Tulu oral traditions. Culture Medicine Psychiatry 3:29–52, 1979.

Spirit possession in South India is not a "natural" cultural explanation of psychosis, and belief in supernatural beings is not a necessary condition for the phenomenon. The psychological and sociological preconditions sometimes identified as the causes of possession may only be secondary features. In order for psychic states to be interpreted as possession, and in order that sociological preconditions set the stage for such states, there must be precise ideological correlates that anticipate precipitation of the phenomenon. Looking at spirit possession in the wider cultural context allows us to understand how the subject is cured by controlling the ritual context and accentuating the expression of the spirit.

221. Clay BJ: Pinikindu: Maternal Nurture, Paternal Substance. Chicago, U. of Chicago Press, 1977.

Among the Mandak people of Papua New Guinea, maternal nurture coincides with sharing of social identity and with continued nourishment, and complements paternal substance (providing shelter, wealth, magic, and protection). Sorcery is common.

222. Coan RW: Hero, Artist, Sage, or Saint? New York, Columbia U. Press, 1977.

Historical and modern views on mental health, normality, maturity, self-actualization, and human fulfillment are presented.

223. Cochrane R: Mental illness in immigrants to England and Wales: an analysis of mental hospital admissions, 1971. Social Psychiatry 12:25–33, 1977.

Where migration is easy the less stable members of a population self-select for migration, but where migration is relatively difficult only the most stable individuals can achieve migration.

224. Cochrane R: Psychological and behavioural disturbances in West Indians, Indians, and Pakistanis in Britain: a comparison of rates among children and adults. Brit J Psychiatry 134:201–10, 1979.

Asian children have lower rates of behavioral deviance and mental hospital admissions than do British children. Children of West Indian immigrants show no more behavioral deviance in schools than British children, but have considerably higher rates of admission to mental hospitals. The pattern for adults is similar to that shown by children.

225. Cochrane R, Hashmi J, Stopes-Roe M: Measuring psychological disturbance in Asian immigrants to Britain. Social Science Medicine 11:157–64, 1977.

Where comparisons are to be made between levels of psychological disturbance of Asian immigrants and natives, the Langer 22 Item Scale is to be preferred over the Goldberg General Health Questionnaire.

226. Cockerham WC: Drinking attitudes and practices among Wind River Reservation Indian youth. J Stud Alcohol 36(3):321–26, 1975.

Despite the possibility of getting into trouble for illegal drinking, Wind River Reservation Indian adolescents (mostly Arapahoe and Shoshone) have positive attitudes toward drinking. Boys begin drinking at an earlier age than girls.

227. Cockerham W, Forslund M, Raboin R: Drug use among white and American Indian high school youth. Intl J Addictions 2:209–20, 1976.

Indian youth have a more favorable attitude toward the use of marijuana and other drugs than white youth. Indian youth are also more likely than white youth to try using marijuana and other drugs, but no more likely than whites to continue using such drugs after having tried them.

228. Cohen CI, Sokolovsky J: Schizophrenia and social networks: ex-patients in the inner city. Schizophrenia Bull 4:546–60, 1978.

Analysis of ex-mental patients residing in a large Manhattan hotel indicates that schizophrenics have significantly fewer linkages than nonpsychotics, but even the most impaired schizophrenics are not totally isolated. Within the schizophrenic spectrum there are differences with respect to network size, complexity, directionality, and interconnectedness. Rehospitalization is dependent upon two factors, degree of psychopathology and hotel network size.

229. Cohen CI, Sokolovsky J: Clinical use of network analysis for psychiatric and aged populations. Comm Ment Health Journal 15:203–13, 1979.

Despite a recent renewal of interest in natural community support networks and self-help groups, there currently exist no systematic therapeutic approaches for working with network systems.

230. Cohen J: German and American workers: a comparative view of worker distress. Intl J Mental Health 5:138–47, 1976.

There is a generally higher level of felt discomfort among German workers than among American workers, in spite of the Germans being subjected to less environmental stress because of the threat of job displacement.

231. Cohn H: Suicide in Jewish legal and religious tradition. Mental Health Society 3:129–36, 1976.

Jewish law takes cognizance of only two kinds of suicide: one that is permissible by reason of its motivation and that may even be highly laudable, and one that is the outcome or symptom of mental disturbances or otherwise legally excusable. Law relating to suicide is not the only instance in which Jewish jurisprudence succeeded in neutralizing threats of divine punishment by human justifications.

232. Cohn N: Europe's Inner Demons. New York, Basic Books, 1975.

Medieval witch-hunts in Europe are best explained in terms of political, religious, and ideological history, rather than individual psychopathology. Assertions about witches created a corpus of concepts that were believed because they were repeated so often, especially by high religious authorities.

233. Cole D, Rodriguez J, Cole S: Locus of control in Mexicans and Chicanos: the case of the missing fatalist. J Consulting Clin Psychology 46:1323–29, 1978.

Mexican and Chicano students were studied to determine if the perception of their being fatalistic was true. The Mexican university students proved to be more internally oriented—and therefore less fatalistic—than students from Ireland, West Germany, and the United States. A comparison of Anglo and Chicano high-school seniors showed that only the Chicano males not planning to enter college had a tendency toward a more external locus of control.

234. Coles R: Eskimos, Chicanos, Indians: Children of Crisis. Boston, Little, Brown & Co., 1978.

The thoughts and feelings of children in crisis are described.

235. Coles R: Privileged Ones: Children of Crisis. Boston, Little, Brown & Co., 1978.

Children of wealthy parents present their world views and discuss their narcissistic entitlement.

236. Colletta NJ: American Schools for the Natives of Ponape. Honolulu, U. Press of Hawaii, 1980.

The Micronesian example demonstrates the impact of policies and practices of transplanted neocolonial education systems on indigenous peoples.

237. Collins AH, Pancoast DL: Natural Helping Methods. Washington, D.C., Natl. Assn. Social Workers, 1975.

Small neighborhood networks meet informally and naturally to provide service needs. Social workers should support these networks and encourage them to broaden their scope.

238. Collomb H: Witchcraft-anthropophagy (genesis and function). Transcult Psych Res Review 15:185–88, 1978.

Witchcraft beliefs in Africa, particularly in Senegal, cast light on a fundamental characteristic of mankind—the primal aggressive trends on which social order is founded. Witchcraft-anthropophagy is a part of a structured whole that orders human relations and accounts for social organization and individual diseases at the same time.

239. Collomb H: De l'ethnopsychiatric a la psychiatrie sociale. Canadian J Psychiatry 24:459–70, 1979.

In traditional African cultures mental illness is integrated into social order and cosmic order. Each member of the culture has precise conceptual and operational models for the causes of the illness. Medical models as imported from France have proved inefficient.

240. Comaroff J: Healing and the cultural order: the case of the Barolong boo Ratshidi of southern Africa. Amer Ethnologist 7(4):637–57, 1980.

Healing in a southern African society entails the manipulation of multivocal symbolic media, seeking to reintegrate the physical, conceptual, and social universe of sufferers and community. In rapidly changing societies, healing reveals how existing symbolic categories subsume chaotic experience and also how perceptions of an expanding sociocultural domain may transform these categories themselves.

241. Comas J: The international fight against racism: words and realities. Human Organization 37:334–44, 1978.

It is clear that the results of a systematic, organized, and scientifically based struggle against racial discrimination have been minimal; there has been a lot of talk, writing, and legislation, but these forms of expression have been speculative and ineffective.

242. Comay M: Political terrorism. Mental Health Society 3:249–61, 1976.

The main aim of international terrorism is to spread fear and undermine morale to achieve political blackmail. In self-protection the free world must combine against terrorist attacks on innocent civilians, taking of hostages, hijacking of aircraft, and involvement of third-party countries.

243. Comer JP: What happened to minorities and the poor? Psychiatric Annals 7(10):79–96, 1977.

Minority and low-income communities suffer from the polarization within our discipline concerning what is an appropriate psychiatric undertaking and from our failure to address systematically the problem of working effectively with minorities and low-income people.

244. Comer JP, Poussaint AF: Black Child Care. New York, Simon and Schuster, 1975.

Black children must be taught to approach racism, school, peer relationships, punishment, sex, violence, and other issues from a basis of knowledge, skill, and confidence.

245. Comfort A: On healing Americans. J Operational Psychiatry 9(2):25–36, 1978.

Modern, project-oriented medicine focuses on treatment of disease but not on healing. Healing, as a reordering of self, acceptance of responsibility for health, and a reconciliation to death as part of the life cycle, can be aided or impeded by how the physician communicates with the patient.

246. Comfort A: I and That: Notes on the Biology of Religion. New York, Crown, 1979.

Religion deals with the relationship between "I" (self) and "That" (other people, nature, gods); its meaning derives from brain function.

247. Comfort A: Is sociobiology real? J Operational Psychiatry 10:5–11, 1979.

The emphasis of sociobiology is on vestigial genetic predisposition rather than on the transition from genetic to cultural transmission of behaviors and the remolding of older automatisms by this continuous cultural evolution.

248. Coney JC: The Precipitating Factors in the Use of Alcoholic Treatment Services: A Comparative Study of Black and White Alcoholics. San Francisco, R & E Research Assoc., 1977.

The circumstances under which black and white alcoholics utilize a community health center alcoholism program in Massachusetts are examined. Although race accounts for some of the utilization differences between groups, religious preference and geographical background are important factors. Average black users are younger than whites. Seventy percent in the study actively made the decision to use treatment.

249. Coney JC: Exploring the Known and Unknown Factors in the Rates of Alcoholism Among Black and White Females. San Francisco, R & E Research Assoc., 1978.

When biases are eliminated, the proportion of black and white female alcoholics is almost equal. Researchers more often define black women's cultural drinking patterns as alcoholic. When police arrest or liver cirrhosis rates are used to determine the scope of alcoholism, black women are overrepresented. The rise in rates of female alcoholism reported in the literature is due to increased visibility of female alcoholics.

250. Connor J: Joge kankei: a key concept for an understanding of Japanese-American achievement. Psychiatry 39:266–79, 1976.

The Japanese concept of *joge kankei,* or an emphasis on superior-inferior relationships, is a valuable tool in understanding Japanese achievement when seen in conjunction with socialization practices that lead to an ego structure that is highly sensitive to the opinions of significant others. This all-pervasive awareness of ranking leads to competition resulting in Japan's remarkable economic growth during the last two decades. The concept of hierarchy or ranking also explains the rapid rise of Japanese-Americans to middle-class status.

251. Connor JW: The social and psychological reality of European witchcraft beliefs. Psychiatry 38:366–80, 1975.

In terms of the culture and belief structure of late-medieval and post-reformation Europe, a belief in witchcraft was neither irrational nor a delusion; it did, in fact, make good sense.

252. Connor L: Corpse abuse and trance in Bali: the cultural mediation of aggression. Mankind 12:104–18, 1979.

During Balinese cremation rituals the crowd may carry off and tear apart the decomposed corpse.

253. Cooper J, Sartorius N: Cultural and temporal variations in schizophrenia: a speculation on the importance of industrialization. Brit J Psychiatry 130:50–55, 1977.

Social and family structures found historically in preindustrial societies and currently in developing countries exert a benign effect upon patients with schizophrenia, and these effects are lost by (1) the rapid increase in size of towns and communities; (2) changes in parental and infant mortality and morbidity; and (3) changes in family structure during and after industrialization.

254. Cooperstock R: A review of women's psychotropic drug use. Canadian J Psychiatry 24:29–34, 1979.

Women are more likely than males to be frequent and particularly steady users of psychotropic drugs. Women are more willing to discuss their problems with their network of intimates, to visit physicians because of these problems, and to request drugs. Physicians are more likely to offer tranquilizers to women than to men presenting with the same complaints.

255. Cordry D: Mexican Masks. Austin, U. of Texas Press, 1980.

Indian ritual dance masks have shamanistic, symbolic, and social functions.

256. Corin E: A possession psychotherapy in an urban setting: zebola in Kinshasa. Social Science Medicine 13B(4):327–38, 1979.

The zebola ritual is one of the possession therapies in the great possession complex of northwest Zaire. The intervention of zebola spirits as protectors of the person suffering from interpersonal conflicts permits that person to remove herself somewhat from the pressures of a milieu that is sometimes difficult to live in, particularly for women.

257. Corin E, Bibeau G: De la forme culturelle an vecu des troubles psychiques en Afrique. Propositions methodologique pour une etude enterculturelle du champ des maladies mentales. Africa 43:280–315, 1975.

Psychiatric researchers in Africa need to discover, through the use of ethnoscientific practices, the names and underlying classificatory principles of native diseases. The three most common African etiological explanations for diseases are the actions of spirits, disturbances in interpersonal relations, and infractions committed by the patient. There seem to be no African therapeutic rituals specifically devoted to mental illness.

258. Corin E, Bibeau G: Psychiatric perspectives in Africa: part II: the traditional viewpoint. Transcult Psych Res Review 17:205–33, 1980.

Researchers of African ethnopsychiatry analyze the ways in which healers are specialized, examine disease concepts, and explore African ways of perceiving individuality. The significance of a disease in any individual is often grasped by the African in terms of interpersonal relationships or of a threat to a group, and treatment may embrace the social context as well as the person. Etiological categories include witchcraft, sorcery, spirits, and magic. Therapeutic principles include suggestion, confession, ritual symbolism, and attention paid to the body, e.g., massage, dance, and fumigation. Possession cults provide aid by relieving tension and anxiety, by supporting an individual's demands on his family milieu by attributing them to a spirit, by increasing the social status of the possessed person, and by serving as a channel for social inability, e.g., by allowing the voices of women to be heard in male-dominated societies.

259. Corin E, Murphy HBM: Psychiatric perspectives in Africa: part I: the Western viewpoint. Transcult Psych Res Review 16:147–78, 1979.

Prior to 1957 it was thought that affective psychoses were rare in Africa. Low suicide rates may reflect the communalism of African society, which restrains the expression of aggression. Bouffee delirante—acute reactive psychosis—is a typical syndrome. Culture-bound syndromes include pobough lang (geophagia, pallor, depression, and social isolation) and nit-ku-bon (failure to thrive in children who relate poorly to others, refuse the breast, seldom speak, and occasionally hallucinate) in Senegal, bon ba nsinga (similar to nit-ku-bon) in the Cameroons, and brain fag (school-related memory loss, headaches, and inability to study) in Nigeria and Uganda. Pueperal psychoses are common, and epidemic hysteria has been reported. Etiological, culture-linked themes include child-rearing practices, somatization, interaction of individual and community, and persecution. Ethnopsychoanalytic themes have been applied widely to Africa. Group therapy and therapeutic villages linked to mental hospitals are significant trends.

260. Cornfield RB, Fielding SD: Impact of the threatening patient on ward communications. Amer J Psychiatry 137:616–19, 1980.

Strained communication patterns are often provoked in the patients and staff by the presence of potentially violent or destructive patients on the ward. Staff need to overcome their resistance to the signals from frightened patients for effective management of the situation.

261. Costello RM: Chicano liberation and the Mexican-American marriage. Psychiatric Annals 7(12):64–73, 1977.

Mexican-American women today are more likely to seek revenge for their husband's abuses and are less likely to seek to maintain the family by "curing" the husband through witchcraft and curanderismo. If the wife seeks a divorce, she is likely to incur the wrath of the relatives. The response to such stress placed on the woman can be very flamboyant and can cause a great deal of anxiety in the indigenous personnel of the mental health clinic. While hospitalization for psychotic behavior and suicide gestures is sometimes indicated, most often a consultive approach that stresses discussion of cultural traditions and community values is sufficient to lower the tension.

262. Cox JL: Aspects of transcultural psychiatry. Brit J Psychiatry 130:211–21, 1977.

Transcultural topics of increasing relevance for British psychiatrists include migration and mental illness, acculturation, culture shock, communication, interpreters and psychiatric services, training of overseas psychiatrists, and research on reliable cross-cultural definitions of mental illness.

263. Cox JL: Postgraduate training in Britain for psychiatrists from East Africa. Mental Health Society 4:152–55, 1977.

Overseas students whose psychiatric training is in Britain need specific assistance to maximize the advantages and minimize the disadvantages of such training. The opportunity to learn aspects of transcultural psychiatry now of relevance for the British graduate is best taught and assimilated in a multicultural learning environment.

264. Cox JL: Amakiro: a Ugandan puerperal psychosis? Social Psychiatry 14:49–52, 1979.

Despite proximity to a modern teaching health center, the majority of the Ugandan women interviewed were familiar with amakiro (puerperal psychosis) and could readily identify its symptoms. Beliefs concerning amikiro are held by the majority of Ugandan women, with such beliefs showing a surprising consistency and internal coherence.

265. Cox JL: Psychiatric morbidity and pregnancy: a controlled study of 263 semirural Ugandan women. Brit J Psychiatry 134:401–5, 1979.

There is increased frequency of psychiatric morbidity in pregnant Ugandan women compared with nonpregnant women. Separated pregnant women are at higher risk. There is no relationship between antenatal psychiatric morbidity and age, gravidity, number of cowives, or the duration of the pregnancy.

266. Cramer M: Psychopathology and shamanism in rural Mexico: a case study of spirit possession. Brit J Med Psychology 53:67–73, 1980.

The personification of personal problems in the motif of spirit possessions enables some persons to maintain a measure of self-esteem, social status, and personality integration.

267. Crapanzano V: Saints, jnun, and dreams: an essay in Moroccan ethnopsychology. Psychiatry 38:145–59, 1975.

The appearance of saints and jnun in the dreams of Moroccans helps with the articulation of conflict and its resolution. Saints and jnun are symbolic-interpretive elements, believed to be external to the individual, which formulate conflict, the fact and terms of which may or may not be acceptable to the individual. The conflict is thereby removed from the individual-particularistic level to the cultural-universalistic level and is structured in terms of the "logic" of saints and jnun.

268. Crapanzano V: Tuhami: Portrait of a Moroccan. Chicago, U. of Chicago Press, 1980.

A Moroccan informant describes his life, including marriage to a spirit and cures from illness.

269. Crapanzano V, Garrison V: Case Studies In Spirit Possession. New York, Wiley-Interscience, 1977.

Detailed case studies of spirit possession include Anglo-American spiritists; the Wolof; Morocco; the Ethiopian Wuquabi cult group; zar experiences in Egypt; Sri Lanka; Kelantanese Malay spirit seances; Brazilian Umbamba spirit mediums; and Puerto Ricans.

270. Creyghton M: Communication between peasant and doctor in Tunisia. Social Science Medicine 11:319–24, 1977.

The lack of communication between doctor and peasant is due to ignorance of the healing paradigm that the other party more or less takes for granted.

271. Crocker JC: The mirrored self: identity and ritual inversion among the Eastern Bororo. Ethnology 16:129–45, 1977.

The Bororo self is created, defined, and systematically transformed by other selves; the person does not exist except as it is reflected by these. The Bororo self is not a cultural idea nor a tangible thing. It is only a social and symbolic process and a structure of transactions between social categories.

272. Crocket R: "Real" and "abstracted" network relationships in social psychiatry. Psychotherapy Psychosomatics 25:267–71, 1975.

The examination of social network relationships may allow for such improvements in social psychiatry as the classification of different treatment units in terms of their structure, the creation of experimental structural networks, and the comparison of two or more treatment networks as to their gross therapeutic outcomes.

273. Cromwell VL, Cromwell RE: Perceived dominance in decision-making and conflict resolutions among Anglo, Black and Chicano couples. J Marriage Family 40:749–59, 1978.

Stereotypic labeling of black families as matriarchal and of Chicano families as patriarchal is questionable. Ethnicity by itself, controlling for social class, is not sufficient to account for the variance in self-perceptions of either conjugal decisionmaking or conflict resolution.

274. Cutler DL, Madore E: Community-family network therapy in a rural setting. Comm Mental Health J 16:144–55, 1980.

Community network therapy is designed to open lines of communication between family members and significant community persons and to keep them open so as to prevent further dissolution and crisis and to facilitate positive efforts for all family members and agency persons.

275. Dalen P: Maternal age and incidence of schizophrenia in the Republic of Ireland. Brit J Psychiatry 131:301–5, 1977.

The excess incidence of schizophrenia in Ireland may be due to the relatively older ages of mothers at childbirth.

276. Danesh HB: The authoritarian family and its adolescents. Canadian Psychiatric Assn J 23:479–85, 1978.

Authoritarian families possess characteristics similar to those of the authoritarian personality. Adolescents in authoritarian families are deprived of their basic needs for stability, flexibility, and guidance.

277. Daneshmand L: A study on the personality characteristics of Iranian addicts. Intl J Social Psychiatry 26:142–44, 1980.

Therapeutic methods should be based on an understanding of the personality characteristics of addicts within their own cultural setting, instead of basing methods on the characteristics of addicts living in an entirely different culture.

278. Danna JJ: Migration and mental illness: what role do traditional childhood socialization practices play? Culture Medicine Psychiatry 4:25–42, 1980.

Evidence from cross-cultural studies indicates that certain areas of child-rearing practices (discipline, independence-dependence training, distance of child from parent of same sex, etc.) influence the degree of psychological differentiation that develops in the cognitive, perceptual, and personality domains of behavior. The hypothesis that harsh and restrictive childhood socialization practices foster the development of a cognitive personality orientation that increases the likelihood of maladaptive responses to culture change is illustrated by anthropological and psychological data obtained from Sicilians living in Sicily, the United States, and Australia.

279. Dasen PR: Concrete operational development in three cultures. J Cross-Cultural Psychology 6:156–72, 1975.

The rate of development of concrete operations among Canadian Eskimos, Australian Aborigines, and Ebrie Africans may be partly determined by ecological and cultural factors. Rates of development are not uniform across different areas of concrete operations, and these rates may reflect the adaptive values of the concepts concerned.

280. Dasen PR (ed): Piagetian Psychology: Cross-Cultural Contributions. New York, Gardner, 1977.

Piagetian assumptions and hypotheses about cognitive development are tested in such diverse cultural groups as the Themne, Kamba, Rwanda, French Canadians, Jordanians, Ga, and Zincantecos. Surveys from Africa, America, Asia, and Oceania indicate that all normal human beings have the childhood potential to operate cognitively at two levels during each stage of the developmental sequence. The first is a base level, while the second is an environmentally supplemented level.

281. Davey AG: Racial awareness and social identity in young children. Mental Health Society 4:255–62, 1977.

Racial awareness and even racial repugnance can be well developed in children of four or five years of age. The development of prejudice in children is a product of the normal, necessary, and rational process of progressively ordering the environment into manageable categories and trying to comprehend a place within it.

282. Davey AG, Mullin PN: Ethnic identification and preference of British primary school children. J Child Psychol Psychiat Allied Disciplines 21:241–51, 1980.

Minority children do not differ significantly from white children in the extent to which they identify with their own group, but their ethnic preferences demonstrate that they perceive the advantages of being white.

283. Davidson AR, Thomson E: Cross-cultural studies of attitudes and beliefs. In Handbook of Cross-Cultural Psychology, edited by HC Triandis and RW Brislin, 5:25–71. Boston, Allyn and Bacon, 1980.

Based on the conceptual framework, a person acquires belief about an object on the basis of life experiences. The affective value of these beliefs influences the person's attitude in a positive or negative direction. The attitude, in turn, is related to the favorableness of the individual's set of behaviors concerning the object. The greatest hindrance to the development of an integrated and cumulative cross-cultural body of knowledge related to attitudes and beliefs is not the lack of application of adequate methodology but the lack of application of adequate theory.

284. Davidson GR, Klich LZ: Cultural factors in the development of temporal and spatial ordering. Child Development 51:569–71, 1980.

A majority of desert aboriginal children from nine to sixteen years show a preference for spatial over temporal order in free-recall tasks. This preference does not decrease significantly with age.

285. Davidson GR, Nurcombe B, Kearney GE, Davis K: Culture conflict and coping in a group of aboriginal adolescents. Culture Medicine Psychiatry 2:359–72, 1978.

Aboriginal adolescents from Elcho Island mission in Australia are part of a complex environment where choice behavior is mediated by specific and broader situational characteristics of the social environment. There is a relationship between conflict responses and orientation to traditional values and skills, but no apparent relationship between conflict responses and modern value orientation or psychopathology variables. Males are less involved in mission and traditional activities and are more restricted by traditional social expectations than females.

286. Davidson L: Ethnic roots, transcultural methodology and psychoanalysis. J Amer Acad Psychoanalysis 8:273–78, 1980.

Transcultural and cross-cultural methodology must pay closer attention to what patients are saying about their generational networks and how these networks affect them not only in the past but also in the present.

287. Davis C, Glick ID, Rosow I: The architectural design of a psychotherapeutic milieu. Hosp Community Psychiatry 30:453–60, 1979.

Reconciling the architectural needs of a psychotherapeutic milieu with code and budgetary restrictions is possible through creative and flexible design if treatment, training, and research objectives are clearly formulated in advance, and if all those affected are genuinely involved in the planning and design process.

288. Davis G: Childhood and History in America. New York, Psychohistory, 1976.

Methods of child rearing influence the later actions of society's leaders.

289. Davis W: Dojo: Magic and Exorcism in Modern Japan. Stanford, Calif., Stanford U. Press, 1980.

Sukyo Mahikari are exorcistic religious sects in Japan; misfortune and illness are attributed to possession by spirits.

290. Dean A, Kraft AM, Pepper B: The Social Setting of Mental Health. New York, Basic Books, 1976.

Readings include such topics as deviance, labeling, social control, and treatment settings as social systems.

291. Dean RS: Distinguishing patterns for Mexican-American children on the WISC-R. J Clin Psychology 35:790–94, 1979.

WISC-R subtest scores may be employed in an attempt to differentiate between specific learning problems and language deficiencies with Mexican-American populations.

292. De Dellarossa GS: The professional of immigrant descent. Intl J Psychoanalysis 59:37–44, 1978.

Immigrants must successfully undergo a mourning process for what was left behind in order to accept their new country. If this process is not worked through, it will fall upon the succeeding generations to do this, as illustrated in the case presented.

293. de Figueiredo JM: Interviewing in Goa: methodological issues in the study of a bilingual culture. Social Science Medicine 10:503–8, 1976.

Important steps in the methodology of a transcultural field study are the construction of an instrument and its use for the collection of data.

294. de Figueiredo JM: Some methodological remarks on transcultural interviewing on psychopathology. Intl J Social Psychiatry 26:280–92, 1980.

When the investigator is not a native of the region he is studying, he should live in it for a period of time so as to gain the confidence of the natives.

295. de Figueiredo JM, Lemkau PV: The prevalence of psychosomatic symptoms in a rapidly changing bilingual culture: an exploratory study. Social Psychiatry 13:125–33, 1978.

The most difficult task in health education is to change those cultural elements that stand as symbols of the dominant sentiments governing interpersonal conduct. The sudden Indian takeover of what was once a Portuguese settlement (Goa) shows that planning related to sociocultural change should take into account both the quantity of change over time and the quality of change.

296. de Figueiredo JM, Lemkau PV: Psychiatric interviewing across cultures: some problems and prospects. Social Psychiatry 15:117–21, 1980.

Approximately fourteen million Americans receive inadequate mental health care, largely because of linguistic and cultural barriers.

297. Degler CN: At Odds. Oxford and New York, Oxford U. Press, 1980.

The size, structure, and social function of the American family and women's lives have been slowly separating and developing independent existences over the past two centuries.

298. De La Fuente JR, Alarcon-Segovia D: Depression as expressed in pre-Columbian Mexican art. Amer J Psychiatry 137:1095–98, 1980.

Depression is depicted in ceramic figures of pre-Columbian Mexican art.

299. Dennis PA: The role of the drunk in a Oaxacan village. Amer Anthropologist 77:856–63, 1975.

Drunks in Oaxacan villages may shout insults, speak the truth, intrude uninvited into social gatherings, and behave in usually unacceptable ways. Apart from alcohol intake, which is its ostensible cause, such behavior is a creation of the villagers' conceptions.

300. Deregowski JB: Perception. In Handbook of Cross-Cultural Psychology, edited by HC Triandis and W Lonner, 3:21–115. Boston, Allyn and Bacon, 1980.

Cross-cultural studies of perception are a caricature of Western studies; that is, in the non-Western studies the trends and tendencies present in the studies in the West are accentuated and exaggerated and the elements that are "secondary" in the West are muted and sometimes entirely ignored.

301. De Rios MD: The Wilderness of Mind: Sacred Plants in Cross-Cultural Perspective. Beverly Hills, Calif., Sage, 1976.

Hallucinogenic plants have been used by Australian Aborigines, Liberian herdsmen, Huichol Indians, New Guinea Highlanders, the Fang, the Aztecs, the Incas, and the Mayas. Music often accompanies hallucinogenic rituals and provides a form of structure for a potentially chaotic experience.

302. De Rios MD, Smith DE: Drug use and abuse in cross-cultural perspective. Human Organization 36:14–21, 1977.

The major danger of certain patterns of ritualistic drug use in American society is that the individual may be arrested for violating laws based on sociocultural norms that derive from ambiguous negative health considerations. Drug use among American youth may be of value to individuals in their interacting group.

303. Der-Karabetian A: Relation of two cultural identities of Armenian-Americans. Psychological Reports 47:123–28, 1980.

The ethnically more involved and the recent immigrants show a greater gap in their American and Armenian identities than the ethnically less involved and the native-born, respectively.

304. des Pres T: The Survivor: An Anatomy of Life in the Death Camps. Oxford and New York, Oxford U. Press, 1976.

Survival in the Nazi death camps required action on both the communal and the individual level that was often the product of naked and savage self-interest.

305. Deutsch A: Observations on a sidewalk ashram. Arch Gen Psychiatry 32:166–75, 1975.

A psychological characteristic of the devotion to a guru is a strong underlying wish for union with a powerful object. Psychedelic drugs contribute to this devotion.

306. Deutsch A: Tenacity of attachment to a cult leader: a psychiatric perspective. Amer J Psychiatry 137:1569–73, 1980.

Devotees remain loyal to their cult leader because of his purported closeness to God, his radical teachings, and his embodiment of a countercultural ideal of freedom. They use denial, rationalization, and other defenses to maintain their fantasy that the leader is acting for their benefit.

307. Devereux G: Ethnopsychoanalysis. Berkeley, U. of California Press, 1978.

The separate sciences of psychoanalysis and anthropology are complementary.

308. Devereux G: The nursing of the aged in classical China. J Psychol Anthropology 2:1–10, 1979.

The Oedipus complex resurfaces at an oral level in senility. Breast feeding of the aged in ancient China transformed the nurse into a mother, making sexual relations incompatible due to castration anxieties and an unconscious fear that "mother's" milk, as a final product of one's own sexual act, may turn into poison.

309. Devereux G: Basic Problems in Ethnopsychiatry. Chicago, U. of Chicago Press, 1980.

Culture from a psychoanalytic perspective is presented in essays on the psychopathology of shamans, normality and abnormality, pathogenic dreams in non-Western societies, therapy with Native Americans (Mohave), and primitive psychiatric diagnosis.

310. Devos G: A Rorschach comparison of delinquent and non-delinquent Japanese family members. J Psychol Anthropology 2:425–41, 1979.

The Rorschach test reveals that nondelinquent individuals resolved or reacted to stimuli by internal processes before demonstrating overt behavioral responses, while delinquency-prone individuals behaved more externally toward stimuli. Delinquent families differed most from nondelinquent families by the absence of such affect responses as positive sensual feeling and responses suggesting active striving.

311. deVries M, Super CM: Contextual influences on the Neonatal Behavioral Assessment Scale and implications for its cross-cultural use. Monographs Society Research Child Devel 43:92–101, 1978.

Using the Neonatal Behavioral Assessment Scale outside the standard hospital setting introduces variations in the physical and social context that influence scores on some of the behavioral items. Interactions between the examiner and the mother, the mother and the baby, and all parties with the physical and cultural context play significant roles, in addition to the interaction of usual interest between the examiner and infant.

312. DeWalt BR: Drinking behavior, economic status, and adaptive strategies of modernization in a highland Mexican community. Amer Ethnologist 6:510–30, 1979.

In the Temascalcingo region of Mexico there is no support for the general contention that heavier drinkers are less likely to be modernizing their productive activities. Heavy drinkers are less likely to be interested in some modernization strategies (specifically animal improvement) and more likely to be interested in others (use of tractors). Alcohol use does contribute significantly to an understanding of sociocultural dynamics in the Temascalcingo region.

313. D'Hondt W, Vandewiele M: Adolescents' groups in Senegal. Psychological Reports 47:795–802, 1980.

Despite the unquestionable influence of Western culture in the groups' names, the prevailing aspirations in the choice of names are symptomatic of the shaping of adolescents' identity: the appeal to unity and brotherly solidarity, the assertion of their youthfulness, and the expression of their black personalities.

314. D'Hondt W, Vandewiele M: Senegalese secondary school students' preferences between living in town and living in the countryside. Psychological Reports 47:731–37, 1980.

Peasants' sons wish to stay in the country while richer students feel more at ease living in town. The socioeconomic status of young Senegalese has a decisive effect on the choice of a way of living.

315. Di Angi P: Barriers to the black and white therapeutic relationship. Perspectives Psychiatric Care 14:180–83, 1976.

Because of the black man's three hundred years of oppressive experience with the white man, the black client enters the therapeutic interview with a set of attitudes and behaviors that, if not acknowledged, will negatively affect the exchanges and outcomes of the relationship. But just as there are problems and resistances in this situation, it can be expected that there are problems in the reverse situation of black therapist and white client.

316. Di Angi P: Erikson's theory of personality development as applied to the black child. Perspectives Psychiatric Care 14:184–85, 1976.

The black adolescent's inability to resolve his identity crisis results in role diffusion and role confusion. If the adolescent is convinced that he is unable to fulfill the roles expected of him from his family and community, he may turn toward a negative group identity or withdraw from society.

317. di Leonardo M: Methodology and the misinterpretation of women's status in kinship studies: a case study of Goodenough and the definition of marriage. Amer Ethnologist 6(4):627–37, 1979.

Goodenough's assumption that women's low status is universally unproblematic is central to his cross-cultural definition of marriage but does not correspond to the evidence of his own sources. It is possible that other models of kinship processes may be similarly inadequate. Appropriate methodology should be used in future construction of such models.

318. Dimitriou EC, Kokantzis NA, Ierodiakonou CS: The family and the psychiatric child patient in Greece. Intl J Social Psychiatry 25:82–83, 1979.

Misconceptions about mental illness, which are widespread in Greece, and the socioeconomic status of the Greek family determine to a great extent the mode of the family's reaction to the child's condition.

319. Dimsdale JE (ed): Survivors, Victims, and Perpetrators. Washington, D.C., Hemisphere, 1980.

Psychosocial studies underscore the enormous damage to the mental health of victims of the Nazi holocaust and provide insight into the behavior of the perpetrators.

320. Dinges NG, Trimble JE, Hollenbeck AR: American Indian adolescent socialization—a review of the literature. J Adolescence 2:259–96, 1979.

Studies of the American Indian adolescent have gone from early research on tribal personality to present-day examinations of the effects of education and a defining of social problems. In the face of recent social changes and an increasingly large adolescent group, a more thorough understanding of the socialization of Indian adolescents is needed to provide programs and services to serve their needs. An integrated model of socialization based on evidence acquired by programmatic research will advance this understanding.

321. Dinnen A: No speak much English: (or how I stopped worrying about the theory and began treating the indigent Greek). Mental Health Society 4:26–35, 1977.

From working with a group of lower-class Greek immigrant patients with chronic psychiatric illness over three years, it is concluded that group psychotherapy techniques can be applied irrespective of class, culture, or language of the group.

322. Diop B, Collignon R: Aspects ethiques et culturels de la psychiatrie en Afrique. Social Science Medicine 13B(3):183–90, 1979.

The contradiction inherent in the African psychiatrist's dual function (the therapeutic contact with his patient and his social mandate for protecting society, which situates him as one part of the centralized power apparatus) invites him to question his working conditions and the final aim of his function.

323. Doane JA: Family interaction and communication deviance in disturbed and normal families: a review of research. Family Process 17:357–76, 1978.

Several measures reliably discriminate disturbed from normal families. Measures designed or modified specifically for use with families, rather than small-group process measures of verbal activity, yield more meaningful and consistent results.

324. Donelson E, Gullahorn J: Women: A Psychological Perspective. New York, Wiley, 1977.

Both biological and sociological factors contribute to what is unique in female psychology.

325. Dore A: Laotian hysterical symbolism, a Phi-pop case. Ethnopsychiatrica 2:49–77, 1979.

The Lao believe that Phi-pop is one of the most dangerous spirits, which can kill its victims by devouring their livers if not chased away quickly. Carriers of the spirit are immune and are thought to have acquired Phi-pop through heredity, by possessing an object belonging to a Phi-pop carrier, or through a failure to perform magic initiation rites. The victims of Phi-pop, usually females, fall into a trance followed by amnesia and then point out the carrier from which they acquired the disease, who is then attacked and ostracized. The carriers move to special Phi-pop colonies.

326. Dore A: Mrs. Chanthi, a psycho-pathological case in a traditional Lao environment. Ethnopsychiatrica 2:37–47, 1979.

A 46-year-old Laotian woman had one-day psychotic reactions during her menstrual periods for seven years. She developed persecutory ideas, exhibitionism, and aggression toward her family. The Buddhist meditation techniques of her family failed to cure her. Only with treatment by lower-class traditional magical practices were her symptoms relieved.

327. Dor-Shav NK: On the long-range effects of concentration camp internment on Nazi victims: 25 years later. J Consult Clinical Psychology 46:1–11, 1978.

Survivors of the Nazi concentration camps twenty-five years later showed evidence of impoverished and constructed personalities and appeared to be less accessible and more emotionally labile. Their perceptive-cognitive functions were more global and less complex than the norm and showed indications of breakdown of ego boundaries. Earlier incarceration seemed to lead to more severe impairment.

328. Dor-Shav NK, Dor-Shav Z: Cross-cultural study of ratings of phenomenological experience of emotion. Psychological Reports 42:583–90, 1978.

There is a great deal of cross-cultural agreement with regard to ratings of emotional phenomenology.

329. Dow MGT, Ledwith J, Fraser WI, Bhagat M: The usefulness of the semantic differential with "mild grade" mental defectives. Brit J Psychiatry 127:386–92, 1975.

Mild-grade retardates in comparison to subjects of average intelligence show less discrimination in the use of the semantic differential; such discriminative deficiencies in turn predispose toward a polarized response bias among the retarded.

330. Draguns JG: Psychological disorders of clinical severity. In Handbook of Cross-Cultural

Psychology, edited by HC Triandis and JG Draguns, 6:99–174. Boston, Allyn and Bacon, 1980.

Culture exerts a noteworthy influence upon manifestations of psychopathology in its overtly observed expressions and subjectively reported experiences. Psychopathology may have some unique features that, for lack of cross-cultural perspective of most investigators and practitioners, have so far gone unrecognized. Potentially, however, the quest for the cultural uniqueness of psychopathology in style, content, and patterning of expression does not appear to be an unrealistic undertaking.

331. Dube KC: Nosology and theory of mental illness in Ayurveda. Comp Med East West 6:209–28, 1978.

Ayurveda, the ancient Indian system of medicine, contains details of etiology, symptoms, diagnosis, and therapy of afflictions in humans and animals.

332. Dunbar C, Edwards V, Gede E, Hamilton J, Sniderman MS, Smith V, Whitfield M: Successful coping styles in professional women. Canadian J Psychiatry 24:43–46, 1979.

There are conflicts for professional women in Canada in the major areas of competition, dependency needs, economic success, and the search for role models.

333. Dundes A: Heads or tails: a psychoanalytic study of potlatch. J Psychol Anthropology 2:395–424, 1979.

The dynamics of the potlatch ritual are closely related to the anal erotic character traits of the Kwakiutl of the Pacific Northwest. The Kwakiutl view power as being achieved by participating in the "normal movement" from head to tail; interruption of this movement by the potlatch ritual can harm or dismay an enemy or rival.

334. Dunham HW: Society, culture, and mental disorder. Arch Gen Psychiatry 33:147–56, 1976.

One of the difficulties of isolating sociocultural factors that eventually emerge as mental disorders is the uncertainty as to whether functional mental illness can be differentiated into several qualitatively distinct syndromes or whether it forms a unity of a more generic character. The other difficulty is the failure to formulate a valid social-psychological theory that can demonstrate that selected sociocultural factors contribute to the molding of a mental illness observed in the phenotype.

335. Dunkas N, Nikelly AG: Group psychother-apy with Greek immigrants. J Group Psychotherapy 25:402–9, 1975.

Group therapy offers a unique solution for psychological problems due to culture stress and conflict among Greek immigrants to the United States. Greek immigrants are exposed to the inadequacies of their defenses and coping mechanisms in a "foreign" culture. Therapy begins with dependency and resentment toward the therapist, who is perceived as authoritarian, but moves toward independence, equality, increased flexibility, and the ability to cope with cultural differences.

336. Durand-Comiot M: La psychose puerperale? Etude en milieu Senegalais. Psychopathologie Africaine 13:269–336, 1977.

Many Senegalese women show symptoms of a psychotic nature in connection with maternity. From a psychoanalytic viewpoint these so-called "puerperal psychoses" are neither puerperal nor necessarily a psychosis. Rather, they may result from many unresolved conflicts over incomplete resolution of the introduction process of the pregnant woman and her own mother.

337. du Toit BM: Configurations of Cultural Continuity. Rotterdam, A. A. Balkema, 1975.

As exemplified by cultures in Africa and Oceania, there are many common features in life-cycle ceremonies and in the recruitment and indoctrination procedures of adjustment movements.

338. du Toit B (ed): Drugs, Rituals, and Altered States of Consciousness. Rotterdam, A. A. Balkema, 1977.

Drugs that cause altered states of consciousness are often taken in a secular ritual context. For the Aymara of Peru and Bolivia, drink and drunkenness are part of the sacred and beyond criticism.

339. Dwyer DH: Ideologies of sexual inequality and strategies for change in male-female relations. Amer Ethnologist 5:227–40, 1978.

In the social sciences, an identity of beliefs about maleness and femaleness among the male and female portions of any society has typically been assumed. Moroccan and other data demonstrate that this presumption of ideological homogeneity constitutes another Western ethnocentrism. Similarly, the political methods that have been utilized in the West in order to implement change in no way emerge as inevitably appropriate for all sexually inegalitarian social systems.

340. Dwyer DH: Images and Self-Images: Male and Female in Morocco. New York, Columbia U. Press, 1978.

Moroccan women maintain and control their own subordination through an ideology and set of symbolic representations that promote sexual inequality.

341. Dyson-Hudson R, Smith EA: Human territoriality. Amer Anthropologist 80:21–41, 1978.

Variations in territorial responses for the Ojibwa, Basin-Plateau Indians, and Karimojong seem to accord with the predictions of the economic dependability model.

342. Earls F, Richman N: Behavior problems in pre-school children of West Indian-born parents: a re-examination of family and social factors. J Child Psychol Psychiat Allied Disciplines 21:107–17, 1980.

The prevalence and pattern of behavior problems, and their associated social and familial characteristics, are similar for both West Indian-born and British-born families.

343. Easson WM: Child psychiatry in the Soviet Union: a preliminary report. J Amer Acad Child Psychiatry 14:515–22, 1975.

Soviet and American child psychiatrists can increase their understanding of each other's society by collaborating in such areas as schizophrenia, adolescent psychiatry, and the patterns of health and emotional illness.

344. Easterlin RA: Birth and Fortune. New York, Basic Books, 1980.

A substantial amount of a person's good or bad fortune is due to the size of the generation or birth cohort into which he or she is born. Generation size has implications on family life, stress, women's roles, birth control, and symptoms of social disorganization such as crime and suicide.

345. Eastwell HD: Projective and identifactory illness among ex-hunter-gatherers: a seven-year survey of a remote Australian aboriginal community. Psychiatry 40:330–43, 1977.

The defense mechanisms of projection and identification persist and assist in the adjustment of the individual and the group in small-scale societies of the Aboriginal tribes of Australia. The model defenses of the people in these societies have not changed over the years, and, under the intensified stresses of modern-day living, these defenses shape the psychiatric illnesses of today.

346. Eastwell HD: A pica epidemic: a price for sedentarism among Australian ex-hunter-gatherers. Psychiatry 42:264–73, 1979.

Pica (clay eating) has become a conspicuous behavior in isolated Aboriginal coastal towns in north Australia. Pica is observed among adult women past childbearing age; a change in diet and in eating customs in nomadic Aboriginals settled in townships, plus other abrupt changes in social roles, seem to be responsible for the recent wave of pica epidemic.

347. Eaton WW, Lasry JC: Mental health and occupational mobility in a group of immigrants. Social Science Medicine 12(A):53–58, 1978.

Job stresses among immigrants who are involved in upward mobility can lead to mild psychiatric symptoms.

348. Ebling FJ (ed): Racial Variation in Man. New York, Halsted, 1975.

The concept of race defies definition and is of limited value in the study of human biosocial variability.

349. Ede A: Koro in an Anglo-Saxon Canadian. Canadian Psychiatric Assn J 21:389–92, 1976.

Clinical manifestation of the koro syndrome as observed in Southeast Asia and in the West are not identical. The koro syndrome as described among Southeast Asians is more often associated with a neurosis, while the atypical koro syndrome as described in the West is more often associated with a psychosis.

350. Edel L: The madness of art. Amer J Psychiatry 132:1005–12, 1975.

The madness of art is the need to transform personal experience by artistic expression, as shown in the lives and works of many great artists. Psychotherapy may be used or rejected by artists to overcome their sadness at aging.

351. Edgerton RB: Alone Together: Social Order on an Urban Beach. Berkeley, U. of California Press, 1979.

The social order on a public beach in California does not result from a sense of community but rather from a limited police presence, selective inattention to trouble, and behavior that encapsulates beachgoers from each other.

352. Edgerton RB: Traditional treatment for mental illness in Africa: a review. Culture Medicine Psychiatry 4:167–89, 1980.

Some aspects of the pattern of belief responsible for the rapid recovery of schizophrenics in Sri Lanka and other parts of the nonindustrialized world (WHO study) are also present among the Yoruba. Yoruba beliefs and expectations about mental illness play some part in the treatment of a mentally ill person. There is complete neglect of social and cultural factors in the International Pilot Study of Schizophrenia, and a study of social and cultural phenomena would help us to understand the reasons for the rapid recovery of schizophrenics in nonindustrialized countries.

353. Ehrenwald J: Possession and exorcism: delusion shared and compounded. J Amer Acad Psychoanalysis 3:105–19, 1975.

The therapist must keep an open mind to the possibility that genuine PSI elements may be involved in the clinical picture. He must allow for the fact that in such a case their very emergence may serve the patient as indications of his sanity and as a vindication of his mental health.

354. Ehrenwald J (ed): The History of Psychotherapy. New York, Jason Aronson, 1976.

The history of psychotherapy is reviewed from healing magic to religion to science and, finally, to new solutions.

355. Eibl-Eibesfeldt I: The Biology of Peace and War. New York, Viking, 1979.

War is a mechanism of spacing out and dividing up resources between human populations and accelerates the rate of both biological and cultural evolution. Cultural evolution, copying biological evolution, is resulting in a ritualization of conflict that is a partial solution to the problem of destructive human conflict.

356. Eibl-Eibesfeldt I: Human ethology. Behavioral Brain Sciences 2:1–57, 1979.

Similar selection pressures have shaped both culturally and phylogenetically evolved patterns. Nonverbal and verbal behaviors can substitute for one another, thus opening the way for the study of a grammar of human social behavior.

357. Einstein S, Feig D: Drug contagion in Jerusalem: a pilot investigation of the Israeli drug use scene. Intl J Addictions 14:423–36, 1979.

The majority of drug users do not initiate anyone else into drug use, and those who do initiate others do not report any monetary gains.

358. Eissler R, Freud A, Kris M, Neubauer P, Solnit AJ: The Psychoanalytic Study of the Child, Vol. 32. New Haven, Conn., Yale U. Press, 1977.

Essays on narcissism as a function of culture, on the treatment of a refugee child, on comic book superheroes, and on the myth of Peter Pan are presented.

359. El-Fatatry M, El-Kashlan K, El-Garem O, Ghazi A: Psychiatric patients of Egyptian culture in Alexandria. Intl J Social Psychiatry 26:69–71, 1980.

Hysteria is not overrepresented in less intelligent, illiterate Egyptian patients.

360. Eliade M: Occultism, Witchcraft, and Cultural Fashions. Chicago, U. of Chicago Press, 1976.

European witchcraft derived from an older, pre-Christian set of practices that changed following the Inquisition. Cultures provide images of journeys after death and allay anxiety about mortality. In many religious systems, the sun and its light are linked with both the "spirit" and with semen.

361. El-Islam MF: Culture-bound neurosis in Qatari women. Social Psychiatry 10:25–29, 1975.

Qatari women are highly susceptible to neurosis because they can achieve sociocultural adequacy only by having a husband and producing children.

362. El-Islam MF: Transcultural aspects of psychiatric patients in Qatar. Comp Med East West 6:33–36, 1978.

Failure to report symptoms in an abstract fashion is characteristic of Qatari patients. The cultural and religious heritage absorbs many behaviors that would otherwise be considered symptomatic of psychiatric disorder.

363. Elmendorf ML: Nine Mayan Women. New York, Halsted, 1977.

Modernization has changed greatly the lives and roles of Mayan women.

364. El Rahmed SA: Some characteristics of mania in an Arab country. Transcult Psych Res Review 15:81, 1978.

Mania in Saudia Arabia is characterized by the absence of hypomania in the premorbid personality and by the absence of pathological elation and flight of ideas.

365. El Sendiony MFM: The problem of cultural specificity of mental illness: a survey of comparative psychiatry. Intl J Social Psychiatry 23:223–30, 1977.

Most of the allegedly "specific" mental illnesses, which reflect in their behavior the specific cultural content of the victim's society, are simply local varieties of a common disease process to which human beings, as such, are vulnerable.

366. El Sendiony MFM, Abou-El-Azaem MGM, Luza F: Culture change and mental illness. Intl J Social Psychiatry 23:20–25, 1977.

The relationship of culture change to the frequency of mental illness in an outpatient clinic in the city of Cairo indicates that rapid industrialization tends to produce significantly higher rates of patients who are judged to have serious symptoms of depression, especially among village immigrants who move from their villages to work in the city's factories.

367. Emovon AC: The relationship between marital status and mental illness. Mental Health Society 3:10–21, 1976.

In Nigeria, single persons have the largest number of referrals, followed closely by married persons, to psychiatric hospitals. The widowed and divorced have a relatively small number of referrals, and there are more male than female patients. There are also sex and age variations in the type of mental disorder. These findings are related to the social structure of the population and to the legal and social definitions of the concepts of marriage and divorce in Nigeria.

368. Emovon AC, Lambo TA: A survey of criminal homicide in Nigeria. Intl J Social Psychiatry 21:214–19, 1975.

The killer/victim relationship is a social relationship, and one should expect it to take place in terms of culture. Therefore, one may expect to find variation in rates of homicide among the different ethnic groups in Nigeria.

369. Engel GL: The clinical application of the biopsychosocial model. Amer J Psychiatry 137:535–44, 1980.

Use of the biopsychosocial model is very practical in the understanding and care of a patient. It is a scientific model that takes into account the missing dimensions of the biomedical model and helps in defining the place of psychiatrists in the education of physicians of the future.

370. Epstein CF: Women's attitudes toward other women—myths and their consequences. Amer J Psychotherapy 34:322–33, 1980.

When women act negatively toward other women, they reflect the cultural view that women are not of much worth. The lack of assistance given to women by their male and female professional and business colleagues can be traced to the lack of women in positions of power, to the feeling that the aid cannot be reciprocated, and to personality differences that are not gender specific.

371. Epstein G: Culture, personality, and behavior: a field study in Jerusalem. Mental Health Society 4:36–44, 1977.

Work with Jerusalem's Eastern-Jewish immigrant communities supports the hypothesis that non-Western societies have a theory of disease causation that is at variance with a Western model.

372. Erchak GM: The nonsocial behavior of young Kpelle children and the acquisition of sex roles. J Cross-Cultural Psychology 7:223–34, 1976.

Because of the greater importance of women than men in Kpelle subsistence activities, girls become more self-reliant and responsible than boys at an earlier age.

373. Erickson GD: The concept of personal network in clinical practice. Family Process 14:487–98, 1975.

The concept of personal network holds high promise for becoming a major unifying framework in clinical practice as an analytic viewpoint, as a schema for problem location, and as an arena of practice and research.

374. Erikson KT: Loss of communality at Buffalo Creek. Amer J Psychiatry 133:302–5, 1976.

The survivors of the Buffalo Creek disaster suffered individual trauma as well as loss of communality. With the loss of ties with familiar people and places, the survivors suffered demoralization, disorientation, apathy, and an inability to care for one another. The survivors have difficulty finding personal resources to replace the communal ones.

375. Erinosho OA: Cultural factors in mental illness among the Yoruba. Intl J Group Psychotherapy 27:511–15, 1977.

Yoruba society is still characterized by a high degree of interaction and close interpersonal relations. Belief in the evil machination of significant others through witchcraft is clearly revealed in treated patients. Adherence to a magicoreligious explanation in the etiology of mental illness is seen in the symbolic significance attributed to dreams and the "social" diagnosis of illness by patients and native healers. The overall effectiveness of treatment modalities may be hindered if cultural factors in the etiology of psychiatric disorders are ignored.

376. Erinosho OA: Pathways to mental health delivery-systems in Nigeria. Intl J Social Psychiatry 23:54–59, 1977.

Next of kin are the primary referral source for treated schizophrenic patients. Patients often seek care from native healers, then syncretic churches, before making any contact with modern psychiatric facilities.

377. Erinosho OA: Social background and preadmission sources of care among Yoruba psychiatric patients. Social Psychiatry 12:71–74, 1977.

Patients with diverse backgrounds utilize traditional healers prior to their admission, suggesting that psychiatric disorders are well-placed within the belief system of the Yoruba despite modernizing influences.

378. Erinosho OA: Mental health delivery systems and post-treatment performance in Nigeria. Intl J Social Psychiatry 24:71–74, 1978.

The proliferation of mental health delivery systems in Nigeria may be linked to widespread disagreement on the most effective therapeutic orientation or milieu for the mentally ill.

379. Erinosho OA: Socio-cultural antecedents of magical thinking in a modernizing African society. J Cross-Cultural Psychology 9:201–11, 1978.

Despite the consensual adherence to a magico-mythical orientation in Africa, a deeper fear of bewitchment is likely to exist among persons who have low as opposed to those who enjoy high levels of social functioning.

380. Erinosho OA: The evolution of modern psychiatric care in Nigeria. Amer J Psychiatry 136:1572–75, 1979.

A range of mental health delivery systems is available in Nigeria, including traditional healers and Western-oriented systems. The effectiveness of modern psychiatric care will depend on accommodation of commonly accepted notions of mental illness by professional care agents.

381. Erinosho O, Ayonrinde A: A comparative study of opinion and knowledge about mental illness in different societies. Psychiatry 41:403–10, 1978.

In western Nigeria, most people in urban as well as rural communities are still unaware of the range of symptoms of various psychiatric illnesses in spite of a long exposure to modern psychiatric delivery systems. Heightening of awareness of psychiatric symptoms through nationwide health education is essential in Nigeria for the full utilization of mental health services.

382. Essock-Vitale SM, Fairbanks LA: Sociobiological theories of kin selection and reciprocal altruism and their relevance for psychiatry. J Nerv Ment Disease 167(1):23–28, 1979.

Using the theories of kin selection and reciprocal altruism from sociobiology, it can be shown that individuals with access to kin-support and/or friend-support systems are less likely to be hospitalized with psychiatric disorders than are individuals without access to such systems. Sociobiology may be useful to psychiatry by providing a new focus on the adaptive functions of human behavior, by providing functional predictions to help identify segments of the population that are at more risk of psychiatric disorder than others, and by providing new directions for research.

383. Estroff SE: The anthropology-psychiatry fantasy: can we make it a reality? Transcult Psych Res Review 15:209–13, 1978.

The interface between cultural anthropology and psychiatry has proved to be disappointing. Research results from non-Western areas are not always applicable to the United States. Anthropologists need to do better and more psychiatric fieldwork.

384. Estroff SE: Making It Crazy. Berkeley, U. of California Press, 1979.

A group of deinstitutionalized chronic mental patients describe their life in the community.

385. Ettorre EM: Lesbians, Women, and Society. London, Routledge and Kegan Paul, 1980.

Lesbianism should no longer be considered as an individual genetic quirk, a psychological malfunctioning, a mental illness, an immaturity, an abnormality, or a perversion. Explanations of lesbianism should be rooted in history and based upon a social theory of sexuality that takes into account the patriarchal and capitalist structures of society.

386. Ewing JA, Rouse B (eds): Drinking: Alcohol in American Society. Chicago, Nelson Hall, 1978.

Topics discussed include social controls over drinking and an overview of drinking behaviors and social policies.

387. Fabrega H Jr: Elementary systems of medicine. Culture Medicine Psychiatry 3(2):167–98, 1979.

Among elementary societies, medical specialists treat forms of disease and symptoms that comembers themselves find difficult to understand and control. Practitioners are not concerned with concrete symptoms and signs that are treated by the individual and his family in a direct and often topical manner. Curing rituals for many of the groups take place in a highly social context and are characterized by physical exertion of the major participants who are experiencing altered states of consciousness. Most elementary societies do not regard sorcery from within their own groups as a cause of disease.

388. Fabrega H Jr: Neurobiology, culture, and behavior disturbance: an integrative review. J Nerv Ment Disease 167:467–74, 1979.

In the study of the influence of culture on behavior disturbance, the methods and rationale of the social sciences have been employed and underlying neurobiological factors neglected. A basic question is to know how cultural influences may possibly affect the organization and functioning of the nervous system and, by extension, behavior and its disturbance.

389. Fabrega H Jr, Hunter JE: Beliefs about the behavioral effects of disease: a mathematical analysis. Ethnology 18:271–90, 1979.

The peasant population of Tenejapa, Mexico, has a rich but integrated theory of disease. Behavioral changes signal disease and allow the people to evaluate and monitor its progression.

390. Fabrega H Jr, Manning PK: Illness episodes, illness severity and treatment options in a pluralistic setting. Social Science Medicine 13B(1):41–51, 1979.

Mexican women of Ladino ethnicity report more illnesses that are less severe and of shorter duration than Mayan Indians do. Ladinos of both sexes suffer more from biologically based disease processes than Indians and become more behaviorally impaired when sick, despite their greater utilization of physicians.

391. Fabrega H Jr, Tyma S: Language and cultural influences in the description of pain. Brit J Med Psychology 49:349–71, 1976.

The language and culture of an individual can affect his experiences of pain during disease.

392. Fabrega H Jr, Zucker M: Comparison of illness episodes in a pluralistic setting. Psychosomatic Medicine 39:325–43, 1977.

Episodes of illness in two different groups of women (indigenous and Ladino) of the Highlands of Chiapas, Mexico, can be compared using a longitudinal-panel design. The method of procedure, which reflects a holistic and integrated view of disease, proves flexible, useful, and easily applicable in the field setting.

393. Fagan TJ, Lira FJ: Profile of mood states: racial differences in a delinquent population. Psychological Reports 43:348–50, 1978.

Whites placed in an essentially black population experience the same negative affective responses that have been reported for black citizens attempting to function vocationally and socially within the larger society where whites heavily outnumber blacks.

394. Fahrmeier ED: The effect of school attendance on intellectual development in northern Nigeria. Child Development 46:281–85, 1975.

The difference in school attendance between schooled and unschooled children tends to be constant at all ages rather than increasing as the amount of schooling increases.

395. Fahrmeier ED: The development of concrete operations among the Hausa. J Cross-Cultural Psychology 9:23–44, 1978.

A 50 percent rate of conservation responses is achieved by age twelve among the Hausa of Nigeria.

396. Farber A: Segmentation of the mother: women in Greek myth. Psychoanalytic Review 62:29–47, 1975.

Myths, like dreams, are a window into the psyche, and we may gain a glimpse of some of the hidden, unconscious preoccupations of the Greeks by analysing the themes prevalent in their myths. The frequent appearance of female figures in segmented form is evidence of the Oedipus complex of the ancient Greeks. Disguised in segments, these females represent versions of the relationship with the mother that are acceptable because she cannot consciously be recognized.

397. Farberow NL (ed): Suicide in Different Cultures. Baltimore, University Park, 1975.
Studies on suicide and culture in Norway, Sweden, Finland, Great Britain, the Netherlands, Italy, Austria, Israel, India, China, Japan, Argentina, and among American Indians.

398. Farris JJ, Jones BM: Ethanol metabolism and memory impairment in American Indian and white women social drinkers. J Stud Alcohol 39(11):1975–79, 1978.
American Indian women metabolize a moderate dose of ethanol significantly more rapidly than do white women of similar age, education, weight, and drinking history; however, the two groups demonstrate a similar memory decrement due to ethanol.

399. Fast I: Developments in gender identity: gender differentiation in girls. Intl J Psychoanalysis 10:443–53, 1979.
Gender differentiation is proposed as a model for understanding gender development. It is hypothesized that the differentiation process is patterned similarly to other major developmental differentiations, being initially narcissistic and finally integrating one differentiation product as part of the self. The implications of this hypothesis and of Freud's interpretation of female development are examined.

400. Favazza AR: Feral and isolated children. In Mental Health In Children, edited by DVS Sankar, pp. 411–58. Westburg, N.Y., PJD, 1975.
Cases of children reared in isolation or by animals have been reported from the time of ancient Greece to the present, the most famous being the Wild Boy of Aveyron, Kaspar Hauser, and the Wolf-Children of Midnapore. There is no good evidence that a true feral child has ever existed.

401. Favazza AR: Feral and isolated children. Brit J Med Psychology 50:105–11, 1977.
Amidst a colorful history of children supposedly reared by animals, feral and isolated children found today need not be condemned to a prognosis of pathology, but instead can be viewed as suffering from psychosocial deprivation.

402. Favazza AR: A solution to the German problem. J Operational Psychiatry 8(2):64–69, 1977.
The moral outrage in America resulting from revelation of Nazi atrocities in World War II strongly affected the deliberations of the behavioral scientists of the Joint Commission on Post-War Planning. In retrospect, their idea of transforming the German national character with a rational mental health plan appears to have lacked the objectivity and scientific detachment needed to deal with this emotionally charged issue.

403. Favazza A: Rejoinder to Estroff's "The anthropology-psychiatry fantasy." Transcult Psych Res Review 16:222–25, 1979.
Since anthropology has not yet developed into a clinical science, anthropologists will find it difficult to support themselves financially in an academic department of psychiatry. Cultural psychiatrists must prove to their colleagues that cultural psychiatry is relevant to clinical practice.

404. Favazza AR: Cultural change and mental health. J Operational Psychiatry 11:101–19, 1980.
The study of behavior has four dimensions —biological, psychological, cultural, and social structural. As a culture becomes more complex, the ability of psychiatrists to deal effectively with cultural change and mental health decreases.

405. Favazza AR, Faheem A: The heavenly vision of a poor woman: a case report with commentary. J Operational Psychiatry 10:93–126, 1979.
The case report of a Pentecostal woman's vision from God is discussed. Commentaries by Comfort, Koss, Pattison, Wittkower, and MacLean diagnose the case as hysterical psychosis.

406. Favazza AR, Oman M: Anthropological and Cross-Cultural Themes in Mental Health. Columbia, U. of Missouri Press, 1977.
An annotated bibliography of articles with anthropological and cross-cultural themes in mental health journals from 1925 to 1974.

407. Favazza AR, Oman M: Overview: foundations of cultural psychiatry. Amer J Psychiatry 135:293–303, 1978.
Among the major conceptual foundations of cultural psychiatry are the definition of mental health and illness, child rearing and basic personality, family and social networks, sex roles and behavior, alcohol use, communication, and therapy. Culture may be approached via ethnography, emic and etic studies, cross-cultural and holocultural studies, and subjective culture studies.

408. Favazza A, Oman M: Anthropology and Psychiatry. In Comprehensive Textbook of Psychiatry (3d ed.), vol. 1, edited by HI Kaplan, AM Freedman, and BJ Sadock. Baltimore, Williams and Wilkins, 1980.

The experience of mental illness and the different causative models, diagnostic techniques, and therapeutic approaches to mental disorder cannot be divorced from the complex interrelationships found in cultural and social settings. Topics discussed include national character, cross-cultural studies, emics and etics, ethnography, subjective culture, mental hospitals culture, folk classification, diaprosis, and treatment of mental illnesses (sorcery, witchcraft, spirit possession, spiritism, zar), folk healers, and Christian beliefs about mental illness.

409. Favret-Sanda J: Deadly Words. Cambridge and New York, Cambridge U. Press, 1980.

Witchcraft beliefs and experiences exist in modern Bocage, a rural area of France.

410. Feather NJ, Cross DG: Value systems and delinquency: parental and generational discrepancies in value systems for delinquent and nondelinquent boys. Brit J Social Clinical Psychology 14:117–29, 1975.

Value systems are more discrepant between delinquent boys and their parents and between the parents themselves than for nondelinquents.

411. Felson RB, Gmelch G: Uncertainty and the use of magic. Current Anthropology 20:587–89, 1979.

Tribal man has faith that his magic works; modern man lacks faith but is not taking any chances.

412. Felton RA: The healing ritual. Intl J Social Psychiatry 21:176–78, 1975.

The healing ritual of the shaman healer should not only be regarded as producing a placebo effect in the cure of so-called "psychosomatic" patients, but also should be considered a valuable tool in itself, capable of bringing about dramatic changes in consciousness and being an effective aid to psychotherapy.

413. Fernandez-Pol B: Culture and psychopathology: a study of Puerto Ricans. Amer J Psychiatry 137:724–26, 1980.

An inverse relationship exists between adherence to Latin American family beliefs and the development of psychopathology. This relationship is more apparent among lower-class than middle-class Puerto Ricans.

414. Fernando SJM: A cross-cultural study of some familial and social factors in depressive illness. Brit J Psychiatry 127:46–53, 1975.

A study of familial and social factors among Jewish and Protestant depressives and nonpsychiatric controls indicates that depressives in both groups have (a) a higher rate of psychiatric illness in their families, (b) lower scores on maternal overprotection, and (c) a higher rate of marriage in both groups and both sexes, except in Jewish men. Depression among Jews may be related to mental stress arising from "marginality," and single Jewish men may be particularly vulnerable to depression.

415. Ferreira AG: Alcoholism in Portugal. Intl J Mental Health 5:63–73, 1976.

The dualistic nature of Portuguese society is reflected in two types of alcoholism: that of the urban, industrial regions, typical of a society in development ("the alcoholism of civilization"), and that of the traditional, rural regions. Alcoholism is much more widespread among men than women in Portugal.

416. Ferro-Luzzi GE: The female lingam: interchangeable symbols and paradoxical associations of Hindu gods and goddesses. Current Anthropology 21: 45–68, 1980.

Symbolic associations, as seen in the Hindu religion, are less psychologically determined than Freudian psychoanalysts are accustomed to think. At the same time, symbolic meanings are less arbitrary and also less context-bound than structuralists are accustomed to think. A symbol can evoke associations in its own right; it does not depend on a system of contrasts for its meaning.

417. Figge HH: Spirit possession and healing cult among the Brazilian Umbanda. Psychotherapy Psychosomatics 25:246–50, 1975.

Umbanda is an animistic-spiritistic religion of Brazil that believes in the existence of all kinds of spirits and seeks to give these spirits the temporary opportunity to inhabit human bodies. The spirits are used to make patients think of effective treatment for their ills.

418. Finger S: Child-holding patterns in Western art. Child Development 46:267–71, 1975.

European and American works of art depicting mothers holding their children should be considered only moderately supportive of recent reports that children are held more frequently by the mother on her left side than on her right side.

419. Finkler K: Non-medical treatments and their outcomes. Culture Medicine Psychiatry 4:271–310, 1980.

Spiritualist healers fail more than they succeed in treating their patients. Therapeutic benefits from spiritualist healing occur in four types of disorders—simple diarrheas, simple gynecological disorders, somatized syndromes, and minor psychiatric disorders. Successful treatment outcomes are effected not only by concrete manipulation of physiological symptoms but by symbolic manipulation as well, i.e., for a therapeutic regime to do its job it must confront cultural imperatives and employ cultural symbols relevant to the removal of the sick role. In Mexicans, the cultural imperatives relate to cleaning and to purification, mediated by tactile communication, which serve symbolically to terminate the sick role.

420. Fireside H: Soviet Psychoprisons. New York, W. W. Norton, 1979.

Psychiatric hospitals in the Soviet Union are used to detain political dissidents. Human rights activists, would-be immigrants, and religious dissidents should deal with their psychiatric captors in special ways.

421. Fisher J (ed): Himalayan Anthropology. The Hague, Mouton, 1978.

Wide-ranging studies of peoples of Nepal, Tibet, and northern India are presented, including a descriptive analysis of Nepalese Buddhist pujas as a medical-cultural system with references to Tibetan parallels.

422. Fisher L: On the classification of families. Arch Gen Psychiatry 34:424–33, 1977.

Presently, insufficient data and experience preclude the establishment of a typological classification system that proposes clearly distinct family types that are mutually exclusive and that assume distinct causes.

423. Fishman RG: A note on culture as a variable in providing human services in social service agencies. Human Organization 38:189–92, 1979.

Unless social service policy begins to deal with cultural differences, agency programs will remain ineffective in dealing with large numbers of the population in need of their services.

424. Fitzgerald TK: A critique of anthropological research on homosexuality. J Homosexuality 2:385–97, 1977.

Anthropologists have recorded the range and diversity of homosexual practices and personality types as they existed through the ages and in specific cultural contexts. A berdache (a male or female who assumes the role and status of the opposite sex) may be a transvestite, but a transvestite need not be a berdache; and neither need be homosexual.

425. Flaherty JA, Meagher R: Measuring racial bias in inpatient treatment. Amer J Psychiatry 137:679–82, 1980.

There is racial bias in the treatment of black schizophrenic patients, who receive lower privilege levels, more prn medications and seclusion restraints, and less recreation and occupational therapy. This is because of subtle stereotyping and staff's greater familiarity with white patients.

426. Flandrin JL: Families in Former Times. Cambridge and New York, Cambridge U. Press, 1979.

Conjugal, extended, and multiple-family households coexisted in France in the sixteenth to eighteenth centuries.

427. Fleck S: Family functioning and family pathology. Psychiatric Annals 10(2):17–35, 1980.

It is important that clinicians recognize deficiencies in family functions not only after a severe disturbance has occurred but also early enough so that preventative measures can be instituted and healthful family life promoted. A systems approach to family functioning and family pathology offers such an opportunity.

428. Fleischman PR: Ayurveda. Intl J Social Psychiatry 22:282–87, 1976/1977.

Ayurveda is an indigenous professional system of medicine, based on Sanskrit texts, that exists side by side with allopathic Western medicine in India. There are now more registered practitioners of ayurveda than of allopathy in India, and though its relative strength is apt to diminish in the near future, it remains a major force in the country's health care system, particularly in the treatment of psychiatric and psychosomatic illnesses.

429. Fletcher JM, Todd J, Satz P: Culture-fairness of three intelligence tests and a short-form procedure. Psychological Reports 37:1255–62, 1975.

Culture-fair tests (such as Raven's CPM, IPAT, and the WAIS) may not adequately assess the range of intellectual ability of Costa Ricans without some form of non-Anglo standardization.

430. Flores JL: The utilisation of a community mental health service by Mexican-Americans. Intl J Social Psychiatry 24:271–75, 1978.

Mexican-Americans and other Latins would utilize mental health services if personnel and policies were responsive to bilingual and bicultural needs.

431. Flynn RJ, Nitsch KE: Normalization, Social Integration, and Community Services. Baltimore, University Park, 1980.

Normalization refers to the use of culturally valued and normative means in order to establish, enable, or support behaviors, appearances, experiences, and interpretations that are as culturally valued and normative as possible. Deviancy is not within the person but rather is within imposed social roles, values, and the interpretations of perceivers. Social and other programs to establish a normalization response to deviancy are reported for Denmark and Massachusetts.

432. Forssen A: Psychiatry in Nigeria. Psychiatric Annals 8(6):85–91, 1978.

Communication between patient and physician in Nigeria is made difficult by the diversity of languages spoken in the country, amounting to some 250 different tongues.

433. Foster GM: Disease etiologies in non-Western medical systems. Amer Anthropologist 78:773–78, 1976.

In personalistic medical systems all misfortune and disease are explained in the same way; illness, religion, and magic are inseparable, powerful curers have supernatural and magical powers, and their primary role is diagnostic. In naturalistic medical systems disease causality has nothing to do with other misfortune; religion and magic are largely unrelated to illness, principal curers lack supernatural or magical powers, and their primary role is therapeutic.

434. Foster GN, Anderson BG: Medical Anthropology. New York, Wiley, 1978.

There are strengths and weaknesses associated with both scientific and nonbiomedical medicine. Culture influences sick roles, illness behavior, hospitals, and processes of professionalism.

435. Foulks EF: Comments on Foster's "Disease etiologies in non-Western medical systems." Amer Anthropologist 80:660–61, 1978.

The dichotomy of personalistic versus naturalistic medical systems may undermine a more emic approach. For some people the personalistic-naturalistic "dichotomy" is a unified field that blends the soul with the mechanics of the body.

436. Foulks EF: Interpretations of human affect. J Operational Psychiatry 10:20–27, 1979.

The subject of affect and its disorders is explored by three major approaches. The medical approach is based on basic biological and cognitive universals, the cultural approach is based on variations of affect and its disorders in different societies, and the ethnopsychiatric approach is based on the realities and cognitive systems of a certain cultural group. Information from each may be valuable in assessing affective disorders.

437. Foulks EF: The concept of culture in psychiatric residency education. Amer J Psychiatry 137:811–16, 1980.

The subject of culture warrants a place in the curriculum of psychiatric residency education. It provides unique insights and approaches in patient care. Curriculum approaches include cultural sensitivity groups, olidactic courses, field and clinical experiences, and study groups.

438. Foulks EF: Psychological continuities: from dissociative states to alcohol use and suicide in Arctic populations. J Operational Psychiatry 11:156–61, 1980.

Eskimo motives for alcohol use and suicide share the same basic psychological mechanisms found in the dissociative states of traditional Eskimo society. Alcohol and suicide have replaced the dissociative state as a means of escaping psychological pain.

439. Foulks E, Freeman DMA, Kaslow F, Madow L: The Italian evil eye: mal occhio. J Operational Psychiatry 8(2):28–34, 1977.

The idea of the evil eye as being responsible for medical and psychological illnesses and misfortunes is illustrated by a case of an Italian-American that demonstrates the complicated cultural issues involved in etiology, diagnosis, and treatment of the evil eye, as well as the complex medical-legal issues that can arise.

440. Foulks E, Wintrob R, Westermeyer J, Favazza A (eds): Current Perspectives in Cultural Psychiatry. New York, Spectrum, 1977.

Topics discussed include anthropological theory in psychiatry; transcultural attitudes toward antisocial behavior; psychiatric research issues with American Indians; hex and possession; ethics in cross-cultural research; folk therapy in Surinam; opium addiction in Laos; and social system therapy.

441. Fox N: Attachment of kibbutz infants to mother and metapelet. Child Development 48: 1228–39, 1977.

While reunion behaviors of kibbutz children differentiate between their mothers and their metaplot, their separation protests do not. Both age and birth order of the child are important in understanding the particular attachment responses.

442. Fox RC: Essays in Medical Sociology. New York, Wiley Interscience, 1979.

The premises, values, and emotions that underlie and accompany the lives and work of physicians and patients in Belgium, America, and Zaire are discussed.

443. Frances V, Frances A: The incest taboo and family structure. Family Process 15:235–44, 1976.

Man inherits from his animal forebears the biological imperative of an incest barrier but brings to it his special complexity of psychology and symbolization; incest barrier becomes incest taboo.

444. Frank A, Eisenthal S, Lazare A: Are there social class differences in patients' treatment conceptions? Myths and facts. Arch Gen Psychiatry 35:61–69, 1978.

Social class differences in treatment disposition and outcome cannot be attributed to social class differences in patients' treatment conceptions.

445. Frank JD: Psychotherapy and the Human Predicament. New York, Schocken, 1978.

Placebo effect, faith, patients' expectations of relief, and the cultural context of psychotherapy are important to the healing process.

446. Frankel S: "I am dying of man'': the pathology of pollution. Culture Medicine Psychiatry 4:95–117, 1980.

Agali are illnesses in men that the Huli people of Papua New Guinea ascribe to sexual intercourse at times deemed dangerous. Once the diagnosis is accepted, the choice of action, whether inaction, use of Western medicine, Huli cure, Christian healing, or a combination of these, depends particularly upon the severity and chronicity of the symptoms. Rather than the nature of symptoms being important in assigning the diagnosis, the diagnosis may influence the symptoms. There is some evidence of the molding of symptoms to conform to culturally set expectations.

447. Freeman DMA, Foulks EF, Freeman PA: Child development and Arctic hysteria in the North Alaskan Eskimo male. J Psychol Anthropology 1:203–10, 1978.

A failure to complete the psychological processes of "separation-individuation" contributes to Arctic hysteria.

448. Freeman H: Mental health and the environment. Brit J Psychiatry 132:113–24, 1978.

Attention should be paid to psychological conservation of the environment in the same way that physical conservation areas have been established in Britain. In this way, the social matrix that forms the identity of place and that is also related to the identity of person and group can be preserved or restored.

449. Freeman JM: Untouchable: An Indian Life History. Stanford, Calif., Stanford U. Press, 1979.

Among the topics discussed in this ethnography of a member of the untouchable Bauri caste in Orissa (India) are possession trance, family structure, marriage customs, sexual exploitation of women, and male prostitutes.

450. Freidin M, Ho R: Cultural change and psychopathology. Transcult Psych Res Review 15:201–2, 1978.

Problems encountered by the children of Chinese immigrants to the United States arise from the clash between the traditional Chinese values held by their parents and the American values they encounter outside the home. One effect of acculturation on the children is an alteration of mental defense mechanisms.

451. French L: Social problems among Cherokee females: a study of cultural ambivalence and role identity. Amer J Psychoanalysis 36:163–69, 1976.

The Cherokee female has a greater chance of being involved in social problems because she is disproportionally represented in the Cherokee society, is often a victim of Cherokee male violence, and is the major socializing agent of Cherokee children, almost always emerging as head of household in family breakups and, therefore, being directly involved with problematic children of both sexes.

452. Fried MN, Fried MH: Transitions. New York, W. W. Norton, 1980.

The rituals that surround birth, adolescence, marriage, and death have changed in the modern world.

453. Friedl E: Women and Men: An Anthropologist's View. New York, Holt, Rinehart & Winston, 1975.

The determinants of sex roles are both biological and sociocultural and may be studied by examining child rearing, symbolism, power, and subsistence technology.

454. Friedman RC: Critique of a hypothesis of dominance and sexual behavior. Amer J Psychiatry 132:967–69, 1975.

The hypothesis that male dominance facilitates heterosexual copulatory behavior while female dominance inhibits it is examined. Such unitary-cause hypotheses applied to complex behaviors may be reductionistic and less helpful than intended.

455. Frieze IH, Parsons JE, Johnson PB, Ruble D, Zellman G: Women and Sex Roles. New York, W. W. Norton, 1978.

Areas discussed include determinants of sex roles, life-cycle issues, reproduction, sexuality, psychological disorders in women, and power.

456. Fritz WB: Psychiatric disorders among natives and non-natives in Saskatchewan. Canadian Psychiatric Assn J 21:393–400, 1976.

In psychiatric disorders diagnosed among Indian, Metis, and nonnative psychiatric inpatients in psychiatric treatment centers in Saskatchewan, there is a significant relationship between the patients' ethnic status and the type of psychiatric diagnosis. Indian and Metis inpatients are more frequently diagnosed as having psychoneurotic and personality/behavior disorder. Indian people with psychiatric disorders are less likely to receive treatment in a psychiatric center.

457. Fritz WB: Indian people and community psychiatry in Saskatchewan. Canadian Psychiatric Assn J 23:1–7, 1978.

There has been an increase in inpatient admissions as compared to outpatient contacts of Treaty Indians in Saskatchewan from 1967 to 1976. This increase represents a contradictory effect to the intention of the community psychiatry program of the province's government.

458. Fruzzeti LM: The Gift of a Virgin. New Brunswick, N.J., Rutgers U. Press, 1980.

Marriage and other rituals in Bengali society are a reality and not merely an idiom for expressing reality for women.

459. Fry CL: Aging in Culture and Society. Brooklyn, N.Y., J. F. Bergin, 1980.

Current policy and theory in the field of adult behavior are often based on profoundly culture-bound conceptions of what is natural, necessary, normal, or optimum. Among the groups studied are the Masai, Garifuna (Black Caribe), Native Americans, Corsicans, Polish-Americans, Indians, and Chinese.

460. Fuchs A: Coca chewing and high-altitude stress: possible effects of coca alkaloids on erythropoiesis. Current Anthropology 19:277–91, 1978.

Indian coca chewers in the Andes cite a variety of reasons for their use of the drug, e.g., alleviating symptoms of hunger, thirst, fatigue, cold, and pain. In addition, the antimuscarinic ingredients in the coca leaf act upon critical areas of the posterior hypothalmus to depress erythropoiesis.

461. Fuchs E: Cross-cultural perspectives on adolescence. J Amer Acad Psychoanalysis 3:91–104, 1975.

Problems of adolescence are in good measure reflective of the problems of the entire world. Scarcely any people of our time have remained untouched by a vastly accelerating pace of culture change. The larger society must assume the social responsibility that adults have assumed throughout history—the responsibility to provide opportunity for participation as productive members of society as young people advance in age.

462. Fuchs E (ed): Youth in a Changing World. Chicago, Aldine, 1976.

Cross-cultural studies reveal that the major influences upon adolescents throughout the world are formal education, the mass media, and changing sexual mores.

463. Fugelli P: Milieu and mental health in a Norwegian fishing community. Psychotherapy Psychosomatics 32:60–64, 1979.

A morbidity study of Norwegian fishing communities was conducted with special reference to factors in the local milieu influencing the morbidity pattern, such as deep insecurity with regard to the future of their home location. Fishermen's wives sought psychiatric help when their husbands were home at double the rate of when their husbands were at sea.

464. Furnham A: Assertiveness in three cultures: multidimensionality and cultural differences. J Clin Psychology 35:522–27, 1979.

There is a significant difference among African, Indian, and European groups on self-reported measures of assertiveness. Many American and European psychological concepts are inapplicable and meaningless in African culture.

465. Furst PT: Hallucinogens and Culture. San Francisco, Chandler and Sharp, 1976.

The institutionalization of hallucinogenic agents affects the social structure of the peoples who use them.

466. Fuse T: Some characteristics of suicide in Japan. Psychiatric J University Ottawa 5:89–94, 1980.

Japan is one of the most suicide-prone countries in the world, with rising rates since World War II. Plural suicides and pacts among lovers and family members (Shinju) are unique to Japan. Theories advanced for suicide in Japan include a character vulnerability fostered by excessive dependency, sudden frustration of a need for social recognition resulting from a narcissistic preoccupation with status and social role, and the Japanese philosophy that judges death by fate or debilitation to be unaesthetic and sees suicide as a means of affirming life. Suicide may also be a cry for help during interpersonal crises, as occurs in the West.

467. Fuse T: Suicide and culture in Japan: a study of seppuku as an institutionalized form of suicide. Social Psychiatry 15:57–63, 1980.

Seppuku, a ritualized form of suicide by disembowelment, is presently outlawed in Japan but is still practiced. Seppuku is viewed as altruistic suicide, in which the individual sacrifices his life for his social role. Zen Buddhism, with its emphasis on transcending life and death, and Confucianism have had an influence on the Bushido code that governs the Samurai's life.

468. Gadpaille WJ: Cross-species and cross-cultural contributions to understanding homosexual activity. Arch Gen Psychiatry 37:349–56, 1980.

Homo sapiens is the only species in which adult preferential or obligatory homosexuality occurs naturally. Preferential or obligatory homosexuality in adulthood, in the presence of available and receptive heterosexual partners, is qualitatively rather than quantitatively distinct from all other manifestations of homosexual activity.

469. Gaines AD: Definitions and diagnoses: cultural implications of psychiatric help-seeking and psychiatrists' definitions of the situation in psychiatric emergencies. Culture Medicine Psychiatry 3:381–418, 1979.

Variation in psychiatrists' conceptions of diagnostic entities and situations are of considerable importance in accounting for diagnostic variability and, hence, unreliability. Differences in diagnostic styles may be attributable to the differing definitions of the situation that psychiatric residents bring to their work and that lead them to emphasize one or another of the component features of the psychiatric emergency picture. The lack of a coherent ideology in society at large produces the lack of consensus in psychiatry because psychiatric etiological ideas are cultural ideas in a scientific guise.

470. Galanter M: Psychological induction into the large-group: findings from a modern religious sect. Amer J Psychiatry 137:1574–79, 1980.

Persons joining the Unification church have relatively weak ties to family and peers outside the sect. There is lower mean general well-being scores among the new joiners than longstanding members, but both groups have lower scores than a comparison group outside the sect.

471. Galanter M, Buckley P: Evangelical religion and meditation: psychotherapeutic effects. J Nerv Ment Disease 166(10):685–91, 1978.

In the members of the religious sect "Divine Light Mission," the incidence of neurotic symptoms and of alcohol and drug use declines from the period prior to joining to that immediately after joining. Symptom decline correlates significantly with group-related activities and attitudes and with specific aspects of the ritual meditation.

472. Galanter M, Rabkin R, Rabkin J, Deutsch

A: The "Moonies": a psychological study of conversion and membership in a contemporary religious sect. Amer J Psychiatry 136:165–70, 1979.

Converts to the Unification church experienced emotional distress before joining. Affiliation with the church provided considerable and sustained relief from neurotic distress in proportion to the amount of religious commitment. Relief of neurotic distress plays an implicit role in continued membership.

473. Galey ME: Ethnicity, fraternalism, social and mental health. Ethnicity 4:19–53, 1977.

Immigrants who settled in ethnic communities at the turn of the century established ethnic fraternal associations that uniquely combined principles of representative government, fraternalism, and ethnic exclusivity. Before establishing new community-based health centers to serve multiethnic populations, a concerted effort should be made to gather information on the sociocultural background and the role of community institutions.

474. Garcia C, Levenson H: Differences between blacks' and whites' expectations of control by chance and powerful others. Psychological Reports 37:563–66, 1975.

Amount of income is related to perceptions of control by chance. People who live on a "mere existence" income are often affected by circumstances that are usually interpreted as being beyond anyone's control. Therefore, such people can identify externality with perceptions of a chaotic and unordered world rather than with control by powerful others.

475. Gardner RE, Podolefsky AM: Some further considerations on West Indian conjugal patterns. Ethnology 16:299–308, 1977.

Among the lower economic stratum of Dominican society, marriage is often delayed until the middle to later years of life. West Indian peasants and proletariats are characterized by a common regard for Christian marriage.

476. Garrison V: Dr. Espiritista, or psychiatrist?: health seeking behavior in a Puerto Rican neighborhood of New York City. Med Anthropology vol. 1, no. 2, part 3, 65–180, 1977.

Spiritist centers are often frequented by Puerto Ricans for relief from somatic symptoms, interpersonal conflicts, and psychological complaints (often of a neurotic nature). Spiritism, Santeria, and witchcraft may be practiced at these centers.

477. Garrison V: Support systems of schizophrenic and nonschizophrenic Puerto Rican migrant women in New York City. Schizophrenia Bull 4:561–96, 1978.

Analysis of the social networks and support systems of Puerto Rican migrant women with emotional disturbance indicates that there is greater reliance upon neighbors, friends, and other nonkin than upon family among the schizophrenic women who lead their lives relatively successfully within the community. These nonkin supports should be used in natural network therapy to reintegrate or maintain chronic schizophrenic patients in the Puerto Rican migrant community.

478. Gatere S: Internal migration and cross-cultural conflicts. Mental Health Society 4:212–14, 1977.

Two societies live side by side in African countries today; the traditional African society living in the rural areas and the modern Westernized African society living in the cities and towns. There is much internal migration from the rural to the urban areas. The problems of a modern doctor working with these cultures are outlined with some suggestions to overcome the problems.

479. Gaviria M, Wintrob RM: Supernatural influence in psychopathology: Puerto Rican folk beliefs about mental illness. Canadian Psychiatric Assn J 21:361–69, 1976.

Puerto Ricans living in urban areas of the northeastern United States differ very little in their conception of the causes of mental illness. Puerto Ricans distinguish two broad categories —"craziness" (or psychotic behavior) and "nervousness" (bad nerves) and consider supernatural or natural factors as causative. Spiritism, witchcraft, and fate are believed to be the most important causes of mental illness.

480. Gaviria M, Wintrob R: Spiritist or psychiatrist: treatment of mental illness among Puerto Ricans in two Connecticut towns. J Operational Psychiatry 10:40–45, 1979.

The unique cultural, social, and linguistic characteristics of the Hispanic population present difficulties in the design of mental health services for Puerto Rican patients. Folk healers play a vital role as therapists because they utilize cultural concepts of the community, they share the same belief systems regarding causes and treatment of mental illness, and they are not associated with the stigma of psychiatry.

481. Geha R: For the love of Medusa: a psychoanalytic glimpse into gynecocide. Psychoanalytic Review 62:49–77, 1975.

That the ego can commit gynecocide with permission and insistence from the superego because rescue—in some form—functions as one of the unconscious fantasies helps explain why certain murderers often show a seeming lack of guilt.

482. Gehrie MJ: On the dual perspective of psychoanalytic anthropology as exemplified by interviews with Japanese-Americans. J Psychol Anthropology 1:165–201, 1978.

Two sansei (third-generation) Japanese-Americans demonstrate that what and how they choose to report about their culture in the interview situation are related, in part, to their reactions to the interview situation itself and reflect each individual's experience of his cultural background.

483. Gehrie MJ: Culture as an internal representation. Psychiatry 42:165–70, 1979.

"Internal representation" of culture is a phenomenon internal to the minds of individuals. It is experienced through the life cycle of the emotional attachment to a cultural group. The internal representation of culture plays a role as carrier of values, attitudes, and other such phenomena and has a significant psychological function in individual development.

484. Gelfand DE: Ethnicity, aging and mental health. Intl J Aging Human Development 10:289–98, 1979–1980.

Adaptation of individuals to aging varies by culture, with Spanish-speaking elderly having the greatest fear of dying compared to blacks and whites, Irish elderly using projective defenses to adapt to aging, and Italian aged maintaining a paranoid, aggressive stance, while the opposite is found among Polish elderly. Expanded research is needed in such areas as the impact of the life experience of first-, second-, and third-generation individuals on the mental health of the ethnic group, and the attitudes of the ethnic community toward mental health therapy, in the formulation of new mental health services for the elderly.

485. Gelfand D, Kutzik A (eds): Ethnicity and Aging. New York, Springer, 1979.

Twenty articles deal with ethnic families and the aged.

486. Gelfand M: The infrequency of homosexuality in traditional Shona society. Central African J Medicine 25:201–2, 1979.

Traditional Shona society views marriage as the most essential and happiest institution it possesses and instills in each child proper respect for the opposite sex. In such an atmosphere, while other sexual offenses such as rape, lesbianism, and bestiality are known, homosexuality is rare.

487. Genthner RW, Graham JR: Effects of short-term public psychiatric hospitalization for both black and white patients. J Consulting Clin Psychology 44:118–24, 1976.

Black and white patients do not respond differently to short-term psychiatric hospitalization.

488. George DM, Hoppe RA: Racial identification, preference, and self-concept: Canadian Indian and white schoolchildren. J Cross-Cultural Psychology 10:85–100, 1979.

Both whites and Indians favor the white identification model and indicate a higher rejection at the early stages. Whites follow this pattern at an earlier age level than Indians, suggesting that the race differences found may have simply been differences in the age at which attitude formation commenced.

489. George O: Eskimo Medicine Man. Portland, Oregon Historical Society, 1978.

In notes compiled while traveling in the 1930s, a physician comments on Eskimo mental and physical health.

490. Gergen KJ, Morse SJ, Gergen MM: Behavior exchange in cross-cultural perspective. In Handbook of Cross-Cultural Psychology, edited by HC Triandis and RW Brislin, 5:121–53. Boston, Allyn and Bacon, 1980.

The results of a range of cross-cultural studies relevant to processes of social exchange are examined. Sociological and anthropological work is included along with traditional social psychological research. Exchange theory is a rich and comprehensive framework for understanding behavior in widely divergent cultural settings.

491. Gharagozlou H, Behin MT: Frequency of psychiatric symptoms among 150 opium addicts in Shiraz, Iran. Intl J Addictions 14:1145–49, 1979.

Addicts have more psychiatric symptoms than nonaddicts, with depression being the most frequent symptom.

492. Gharagozlou H, Foulks E, Sherif M, Roknie R: Zar healing in South Iran. Transcult Psych Res Review 17:178–81, 1980.

Zar, a pattern of folk psychotherapy in which diagnosis and treatment are determined while both healer and patient are in a dissociated state, is widely distributed throughout the Middle East. Information is provided both on the cult and on participating patients among the Bandari people of South Iran. Bandari Zar ceremonies, although they feature all the characteristics of Zar elsewhere, primarily involve men and not women. Zar spirits represent the appeasement of political power and the wish to participate in the control of society.

493. Gharagozlou H, Hadjmohammadi M: Report on a three-year follow-up of 100 cases of suicidal attempts in Shiraz, Iran. Intl J Social Psychiatry 23:209–10, 1977.

Suicide attempts can be a way of seeking help and at times contribute to reintegration and a better psychological adaptation.

494. Gibson G: An approach to identification and prevention of developmental difficulties among Mexican-American children. Amer J Orthopsychiatry 48:96–113, 1978.

Early and Periodic Screening Diagnosis and Treatment programs (EPSDT) have the potential both for hurting and for helping Chicanos. It is urgent that their inherent iatrogenic dangers, as well as their potential uses for social control, be recognized and prevented. The potential benefits need to be explored, developed, and exploited.

495. Giel R: Minority conflict: the hijacking of a train by South Molukkan youngsters in the Netherlands. Mental Health Society 4:215–20, 1977.

The hijacking of a train by South Molukkan youngsters in the Netherlands can be analyzed in terms of the generation gap existing between the postfigurative South Molukkan elders and their children who were unsuccessful in their attempts at cofiguration in Holland.

496. Giel R: Problems of transcultural communication. Mental Health Society 4:291–300, 1977.

Both verbal and nonverbal communication occur at various levels of meaning and explicitness. This is most obvious in transcultural exchanges and affects the selection and interpretation of psychological tests administered in countries where the tests were not developed.

497. Giel R: Psychiatry in developing countries. Psychiatric Annals 8(6):92–99, 1978.

Because of his location in a general hospital, the university psychiatrist in a developing country is in a unique position to draw the attention of his students and his colleagues to the important psychosocial aspects of physical illness.

498. Giel R, Harding TW: Psychiatric priorities in developing countries. Brit J Psychiatry 128:513–22, 1976.

Expansion of mental health services in the developing countries will only take place if the task of mental health care is undertaken by a wide range of nonspecialist health workers, including those responsible for primary health care, and if services are directed initially at a very limited range of priority conditions.

499. Giel R, Ormel J: Crowding and subjective health in the Netherlands. Social Psychiatry 12:37–42, 1977.

In the Netherlands, the relationship between dwelling-unit density or crowding and a number of self-reported measures of ill health appears negligible. The proportion of people to rooms may be much too crude a measure to study crowding because it gives no indication of its effects on such factors as personal interaction and privacy.

500. Giel R, Ten Horn GHMM, Ormel J, Schudel WJ, Wiersma D: Mental illness, neuroticism and life events in a Dutch village sample: a follow-up. Psychological Medicine 8:235–43, 1978.

In a five-year follow-up of thirty-two patients identified during a survey of a Dutch village in 1969, about two-thirds were found to have recovered. The persistence of psychiatric problems was related to life experience, as measured by a life-event interview.

501. Gilberg AL: Adolescence: the interface of neurophysiology and cultural determinants. Amer J Psychoanalysis 38:87–90, 1978.

Neurophysiology and culture act as agents to develop a system of normalcy and pathology during adolescence. Cognizance of this interwoven matrix is imperative for all mental health professionals in order to better understand their adolescent patients.

502. Gillies H: Homicide in the west of Scotland. Brit J Psychiatry 128:105–27, 1976.

The salient features of people accused of murder in Scotland are maleness, youthfulness, the causal importance of alchohol, the rarity of suicide after murder, and the high percentage of psychiatrically normal persons.

503. Gilmore MM, Gilmore DD: "Machismo": a psychodynamic approach (Spain). J Psychol Anthropology 2:281–99, 1979.

Machismo, common in lower-class males of many cultures, expresses itself in Spain as hypermasculine sexual aggressiveness. The socioeconomic situation of the lower-class males in Andalusia encourages a father-absent family structure, resulting in an intrapsychic gender identity conflict in young males, who must then stress machismo as a compensatory measure.

504. Gilson BS, Erickson D, Chavez CT, Bobbitt RA, Bergner M, Carter WB: A Chicano version of the Sickness Impact Profile (SIP). Culture Medicine Psychiatry 4:137–50, 1980.

The translated and rescaled Chicano version of the Sickness Impact Profile (SIP) is of great practical use in the field where there is a need for an evaluation instrument in the delivery of health care to the Spanish-speaking population of migrant farm workers and other Spanish-speaking Americans. In the development of the Chicano version of the SIP, there are several issues that may warrant further investigation.

505. Giordano J: Community mental health in a pluralistic society. Intl J Mental Health 5:5–15, 1976.

The reassertion of group identity over the past ten years has pierced the widespread belief that homogenization of culture and institutions and sterilization of group diversity would lead to unity within the individual and society as a whole. A new mental health movement must build and support humanistic and pluralistic institutions and communities.

506. Giordano J, Giordano GP: The Ethno-Cultural Factor in Mental Health. New York, Inst. on Pluralism and Group Identity of the American Jewish Committee, 1977.

Ethnicity affects the prevalence and incidence of mental illness as well as perceptions of illness, utilization of services, and the patient-therapist relationship. Ethnic groups must join to achieve common mental health goals.

507. Glazier S: Pentecostalism, exorcism, and modernization. Transcult Psych Res Review 16:82–83, 1979.

The Pentecostal church in Trinidad has developed an impersonal method of healing with Obeah and spirit possession. Persons who believe themselves to be possessed are encouraged to seek medical attention.

508. Goebel JB, Cole SG: Mexican-American and white reactions to stimulus persons of same and different race: similarity and attraction as a function of prejudice. Psychological Report 36:827–33, 1975.

Mexican-Americans have little to lose and much to gain by viewing whites as similar and by indicating that they would be friendly toward them.

509. Gokay FK: Development of psychiatry in Turkey. Psychiatric Opinion 12:31–35, 1975.

Neuropsychiatry in Turkey and various establishments of Turkish mental health are still in the course of development, which must be supported and accelerated.

510. Gold JH: University students and mental health: Canada, Britain, and Singapore. Intl J Social Psychiatry 25:84–91, 1979.

There are many crucial determinants of the individual outcome and benefit of a university education including the stressful interplay of cultural and socioeconomic factors, which are of growing importance in the inflationary 1970s.

511. Gold JH, Garner JB, Murphy GD, Weldon KL: Youth in transition: mental health problems of black and Micmac students at Dalhousie University. Canadian J Psychiatry 25:49–56, 1980.

Nova Scotia black and Micmac students who are enrolled in the transition-year program at Dalhousie University in Canada have greater anxiety and report more emotional problems than other undergraduates. This anxiety is related to discomfort in the university environment, decreased adherence to religious beliefs and practices, and insufficient encouragement from family and friends.

512. Golden KM: Voodoo in Africa and the United States. Amer J Psychiatry 134:1425–27, 1977.

Hexing practices are a phenomenon of rural isolated communities in the Deep South as well as large urban areas in the northeastern and western United States. The practice of voodoo in the United States is a blend of African voodoo and European witchcraft beliefs.

513. Goldenberg E, Macey T, Sata LS: Socioeconomic factors which influence labeling of mental illness. Psychological Reports 44:1021–22, 1979.

Socioeconomically deprived individuals are more likely to be diagnosed psychotic than are upper-middle-class individuals.

514. Goldstein E: Compulsory treatment in Soviet psychiatric hospitals: a view from the inside. Psychiatric Opinion 12(7):14–20, 1975.

Soviet psychiatry has allowed clinical analysis to be replaced by ideological speculations and people to be incarcerated in hospitals for many years only because they have certain ideas on political reform.

515. Goldstein GS, Oetting ER, Edwards R, Garcia-Mason V: Drug use among Native American young adults. Intl J Addictions 14:855–60, 1979.

Young Native Americans from relatively isolated environments have a higher susceptibility to drugs when they enter an urban culture.

516. Goldstein MC: Pahari and Tibetan polyandry revisited. Ethnology 17:325–37, 1978.

Pahari and Tibetan fraternal polyandry is a functional analog of other wealth-conserving kinship mechanisms such as primogeniture, which operate to reduce the frequency of, or preclude, division of family patrimonies and, in an unperceived and unintended manner, also reduce fertility levels in their respective societies.

517. Gomberg E, Franks V (eds): Gender and Disordered Behavior. New York, Brunner/Mazel, 1979.

Sex differences in psychopathology are common, often because of bias against women.

518. Gomez AG: Some considerations in structuring human services for the Spanish-speaking population of the United States. Intl J Mental Health 5:60–68, 1976.

In the planning and implementing of changes regarding the Spanish-speaking population in the United States, it is essential for the helping professions and services to involve the people themselves, particularly those whom the community considers to be its leaders.

519. Gonzalez R: Mental health services for children in the region of the Americas. Intl J Mental Health 7:39–48, 1978.

Even in the most advanced countries of the Americas, mental health services for children and adolescents are inadequate with respect to both the number of facilities available and the number of competent personnel to operate them.

520. Goodenough WH: Ethnographic field techniques. In Handbook of Cross-Cultural Psychology, edited by HC Triandis and JW Berry, 2:29–55. Boston, Allyn and Bacon, 1980.

Ethnographic field work aims to describe a society's culture. It describes basically two things, what people must have learned in order to participate acceptably in most of the activities of that society, and how members of a society deal with one another.

521. Gordon AJ: Cultural and organizational factors in the delivery of alcohol treatment services to Hispanos. J Alcoholism Related Addictions 15:43–62, 1979.

Data from a Hispanic community in a New England city indicate that service providers, in order to be effective with this community, should emulate the social arrangements of indigenous services.

522. Gorney R, Long JM: Cultural determinants of achievement, aggression, and psychological distress. Arch Gen Psychiatry 37:452–59, 1980.

Levels of achievement, aggression, and psychological distress are partly determined by corresponding levels of competition and interpersonal intensity. However, in the presence of high levels of social synergy, aggression and psychological distress are lowered without affecting the level of achievement.

523. Gottesfeld ML: Countertransference and ethnic similarity. Bull Menninger Clinic 42:63–67, 1978.

The inability of therapists to free themselves from their archaic superegos, which render them inflexible with patients of different cultural backgrounds, can even hamper communication between the therapist and a patient of a similar ethnic background.

524. Gove WR: Sex differences in mental illness among adult men and women: an evaluation of four questions raised regarding the evidence on the higher rates of women. Social Science Medicine 12(3B):187–98, 1978.

In our society, women have higher rates of mental illness than men, and this difference is due primarily to their sex and marital roles. However, it is clear that we know relatively little about the precise nature of the interaction of sex roles, marital roles, socialization, and personality that produces the higher rates in women.

525. Graber RB: Anabaptism: repression or release? J Psychol Anthropology 3:31–32, 1980.

The accusation that sixteenth-century Anabaptism was tied to excessive sensuality and antinomianism—the belief that salvation is through God's grace and one's own works, and that theological and secular laws need not be obeyed—was based on a hostile contemporary source and on relationships between antinomianism and Anabaptism that were historically and culturally nonexistent. Anabaptism has historically shown a significant restriction of sexual and aggressive drives.

526. Graham P: Environmental influences on psychosocial development. Intl J Mental Health 6:7–31, 1977.

In broad terms, social and cultural factors both dictate the criteria by which the presence or absence of psychiatric disorder and behavioral deviance is judged and determine, to a large extent, which people or which children within a particular society will develop such disorder or deviance.

527. Graham P: Intergenerational influences on psychosocial development. Intl J Mental Health 6:73–89, 1977.

The presence of chronic malnutrition and infection in a large section of the population in one culture may result in a pattern of intergenerational continuity with respect to mental retardation that is very different from that in a healthier and better-nourished population living in another culture.

528. Graves PL: Infant behavior and maternal attitudes: early sex differences in West Bengal, India. J Cross-Cultural Psychology 9:45–74, 1978.

Differential maternal attitudes toward boys and girls become marked during the second year of the childrens' lives. This culturally determined change in maternal attitudes leads to insecure attachment among girls.

529. Graves TD, Graves NB: Stress and health: modernization in a traditional Polynesian society. Med Anthropology 3:23–60, 1979.

A study of seventy adult males on Aitutaki (Polynesian Cook Islands) demonstrates that those with the greatest exposure to Western influences experience more conflicts with their friends and family but do not report more physical or mental health problems than those who are more traditionally oriented.

530. Green J (ed): Zuni: Selected Writings of Frank H. Cushing. Lincoln, U. of Nebraska Press, 1979.

A nineteenth-century ethnologist's essays on Zuni include sections on medicine and mythology.

531. Greene LR, Ambramowitz SI, Davidson CV, Edwards DW: Gender, race, and referral to group psychotherapy: further empirical evidence of countertransference. Intl J Group Psychotherapy 30:357–64, 1980.

A greater proportion of female patients are referred to group psychotherapy than are males. White clinicians are more likely to refer patients to groups than minority clinicians. A patient is somewhat more likely to be referred to a group by a clinician of the same sex.

532. Greene PJ: Promiscuity, paternity, and culture. Amer Ethnologist 5:151–59, 1978.

Data from the Human Relations Area Files indicate that paternity uncertainty as measured by female promiscuity is associated with specific marital patterns and kinship terminology systems.

533. Gregory JR: Image of limited good, or expectation of reciprocity? Current Anthropology 16:73–92, 1975.

Expectation of circumstantially balanced reciprocity (ECBR) is a belief that those having more should share with those having less. Whereas the image of limited good involves a zero-sum game—if you have more than others, you have taken something from them—ECBR does not; it simply holds that if you have more than others, you should share it with them.

534. Gregory JR: The modification of an interethnic boundary in Belize. Amer Ethnologist 3:683–708, 1976.

Of Belize's several ethnic groups, the Mopan have been among the last to be drawn into the society's larger institutional system to a significant extent. Although the steadily increasing flow of transactions through a growing number of points of intercultural articulation has resulted in an ongoing process of institutional assimilation, the ethnic assimilation of the Mopan remains problematical.

535. Gregory MS, Silvers A, Sutch D (eds): Sociobiology and Human Nature. San Francisco, Jossey-Bass, 1978.
Sociobiological research has great implications for the human sciences and for the humanities.

536. Griel JZ, Smock AC (eds): Women: Roles and Statuses in Eight Countries. New York, Wiley, 1977.
In Ghana women's and men's domains are separate but equal. In Bangladesh and Egypt women's activities are highly restricted. In France, the United States, and Poland women's options are becoming more equal to those of men.

537. Griffin JDM: Trepanation among early Canadian Indians. Canadian Psychiatric Assn J 21:123–25, 1976.
Evidence indicates that trepanation (cutting a hole in the skull of a living human being for therapeutic reasons) was performed among early Canadian Indians.

538. Griffith EEH, Ruiz P: Cultural factors in the training of psychiatric residents in an Hispanic urban community. Psychiatric Quarterly 49:29–37, 1977.
Therapists need to be familiar with the cultural forces affecting the people they will likely be treating, as illustrated by the case of a Puerto Rican spiritualist.

539. Group for the Advancement of Psychiatry: Mysticism: Spiritual Quest or Psychic Disorder? New York, GAP, 1976.
Mystical experiences are not confined to any one type of personality. Although mysticism may be understood psychoanalytically, some essential features are inexplicable in terms of Western cosmology.

540. Guimera LM: Witchcraft illness in the Evuzok nosological system. Culture Medicine Psychiatry 2:373–96, 1978.
To understand the Evuzok nosological system, it is necessary to grasp the fundamental distinction made between two etiological registers: diurnal and nocturnal illnesses. This opposition implies not only the difference in the status of aggressor, victim, and folk doctor, but also concomitant differences in the relations among them.

541. Guinn R: Self-reported attitudes and behavior of Mexican-American drug use. Intl J Addictions 14:579–84, 1979.
Mexican-American drug users and nonusers differ significantly in attitudes toward drug use and social behaviors. Users tend to be multiple drug users.

542. Guirguis WR: The family and schizophrenia. Psychiatric Annals 10(7):45–54, 1980.
Emphasis on the family rather than on the individual is certainly a useful and practical approach that is applicable not only to the problem of schizophrenia but to all other psychiatric problems as well.

543. Guntern G: Alpendorf tourisme, changement social, stress et problemes psychiatriques. Social Psychiatry 13:41–51, 1978.
Social change transforms rural settlements all over the world into industrialized, and to a certain degree urbanized, international tourist resorts.

544. Gupta GR: Family and Social Change in Modern India. Durham, N.C., Carolina Academic Press, 1976.
While educational level and rate of economic development in different regions are related to variations in family structure, the ideals and affectional bonds in family life influenced by joint family values play a very important part in maintaining the general stability of family life in modern India.

545. Guthrie GM: A social-psychological analysis of modernization in the Philippines. J Cross-Cultural Psychology 8:177–206, 1977.
People in the rural Philippines will often simultaneously hold a variety of both traditional and modern beliefs. Traditional and modern lifestyles are made up of many lowly correlated components, so that an individual can be modern in one activity and traditional in another.

546. Guthrie GM, Tanco PP: Alienation. In Handbook of Cross-Cultural Psychology, edited by HC Triandis and JG Draguns, 6:9–59. Boston, Allyn and Bacon, 1980.
Anyone undertaking cross-cultural research on alienation should specify his or her definition of alienation, adopt measurement techniques that reflect the definition and minimize response biases, and interpret results within the context of the cultural patterns of the people being examined. We cannot assume that our conceptualization of alienation is as appropriate in an alien society as it is in North America. Culturally induced differences in alienation are, after all,

part of the domain of study of cross-cultural psychology.

547. Gynther MD, Lachar D, Dahlstrom LW: Are special norms for minorities needed? Development of an MMPI-F scale for blacks. J Consulting Clin Psychology 46:1403–8, 1978.

Black endorsement patterns agree with only a third of the standard F-scale items of the Minnesota Multiphasic Personality Inventory (MMPI) and show comparable levels of infrequency on only six of thirty-eight supplementary F items. The amount of difference between black and white responses to rarely endorsed items suggests that the MMPI F-scale for blacks will be a more accurate measure of correlates associated with endorsement of deviant items than the standard F-scale.

548. Haavio-Mannila E, Stenius K: Immigrants and natives as mental health care recipients. Mental Health Society 4:171–89, 1977.

There are more mental health problems among immigrants than in the native population in Sweden and in Finland. The immigrant patient rate is high even in socially advantaged groups. Some problems, e.g., paranoia, somatic symptoms, and diffuseness of difficulties, are clearly related to immigration status but others, e.g., alcohol, work, or human relations problems, are connected only with social class or sex, irrespective of immigration status.

549. Hafkin NJ, Bay EG (eds): Women in Africa: Studies in Social and Economic Changes. Stanford, Calif., Stanford U. Press, 1976.

In many respects, the activities of women in Africa have a glowing past, a frustrating present, and an uncertain future.

550. Hahn RA: Aboriginal American psychiatric theories. Transcult Psych Res Review 15:29–58, 1978.

Medicine and healing are thought to be religious activities. Although aboriginal societies reportedly distinguish types of illness, it is not clear whether this distinction is truly explicit in native theory or is ascribed by the scientific observer. Among the illnesses that have been described are tawatl ye sni ("totally discouraged"), susto, pibloqtoq, windigo psychosis, chiyoroso (deafmuteness), and chuvah (acute psychosis). Etiologies include strong emotional experiences, dreams, improper conduct, soul loss, delicts of kin and ancestors, and spirit possession. Therapies include psychoactive drugs, dream interpretation, and healing rituals.

551. Halberstein RA, Saunders AB: Traditional medical practices and medicinal plant usage on a Bahamian island. Culture Medicine Psychiatry 2:177–203, 1978.

The Bimini medical system has historically been efficacious in the treatment and management of many health problems on the islands, partly due to the resourceful utilization of indigenous medicinal plant species. In recent years, the island has experienced a relatively smooth process of medicinal modernization, including the increased availability of Westernized health care and the gradual supplementation of the herbal remedies by imported patent and prescription medications.

552. Haldipur GV: The idea of "cultural" psychiatry: a comment on the foundations of cultural psychiatry. Comp Psychiatry 21:206–11, 1980.

The definition of cultural psychiatry is as elusive as the concept of culture. Conceptual issues such as the individual-culture and culture-environment dichotomies lie at the very foundation of the idea of cultural psychiatry. Hundreds of studies carried out over many years have revealed a significant interrelationship between culture and mental illness.

553. Hall ER, Woods MJ, Joesting J: Relationships among measures of locus of control for black and white students. Psychological Reports 40:59–62, 1977.

The construct of locus of control is multidimensional.

554. Hallpike CR: The Foundations of Primitive Thought. Oxford, Clarendon, 1979.

Primitive thought closely resembles the preoperatory thought of children. While it can solve practical problems of daily living, it is incapable of comprehending modern Western concepts of causality, space, time, realism, abstraction, and introspection.

555. Hamburger S: Profile of curanderos: a study of Mexican folk practitioners. Intl J Social Psychiatry 24:19–25, 1978.

The possibility of utilizing the folk practitioner in an Anglo setting to extend health care to patients may be beneficial to both types of practitioners. The Anglo physician gains a better understanding of the cultural and social problems of his Mexican-American patients, while the curandero extends his usefulness to his people in a setting that is both legally and socially sanctioned.

556. Hamer J: Crisis, moral consensus, and the Wando Magano movement among the Sadama of southwest Ethiopia. Ethnology 16:399–412, 1977.

The Wando Magano movement has not developed into a full-scale revitalization quest because the cultural identity of the Aleta has not been demeaned. Instead, the Aleta have been deprived of a part of their social control system and confronted with alternative values and beliefs pertaining to the exchange system, legitimation of authority, and concepts of justice. The uncertainty created by these events has led to a crisis of moral consensus, but not a cultural breakdown.

557. Hamer J, Steinbring J (eds): Alcohol and Native Peoples of the North. Lanham, Md., University Press of America, 1980.

Beliefs about alcohol and current consumption data are presented for the Inuit (Baffin Island), an Athabaskan group, Algonquin-speaking peoples, and a mixed grouping of urban Native Americans.

558. Hamilton NG: The trickster: the use of folklore in psychoanalytic psychotherapy. Bull Menninger Clinic 44:364–80, 1980.

Insights gained through the application of psychoanalytic principles to folklore can be reapplied to help in the work of psychoanalytic psychotherapy.

559. Hammer M, Makiesky-Barrow S, Gutwith L: Social networks and schizophrenia. Schizophrenia Bull 4:522–45, 1978.

Social-network concepts and methods can provide a unifying framework for social research and schizophrenia. A social-network perspective not only is consistent with a range of other research approaches and findings, but also may help resolve some basic and persistent methodological and conceptual problems.

560. Hamnett MP, Brislin RW (eds): Research in Culture Learning. Honolulu, U. Press of Hawaii, 1980.

The cultural researcher must understand not only the relationship between language and culture but also such concepts as assimilation and field work.

561. Hanemann M: Violence at home: a review of the literature. Amer J Orthopsychiatry 45:328–45, 1975.

A comprehensive theory of violence at home must take into account factors at several social and cultural levels, placing individual functioning within the social group and within the cultural norms by which the group operates. Violence at home occurs when social needs and expectations of the individual are unsupported by either the family or by other social institutions, and when such a mode of expression seems eminently available and legitimate to the individual.

562. Hankins-McNary LD: The effects of institutional racism on the therapeutic relationship. Perspectives Psychiatric Care 17:25–31, 1979.

White educational institutions are not preparing students to provide therapy to black clients. Therapist trainees must be given the opportunity to experience therapeutic encounters with clients who are culturally different from themselves and to explore their negative or inaccurate feelings and perceptions.

563. Hanna JM, Baker PT: Biocultural correlates to the blood pressure of Samoan migrants in Hawaii. Human Biology 51:481–97, 1979.

Samoan adults and children living in Hawaiian urban areas have significantly lower blood pressures than those living in rural areas.

564. Hansen HA: The Witch's Garden. Santa Cruz, Calif., Unity, 1978.

Psychoactive plants have been used by witches and sorcerers for magical flight, prophecy, divination, and poisoning.

565. Harding RK, Looney JG: Problems of Southeast Asian children in a refugee camp. Amer J Psychiatry 134:407–11, 1977.

Vietnamese refugee children who receive strong emotional support from multigenerational Vietnamese families adapt to the new environment. Children separated from their families demonstrate increased emotional vulnerability, and foster placement of children without families presents a serious problem.

566. Harding TW: Psychiatry in rural-agrarian societies. Psychiatric Annals 8(6):74–84, 1978.

There has been a surge of fresh thought and ideas concerning psychiatry in rural-agrarian societies. An approach has emerged, based largely on the work of existing staff in general health services and on community participation, entailing a rigorous selection of priorities.

567. Harding TW, DeArango MV, Baltazar J, Climent CE, Ibrahim HHA, Ladrido-Ignacio L, Murthy RS, Wig NN: Mental disorders in primary health care: a study of their frequency and diagnosis in four developing countries. Psychological Medicine 10:231–41, 1980.

There is a significant rate of psychiatric morbidity in the primary health-care setting of developing countries such as Colombia, India, Sudan, and the Philippines.

568. Harner M: The Way of the Shaman: A Guide to Power and Healing. New York, Harper and Row, 1980.

An anthropologist-shaman describes healing techniques learned from the Jivaro and Carribo (South America), e.g., the quest for a guardian spirit, achieving a spirit state of consciousness, and traveling to the spirit world to retrieve lost souls and to heal.

569. Harper D, Babigian HM, Parris R, Mills B: Migrant farm workers: social conditions, adaptive belief systems, and psychiatric care. Psychiatric Quarterly 51:28–38, 1979.

An examination of two migrant-farm-labor camps shows that laborers are concerned with being exploited, numb about their lives and their place in society, self-critical, distrustful, anxious, and fearful. An understanding of the migrant farm workers' social setting and how they adapt to it is necessary for therapists seeking to diagnose and treat their disorders.

570. Harris GG: Casting Out Anger: Religion Among the Taita of Kenya. Cambridge and New York, Cambridge U. Press, 1978.

Taita religion is a mode of acting in the world rather than a way of thinking about the world and is a means of restoring peace and health. Anger-removal rituals are significant for Taita healing and religion.

571. Harrison GA, Gibson JB (ed): Man in Urban Environments. Oxford and New York, Oxford U. Press, 1977.

The physical environment, human variation, medical and health problems, and behavior and mental health are examined in an evolutionary, biological perspective as adaptations to the urban setting.

572. Harrison I, Cosminsky S: Traditional Medicine. New York, Garland, 1976.

An annotated bibliography (1,135 items, mainly English language) covering ethnomedicine, ethnopharmacology, maternal and child health, mental health, and public health in Africa, Latin America, and the Caribbean; no subject index.

573. Harvey EB, Gazay L, Samuels B: Utilization of a psychiatric-social work team in an Alaskan native secondary boarding school: a five-year review. J Amer Acad Child Psychiatry 15:558–74, 1976.

The mental health team aids the students of an Alaskan secondary school to cope with change by strengthening and enhancing the identity of students and of staff who serve as their role models. As constructive attitudes for coping have developed, there has been a marked decrease in destructive and masochistic behavior.

574. Harvey YK: Six Korean Women. St. Paul, Minn., West, 1979.

The life history accounts of six Korean women who became shamans after being possessed by spirits (Sinboyang) are described.

575. Harwood A: Spiritist As Needed. New York, Wiley, 1977.

Puerto Rican spiritist churches (centro) are a community mental health resource in New York City. Spiritist healers utilize complex diagnostic and therapeutic procedures. Case examples demonstrate cooperation between psychiatrists and spiritist healers.

576. Hasan KZ: Effects on child mental health of psychosocial change in developing countries. Intl J Mental Health 6:49–57, 1977.

Adequate planning for children is limited not only by the general unavailability of financial resources but also by shortages in the supply of trained workers, specialized equipment, school buildings, transport facilities, and cooperation and understanding on the part of teachers, parents, and the children themselves.

577. Hasegawa K: Aspects of community mental health care of the elderly in Japan. Intl J Mental Health 8:36–49, 1979–1980.

Cultural, financial, and various environmental factors must all be taken into consideration in mapping future policy for community care of Japan's mentally disordered elderly, whose number is increasing as the proportion of the elderly in the population increases.

578. Haynes WD: Stress Related Disorders in Policemen. San Francisco, R & E Research Associates, 1978.

Theoretical considerations for a causative relationship between stress and job-related disorders in police work are presented. It is concluded that the recognition of stress as a major factor in job-related disorders for policemen should be an important area of concern for relevant authorities and future research.

579. Hays JR, Smith AL: Comparison of WISC-R and Culture Fair Intelligence Test scores for three ethnic groups of juvenile delinquents. Psychological Reports 46:931–34, 1980.

The Culture Fair Intelligence Test more nearly equates the measured intelligence scores among Mexican-Americans, black Americans, and white Americans. It provides a more reasonable measure of overall intellectual functioning than does the WISC-R.

580. Heacock DR: The black slum child and the problem of aggression. Amer J Psychoanalysis 36:219–26, 1976.

An exposure to violence and life-threatening aggression from many sources causes black children from socioeconomically deprived areas to respond in certain adaptive ways that are appropriate for the culture in which the child is reared. Aggression is displayed directly in an attempt at mastery of the overwhelming frustration and life-threatening aspects of the ghetto. The significance of aggression in the psychotherapeutic relationship between the white therapist and the black child needs to be understood for the therapy to be successful.

581. Heath DB: The sociocultural model of alcohol use: problems and prospects. J Operational Psychiatry 9(1):55–66, 1978.

The sociocultural model of alcohol use focuses on beliefs (and behaviors) about alcohol, its uses, and its effects among members of different populations.

582. Heaven PCL: Authoritarianism and ethnocentrism: a South African sample. Psychological Reports 39:656, 1976.

Authoritarianism and ethnocentrism are slightly evident among white Afrikaans-speaking students in South Africa.

583. Heckel RV: Relationship problems: the white therapist treating blacks in the South. Intl J Group Psychotherapy 25:421–28, 1975.

The white therapist can treat black patients in the southern United States. It is sometimes difficult, occasionally impossible, but often effective if the therapist understands the emerging black value system and the depth of ties that blacks retain with the white culture as well as those ties that have been set aside or abandoned.

584. Heckerman CL (ed): The Evolving Female: Women in Psychosocial Context. New York, Human Sciences, 1980.

Topics include abortion, employment, heterosexual passion, midlife crises, assertive training, consciousness raising, self-help groups, depression, math anxiety, and female mental health.

585. Heiman EM, Burruel G, Chavez N: Factors determining effective psychiatric outpatient treatment for Mexican-Americans. Hospital Community Psychiatry 26:515–17, 1975.

A mental health center offering outpatient services to Mexican-Americans should be centrally located in the Mexican-American community, should have a bicultural and bilingual staff, and should have an informal atmosphere with a minimum number of bureaucratic procedures.

586. Heiman EM, Kahn MW: Mexican American and European American psychopathology and hospital course. Arch Gen Psychiatry 34:167–70, 1977.

Hospitalized Mexican-Americans are not any more severely disturbed than other ethnic groups.

587. Heinrich AC: Changing anthropological perspectives on color-naming behavior. J Psychol Anthropology 1:341–63, 1978.

The development of color-naming behavior, from vague philosophy to rational formulation and empirically based concepts, parallels the development of anthropology as a discipline.

588. Heinrich W: A surface-analysis of German TAT-responses. J Psychol Anthropology 3:17–29, 1980.

The responses of traditional, rural Germans reveal that the mother is viewed as the authoritative center of the family, that the elder man has authority over the younger man, that the female is the center of orientation and the man dependent on her in male-female relations, and that the church has a stronger influence on females than males.

589. Heinrichs HJ: Psychoanalysis and shamanism. Psyche 31:457–75, 1977.

M. L. Leiris, a pioneer of unorthodox social and human science whose work rests on an elementary sensual and analytic base, makes the examination of other cultures a domain for his own personal and cultural-political engagement. Like the practicing psychoanalyst, he regards himself and his knowledge as intertwined with the analytic process. His science offers a chance to develop an engagement against oppression and discrimination.

590. Helgason L: Psychiatric services and mental illness in Iceland. Acta Psychiatrica Scandinavica, supplement 268:1–140, 1977.

Individuals who use psychiatric services are most probably a highly selected sample of those who are mentally ill. The reduction in incidence of patients seeking psychiatric services in late middle age is probably caused by some reduction of mental illness at that age. A growing trend toward treatment of mentally ill patients in facilities other than psychiatric services, and new and more comprehensive psychiatric services, will probably encourage the patient who until now has been reluctant to come for treatment.

591. Helias PJ: The Horse of Pride. New Haven, Conn., Yale U. Press, 1978.

Life in a Breton (France) village is described, including information on sex roles, acculturation, and ethnomedicine.

592. Heller PL, Chalfant HP, Worley MdCR, Quesada GM, Bradfield CD: Socioeconomic class, classification of "abnormal" behaviour and perceptions of mental health care: a cross-cultural comparison. Brit J Med Psychology 53:343–48, 1980.

Class differences are pertinent for both recognition of and recommendations for help regarding behaviors that are commonly considered as "disordered" by professional mental health personnel. These differences are related to conditions of lower-class life, particularly a sense of powerlessness.

593. Henderson DJ: Exorcism, possession, and the dracula cult: a synopsis of object-relations psychology. Bull Menninger Clinic 40:603–28, 1976.

The work of object-relations psychologists has created a synthesis founded on classical tradition that incorporates concepts of "possessing forces." These new possessing forces are the good and bad objects of inner psychic reality.

594. Henderson JH: Psychiatry in Scotland. Psychiatric Opinion 12:27–30, 1975.

In the long run, the real success or failure of psychiatry in Scotland will be judged by the success or failure of services in caring for and managing the patient with long-term mental handicap, disability, or disease.

595. Henderson S: The social network, support and neurosis: the function of attachment in adult life. Brit J Psychiatry 131: 185–91, 1977.

In considering the psychological functions of social networks in terms of attachment theory, it is apparent that social bonds are essential for obtaining support. Individuals have a requirement for affectively positive interaction with others; under stressful conditions this interaction is called support. When support is lacking, psychiatric and medical morbidity rates increase.

596. Henderson S: A development in social psychiatry: the systematic study of social bonds. J Nerv Ment Disease 168:63–69, 1980.

The development in social psychiatry of the systematic study of social bonds has helped with the epidemiological problem of examining individuals' immediate social environment as a principal independent variable. The evidence so far supports the hypothesis that a deficiency in social bonds is a cause of neurosis.

597. Henderson S, Byrne D: Towards a method for assessing social support systems. Mental Health Society 4:164–70, 1977.

The protective function of man's social environment is called "support." The study of support may tap something very fundamental about human social organization with universal applicability irrespective of nationality, social class, or affluence. Careful investigation of "support" promises to be a new development in a social psychiatry that can truly be said to be transcultural.

598. Henderson S, Byrne DG, Duncan-Jones P, Adock S, Scott R, Steele GP: Social bonds in the epidemiology of neurosis: a preliminary communication. Brit J Psychiatry 132:463–66, 1978.

A strong inverse relationship exists between social bonds and the presence of neurotic symptoms; this association is strongest in the case of close affectional ties.

599. Henry EO: A North Indian healer and the sources of his power. Social Science Medicine 11:309–17, 1977.

An understanding of the folk healer's effectiveness requires consideration of the pertinent mental culture, the roles of the curer, and the image of himself that the curer projects.

600. Henscher JE: The role of humor and folklore themes in psychotherapy. Amer J Psychiatry 137:1546–49, 1980.

The effectiveness of humor and of folklore

themes is proportional to the genuineness of the interpersonal relationship and can prove helpful when used judiciously in psychotherapy.

601. Hessler RM: Citizen participation, social organization, and culture: a neighborhood health center for Chicanos. Human Organization 36:124–34, 1977.

A decentralized, nonhierarchical model of citizen participation leads to integration within communities and increased organizational adaptiveness. This is accomplished through the application of elements of local culture to institutional decisionmaking.

602. Hessler RM, Nolan MF, Ogbru B, Kong-Ming New P: Intraethnic diversity: health care of the Chinese-Americans. Human Organization 34:253–62, 1975.

No one pattern of health care usage can be used to characterize the illness behavior of Chinese-Americans. Furthermore, one cannot assume that the normative structure of the community is simple enough to allow one to predict a common utilization pattern knowing specific ethnicity, beliefs, and demographic factors. Chinatowners participate in a complex multifaceted pattern of illness behavior.

603. Hiatt LR (ed): Australian Aboriginal Mythology. Canberra, Australian Inst. Aboriginal Studies, 1975.

Myth and ritual are closely linked. Psychoanalytic interpretations of aboriginal myths have excessive sexual interpretations but may sometimes be valid.

604. Hibbs BJ, Kobos JC, Gonzalez J: Effects of ethnicity, sex, and age on MMPI profiles. Psychological Reports 45:591–97, 1979.

Differences between Mexican-Americans and Anglo-Americans on the MMPI cannot be attributed to ethnicity alone. Ethnicity, sex, age, and their interactions all contribute to these differences.

605. Higginbotham H: Culture and the delivery of psychological services in developing nations. Transcult Psych Res Review 16:7–27, 1979.

Societies undergoing modernization or disintegration place undue stress on their members, with resulting psychological problems and a need for therapeutic resources. Service innovators should not be guided solely by the tenets of Western psychiatry. They must be sensitive to indigenous lifestyles, to socioeconomic barriers,

to absent specialized facilities, training opportunities, and manpower, to problems with community and family acceptance of psychiatry, and to traditional healers. The Ethno-Therapy and Culture Accommodation Scale (ETCAS) may be used to gather and to analyze mental health data.

606. Hippler AE: Culture and personality of the Yolngu of Northeastern Arnhem Land. Part 1: Early socialization. J Psychol Anthropology 1:221–44, 1978.

Cultural description and analysis are integrated with personality dynamics to achieve a perspective on the early socialization of the Yolngu Aborigines. This socialization is reflected in adult life and institutions.

607. Hippler A: Rejoinder to Estroff's "The anthropology-psychiatry fantasy." Transcult Psych Res Review 16:104–7, 1979.

The anthropologist who is not well trained in psychoanalytic development psychology and psychodynamic theories remains a mere collector of unrelated trivia that is often more puzzling than useful.

608. Hippler A, Cawte J: The Malgri territorial anxiety syndrome: primitive pattern for agoraphobia. J Operational Psychiatry 9(2):23–31, 1978.

The Malgri group of disorders—symptoms that occur upon entering new territory—is described among the Lardil and Yolgrau of Australia. The presence of this syndrome in hunters and gatherers may represent an early pattern of agoraphobia.

609. Hirai T: Zen Meditation Therapy. Tokyo, Japan Publications, 1975.

Zen (Zazen) is a therapeutic process. Hishiryo, a state of enlightenment, can be defined in terms of brain-wave activity, cardiac and respiratory rates, and galvanic skin response.

610. Hirokoshi H: Mental illness as a cultural phenomenon: public tolerance and therapeutic process among the Moslem Sundanese in west Java. Indonesia 28:121–38, 1979.

Mental illness results from moral weakness or supernatural fate, which causes an overheating of the mind and an inability to recall God's wisdom and words.

611. Hitch PJ: Culture, social structure, and the explanation of migrant mental illness. Mental Health Society 4:136–43, 1977.

Both the culture of the migrant community and

the cultural, social, economic, and political realities of life in the host community affect the rate of mental illness found in migrants.

612. Hitch PJ, Rack PH: Mental illness among Polish and Russian refugees in Bradford. Brit J Psychiatry 137:206–11, 1980.

In Bradford, England, foreign-born people have substantially higher psychiatric illness rates than native born. Morbidity is higher among Poles than Ukrainians.

613. Hitchcock JT, Jones RL (eds): Spirit Possession in the Nepal Himalayas. Westminster, England, Aris and Phillips, 1976.

The disease forms of Nepalese spirit possession are classified according to their designation in time and space. The training and roles of six shamans are discussed.

614. Ho DYF: The conception of man in Mao Tse-tung thought. Psychiatry 41:391–402, 1978.

The main idea of man in Mao Tse-tung thought can be summarized as follows: (1) human beings are distinguished from all other creatures by virtue of the fact that they alone are capable of exercising the voluntary activist capability that enables them to form conceptual knowledge and to reflect upon this knowledge and to test for its correctness through social practice; (2) in a class society, human nature that transcends class boundaries does not exist; universal human nature can be realized only in a classless society.

615. Hobfoll SE, Kelso D, Peterson WJ: The Anchorage skid row. J Stud Alcohol 41:94–99, 1980.

An Alaskan skid row contains a high percentage of Native Americans. Four groups are identified: highly mobile workers, working residents, semiemployed residents, and the homeless unemployed.

616. Hock-Smith J, Spring A (eds): Women in Ritual and Symbolic Roles. New York, Plenum, 1978.

The relationship of dominant female metaphors and ritual roles to ideas and practices concerning female reproductive and sexual energies is examined in such cultures and religious systems a Scottish Pentecostalism, rural Mexican Catholicism, and the Luvale of Zambia, where spirit possession is important.

617. Hoffman H, Noem AA: Adjustment of Chippewa Indian alcoholics to a predominantly white treatment program. Psychological Reports 37:1284–86, 1975.

Treatment for alcoholism in an integrated program can sometimes help Indian alcoholics.

618. Hojat M, Foroughi D: Iranian subjects' responses as ideal person on the Eysenck Personality Inventory. Psychological Reports 45:499–502, 1979.

Instructions to fake a "nice personality" on the Eysenck Personality Inventory produce a significant decrease in neuroticism and a significant increase in extroversion and lie scales.

619. Hollos M: Logical operations and role-taking abilities in two cultures: Norway and Hungary. Child Development 46:638–49, 1975.

Socially isolated children in both Norway and Hungary perform less well on role-taking tasks but do significantly better on logical operations at all ages than village and town children.

620. Holmes LD, Fallman G, Jantz V: Samoan personality. J Psychol Anthropology 1:453–72, 1978.

Traditional Samoan values of hereditary rank, the functions and privileges of relationship groups, the rights of the village, and the individual as a minor component of the family have persisted, although the youth of American Samoa are increasingly acquiring more modern traits, such as self-reliance and a sense of self-worth.

621. Holter FR: Psychoanalytic questions and methods in anthropological field work. J Psychol Anthropology 1:391–405, 1978.

Psychoanalytic questions and methods are applied in anthropologic field work to investigate the unconscious meaning and forces in human behavior, development concepts, and other areas pertaining to the individual and his society.

622. Holtzman WH: Projective techniques. In Handbook of Cross-Cultural Psychology, edited by HC Triandis and JW Berry, 2:245–78. Boston, Allyn and Bacon, 1980.

Projective techniques are indirect methods of assessment of personality by analyzing the responses of an individual to ambiguous stimuli presented in a standard manner. Attempts to categorize, quantify, and standardize the response variables underlying projective test behavior have met with varying degrees of success. Although the Rorschach has proved to be somewhat refractory to such efforts, a new ink blot method, the Holtzman Inkblot Technique (HIT), yields twenty-two well-standardized scores having high reliability and demonstrated validity.

623. Holtzman WH, Diaz-Guerrero R, Swartz JD: Personality Development in Two Cultures. Austin, U. of Texas Press, 1975.

A cross-cultural longitudinal study of schoolchildren in Mexico and the United States supports the hypotheses that Americans tend to be more active in their style of coping with problems and challenges, more dynamic, technological, and external in the meaning of activity within subjective culture, and more complex and differentiated in cognitive structure, while Mexicans are more family centered, more cooperative in interpersonal activities, and more pessimistic in outlook on life.

624. Hong KM, Townes BD: Infant's attachment to inanimate objects: a cross-cultural study. J Amer Acad Child Psychiatry 15:49–61, 1976.

The phenomenon of attachment to an inanimate object appears to be closely associated with child-rearing practices, especially those related to the time of going to sleep. The incidence of an infant's attachment to inanimate objects is lower in a culture or social group in which infants receive a greater amount of physical contact.

625. Honigmann J Jr, Honigmann I: Responsibility and nurturance: an Austrian example. J Psychol Anthropology 1:81–100, 1978.

There is a close association between responsibility and nurturant behavior in a rural Austrian community.

626. Hood RW, Hall JR: Comparison of reported religious experience in Caucasian, American Indian, and two Mexican American samples. Psychological Reports 41:657–58, 1977.

American Indians and Mexican-Americans report more mystical experiences than either Caucasians or acculturated Mexican-Americans.

627. Hood RW, Hall JR, Watson PJ, Biderman M: Personality correlates of the report on mystical experience. Psychological Reports 44:804–6, 1979.

The person reporting a mystical experience may be described as one who has a breadth of interest and is creative and innovative, tolerant of others, socially adept, and unwilling to accept simple solutions to problems.

628. Horikoshi H: Asrama: an Islamic psychiatric institution in west Java. Social Science Medicine 14(B):157–65, 1980.

The Moslem Sundanese of Java believe that God influences the mind, while Satan influences the flesh. Most illness occurs when excessive heat is absorbed from Satan, and mental illness is thought to occur when the overheated blood affects the mind and allows the victim to be exposed to spirit possession. Thus the folk medicine seeks to reduce excessive heat and restore a balance. Treatment at the Asrama consists of taking cool fluids, eating a bland, cool diet, and talking with the possessing spirit. The second phase of treatment consists of counseling, work therapy, and religious training to rehabilitate the patient.

629. Horowitz RT: Jewish immigrants to Israel: self-reported powerlessness and alienation among immigrants from the Soviet Union and North America. J Cross-Cultural Psychology 10:366–74, 1979.

While personal control dimensions tend to be shared by individuals in all highly industrialized societies, the control ideology tends to be conditioned by factors related to the societal climate and political regime.

630. Howard A: Polynesia and Micronesia in psychiatric perspective. Transcult Psych Res Review 16:123–45, 1979.

The isolated island environments of the region form a strong emphasis on interpersonal harmony, on control of anger, and on shame as opposed to guilt. The key to character development is a pattern of early childhood indulgence followed by harsh socialization. Most problem drinking is indicative of a sense of impotence produced by an inability to master a rapidly changing world. Suicide seems to be an impulsive response to a distressing event and may be contagious. Although persons exhibit little neurosis, they are not free from anxiety and emotional pain. Modernization of the region has resulted in increased psychosomatic ailments.

631. Howells JC: Family diagnosis. Psychiatric Annals 10(7):6–14, 1980.

The aim of family diagnosis is to examine the disorder of the whole family. Only after he arrives at an understanding of the family disorder can the clinician plan effective treatment.

632. Hraba J: American Ethnicity. Itasca, Ill., F. E. Peacock, 1979.

Sociological and psychological perspectives on ethnic relations are reviewed, with emphasis on Japanese-, Chinese-, Mexican-, black, and Native Americans.

633. Hudson RP, Humphrey JA, Kupferer HJ: Regional variations in the characteristics of victims of violence. Intl J Social Psychiatry 26:300–20, 1980.

Explorations of homicidal and suicidal behavior must take into account variations in the sociocultural context of these acts, the variations in the patterns of violence, and the divergent characteristics of the victims of violence.

634. Hufford D: Christian religious healing. J Operational Psychiatry 8(2):22–27, 1977.

Christian religious healing is rapidly increasing among all classes of patients and may be adaptive or maladaptive. In attempting to modify, accommodate, or mobilize this complex cultural phenomenon, the therapist must consider the patient's religious healing system in terms of variations in structure, language, social context, emphasis on physical as opposed to spiritual healing, and empirical base.

635. Humphrey JA, Kupferer HJ: Pockets of violence: an exploration of homicide and suicide. Dis Nervous System 38:833–37, 1977.

When social structural blockage or frustrations are encountered, aggression in the form of homicide or assaultive behavior is a likely consequence.

636. Huntington R, Metcalf P: Celebrations of Death. Cambridge and New York, Cambridge U. Press, 1979.

The symbolic interpretation of funeral rituals is examined in various cultures in Borneo (Berawan, Ma'anyan, Iban), the Celebes (Toradja), Bali, Timor (Mambai), Malagasy, Thailand, Egypt, France, England, and the United States.

637. Hynes K, Werbin J: Group psychotherapy for Spanish speaking women. Psychiatric Annals 7(12):52–63, 1977.

A women's group was formed by a group of Spanish-speaking women in San Mateo County. The group members discussed their feelings of loneliness, their frustrations with their families, and their somatic complaints. The women became strongly supportive of one another. The change that took place is felt to indicate that Spanish-speaking women in the United States can benefit from group psychotherapy.

638. Ibrahim AS: Extraversion and neuroticism across cultures. Psychological Reports 44:799–803, 1979.

Scores from the Eysenck Personality Inventory given to members of three different cultures reveal that Egyptians are the most neurotic and the least extraverted, while Americans exhibit a greater tendency toward extraversion than Britons.

639. Ichilov O, Bar S: Extended family ties and the allocation of social rewards in veteran kibbutzim in Israel. J Marriage Family 42:421–26, 1980.

The proportion of extended family members in a kibbutz's population cannot in itself account for a member's power and influence.

640. Ichiro H: Nihon No Shamanism. Tokyo, Ko-dan-sha, 1977.

Genuine charismatic shamans in Japan are characterized by nervousness, excitability, suggestibility, hallucinations, loss of consciousness, seizures, and active dreaming; hereditary professional shamans achieve their profession by virtue of birth and training. Shamans are not pathological and are able to express universal needs as well as mediate between the sacred and the profane. Shamanism, in disguised form, exists in the styles of Japanese student movements and of political and religious leadership.

641. Iga M: Stress and suicide in Japan. Transcult Psych Res Review 17:243–44, 1980.

The extreme stress of the present-day school examination system is a major cause of the increased incidence of suicide among young people in Japan. This system is a reflection of traditional, philosophical, and cultural attitudes acting within the context of a rapidly modernized industrial society.

642. Iga M, Yamamoto J, Noguchi T, Koshinaga J: Suicide in Japan. Social Science Medicine 12(A):507–16, 1978.

High suicide rates in Japan are the result of an inability of persons to resolve conflicting values.

643. Ikegami N: Growth of psychiatric beds in Japan. Social Science Medicine 14(A):561–70, 1980.

The increase in psychiatric beds in Japan has resulted in large part from the establishment of private hospitals. A further increase in psychiatric beds is necessary if the psychiatric sector is to play a major role in geriatric care.

644. Ikemi Y: Eastern and Western approaches

to self-regulation. Canadian J Psychiatry 24:471–80, 1979.

Japanese zen and some techniques of yoga require modification if they are to be used for medical therapy. Autogenic self-regulatory methods have limitations in treating subjects with severely distorted conditioning in their bodily and mental functions. Naikan therapy can be one of the effective self-analytical and self-regulatory approaches.

645. Ikemi Y, Ishikawa H: Integration of occidental and oriental psychosomatic treatments. Psychotherapy Psychosomatics 31:324–33, 1979.

The oriental way of life can contribute to psychosomatic medicine through its realization of the illusion of mind-body dualism, its development of practical somatopsychic techniques for learning self-control, and its orientation toward realizing one's true nature. A meaningful integration of both standard psychosomatic and somatopsychic techniques is sought by the authors.

646. Ilfeld FW: Current social stressors and symptoms of depression. Amer J Psychiatry 134:161–66, 1977.

Over a fourth of the variance in depressive symptoms are accounted for by five social stressors (marriage, job, neighborhood, parenthood, and economic activity). Depression is most closely related to the social stressors of marriage and parenting, and symptoms increase proportionately to the total numbers of stress areas.

647. Imperato PJ: African Folk Medicine. Baltimore, York, 1977.

The folk medicine of the Bambara is intimately related to African religious beliefs, with a strong Islamic component.

648. Inamura H: The pattern of maladaptation among overseas Japanese: a psychopathological study of culture conflict (in Japanese). Seishin Igaku 22:983–1010, 1980.

In comparison with rates in Japan, Japanese living abroad have higher rates of suicide, neurosis, psychosis, alcoholism, and social phobias. They are often perceived incorrectly to be interested only in business and to be disinterested in local cultures and sensitivities. A general pattern of cultural adjustment consists of periods of transition, discontent, resignation, adaptation, and nostalgia.

649. Inkeles A: Understanding and misunderstanding individual modernity. J Cross-Cultural Psychology 8:135–76, 1977.

Just as the impact of institutions on individuals must be taken as problematic, so should the impact of individual characteristics on the social system be recognized as a matter for study. Confusion is inevitable if discussions are couched in extremely general terms rather than specifying precisely what types and degree of social change are in question.

650. Ionesau-Tongyonk J: The depressive equivalents of Orientals and Occidentals. Transcult Psych Res Review 15:77–78, 1978.

Masked depressions are atypical forms of endogenous depression. In Orientals, the extended family provides some protection against depression. Fewer people in Thailand now consider agitated depressives as being possessed by evil spirits, and even retarded depressives are no longer tolerated by the village communities.

651. Ireland JF, Kahn MW: How fair is the culture IQ test? Intl J Social Psychiatry 25:1–3, 1979.

Considerable caution should be exercised in using the Cattell as a culture-fair method of IQ evaluation with underprivileged delinquent youth.

652. Irfani S: Eysenck's extraversion, neuroticism, and psychoticism inventory in Turkey. Psychological Reports 41:1231–34, 1977.

Turkish students score higher on the lie and psychoticism scales of the Eysenck's PEN inventory than do members of other national groups.

653. Irvine JT: Wolof "magical thinking": culture and conservation revisited. J Cross-Cultural Psychology 9:300–10, 1978.

Cultural conventions governing the organization of talk are more likely to explain the responses of unschooled Wolofs of Senegal than is "magical thinking."

654. Irvine SH, Carroll WK: Testing and assessment across cultures: issues in methodology and theory. In Handbook of Cross-Cultural Psychology, edited by HC Triandis and JW Berry, 2:181–244. Boston, Allyn and Bacon, 1980.

Convergent validity across cultures has to be demonstrated by the inclusion of measures constructed on the principle of stimulus identity along with measures supposed to guarantee conceptual equivalence. Major variations will occur within cultures and across them. The goal of constructing a general science of man might best be furthered, in the context of paper and pencil testing, by recognizing this at the outset of research and theorizing, and by conducting such activities in terms of that recognition.

655. Issacs HL: Iroquois herbalism: the past 100 years. Intl J Social Psychiatry 22:272–81, 1976/1977.

The medical competence of the Iroquois derives mainly from an accumulated store of botanical observations and their application to pharmaceutical experimentation. However, these time-tested treatments have been altered over the years. The conditions of Iroquois life over the past hundred years, specifically the pressures of their position as an enclave within a larger society, have in certain ways affected their pragmatic grasp on reality.

656. Iwai H: East and West. Psychotherapy Psychosomatics 31:357–60, 1979.

Western psychotherapy is very rationalistic, viewing the suppression of desire as the cause of neurosis. Japanese psychotherapy, however, views neurosis as an imbalance that is the weak point of human nature.

657. Iwai H, Homma A, Amamoto H, Asakura M: Morita psychotherapeutic process. Psychotherapy Psychosomatics 29:330–32, 1978.

Morita psychotherapy, established in 1921 by Professor Schoma Morita, is divided into three stages—bed rest, work therapy, and actual life stages. While psychoanalysis based on Western rationalism seeks to obtain insight into human nature by self-analysis, Morita psychotherapy, based on Eastern naturalism, aims to find solutions through the harmony between man and nature.

658. Izard CE: Cross-cultural perspectives on emotion and emotion communication. In Handbook of Cross-Cultural Psychology, edited by HC Triandis and W Lonner, 3:185–221. Boston, Allyn and Bacon, 1980.

Although the expressions and inner experiences that characterize the fundamental emotions are innate and universal, there are numerous cultural differences in attitudes toward emotions and their expressions. Each culture tends to have its own set of display rules, and these norms tend to restrict the expression of emotions in terms of time and circumstance.

659. Jackson A: Na-khi Religion. New York, Mouton, 1979.

Ritual texts on suicide, medicine, healing, and many other areas are presented. The Na-khi are an ethnic minority of 130,000 persons in northwestern China.

660. Jaffee Y, Berger A: Cultural generality of the relationship between sex and aggression. Psychological Reports 41:335–36, 1977.

The positive relationship observed between sexuality and aggression is a cross-cultural phenomenon.

661. Jahoda G: Theoretical and systematic approach in cross-cultural psychology. In Handbook of Cross-Cultural Psychology, edited by HC Triandis and WW Lambert, 1:69–144. Boston, Allyn and Bacon, 1980.

The reasons for the growing importance of theory in cross-cultural psychology are examined, and the general types of theories and models that have been prominent are surveyed, including a broad account of the methods and samples used to test them. A major weakness of current theories is an inadequate operationalization of the concept *culture*.

662. Janakiramaiah N, Subbakrishna DK: Somatic neurosis in Muslim women in India. Social Psychiatry 15:203–6, 1980.

Muslim women with "somatic neurosis" are significantly different from women with anxiety neurosis and depressive neurosis in regard to all variables except age.

663. Janus S, Bess B: A Sexual Profile of Men in Power. Englewood Cliffs, N.J., Prentice-Hall, 1977.

Interviews with elite call girls and madams reveal the proclivity of politicians to frequent prostitutes.

664. Janzen JM: The Quest for Therapy in Lower Zaire. Berkeley, U. of California Press, 1978.

In Kongo society, remedial therapeutic action for medical problems is arranged and sometimes created by the therapy-managing group. Each of the major medical systems—the art of the Nganga, kinship therapy, purification and initiation, and Western medicine—is couched in a social and a cognitive consensus.

665. Jaynes J: The Origin of Consciousness in the Breakdown of the Bicameral Mind. Boston, Houghton Mifflin, 1977.

Primitive man, dominated by input from the right cerebral cortex, developed consciousness when he began to introspect on his destructive behavior.

666. Jegede RO: Outpatient psychiatry in an urban clinic in a developing country. Social Psychiatry 13:93–98, 1978.

Physical complaints dominate the symptomatology in most Nigerian psychiatric patients irrespective of degree of formal education.

667. Jensen GF, Stauss JH, Harris VW: Crime, delinquency, and the American Indian. Human Organization 36:252–57, 1977.

Indian versus non-Indian differences are greatest for alcohol-related offenses, with the Indian arrest rates paralleling the black arrest rates for several different types of offenses.

668. Jessor R, Jessor S: Problem Behavior and Psychosocial Development. New York, Academic, 1977.

The complex psychosocial variables that influence the transitions from childhood to adolescence to young adult life are presented. Problem behavior is associated with adolescents who express great concern for personal autonomy, lack of interest in the conventional goals of church and school, and a jaundiced view of society.

669. Jilek WG: A quest for identity: therapeutic aspects of the Salish Indian guardian spirit ceremonial. J Operational Psychiatry 8(2):46–51, 1977.

The therapeutic aspects of the guardian spirit ceremonial of the Coast Salish Indians of British Columbia and Washington State are described. By ritual death and rebirth, the anomic depression that may result from deculturization under Western influences can be removed.

670. Jilek W: Native renaissance: the survival and revival of indigenous therapeutic ceremonials among North American Indians. Transcult Psych Res Review 15:117–47, 1978.

A contemporary vitality of therapeutic ceremonialism is clearly demonstrated among the Navaho, Iroquois, and Dakota Sioux (Heyoka cult and Yuwipi ritual). The Gourd Dance and the Sun Dance of the Plains Indians and the Winter Spirit Dance of the Northwest Pacific Coast Indians are dance cults with significant therapeutic components. Peyotism is a pan-Indian religious and therapeutic movement. The persistence and revival of indigenous Amerindian healing result from the need for culture-congenial and holistic therapeutic approaches.

671. Jilek WG: The epileptic's outcast role and its background: a contribution to the social psychiatry of seizure disorders. J Operational Psychiatry 10:127–33, 1979.

The prevailing social discrimination against epileptics among the Wapogoro preserves the outcast role. Of the three etiological conceptualizations of epilepsy—sin and punishment, spirit possession, or contagious disease—contagious disease is the most significant in its implications for the social psychiatry of epilepsy.

672. Jilek W, Jilek-Aall L: Massenhysterie mit koro-symptomatik in Thailand. Schweizer Archiv fur Neurologie, Neurochirurgie und Psychiatrie 120:257–59, 1977.

An epidemic of koro occurred in at least 200 patients (most of them Thai) in 1976. All patients recovered after brief symptomatic intervention. Popular opinion and the news media echoed the patients' paranoid projection of viewing the epidemic as a Vietnamese assault through food and tobacco poisoning.

673. Jilek W, Jilek-Aall L: The psychiatrist and his shaman colleague: cross-cultural collaboration with traditional Amerindian therapists. J Operational Psychiatry 9(2):32–39, 1978.

Disease is seen by tradition-oriented, non-Western societies as a supernatural phenomenon with moral implications, while modern Western society sees disease as a natural phenomenon with moral implications. Western therapists have been impressed by the positive psychohygiene and therapeutic role of North Amerindian traditional healers in native cultures.

674. Jilek W, Jilek-Aall L: Rejoinder to Estroff's "The anthropology-psychiatry fantasy." Transcult Psych Res Review 16:108, 1979.

Ethnopsychiatric work continues to be motivated by the ongoing need of Western therapists to understand non-Western patients and their indigenous healers.

675. Jilek W, Roy C: Homicide committed by Canadian Indians and non-Indians. Intl J Offender Therapy Comparative Criminology 20(3):201–16, 1976.

Hypotheses that emerged from a study of prisoners in British Columbia include the following: Canadian Indians (1) are overrepresented in cases of criminal homicide; (2) differ from white homiciders by a lack of purposefulness of the criminal act, by the different nature of victims, by a predominant association of homicide and previous delinquency with alcohol, by deficient preincarceration school and vocational training, and by a different perception of incarceration's benefits, therapeutic opportunities, and lack of intergroup stigma attached to it; and (3) show less deviant sexual adjustment or psychosis than do white homiciders.

676. Jilek-Aall L: The Western psychiatrist and his non-Western clientele. Canadian Psychiatric Assn J 21:353–59, 1976.

Whenever a Western-trained psychiatrist is treating patients from a non-Western society he must acquire sufficient knowledge of that culture in order to distinguish between genuine psychiatric illness and culturally determined states. He must also be able to gauge the degree of acculturation in his patient and to judge whether a therapist or indigenous healer of that very culture would be of more benefit to his patient than Western psychiatry.

677. Jilek-Aall L: Alcohol and the Indian-white relationship. Confina Psychiatrica 21:195–223, 1978.

As exemplified by the Coast Salish Indians, displeasure with mixed AA meetings has led to the formation of all-Indian AA groups that are more attuned to nativistic movements. These AA groups are a form of nonorganized religion such as the Peyote Religion, the Indian Shaker Church, the Ghost Dance, and the Longhouse People.

678. Jilek-Aall L, Jilek W, Flynn F: Sex role, culture and psychopathology: a comparative study of three ethnic groups in western Canada. J Psychol Anthropology 1 (4):473–88, 1978.

Cultural factors are shown to be the most important differentiating criteria of symptom formation among three ethnic groups in western Canada: Doukhobors of both sexes manifest paranoia toward God, the Devil, or legal authority; Salish Indians display prolonged mourning reactions and suicide attempts; and Mennonites manifest guilt and fear of rejection or punishment by God.

679. Johannes A: Many medicines in one: curing in the eastern highlands of Papua New Guinea. Culture Medicine Psychiatry 4:43–70, 1980.

Examination of traditional medical care among the eastern highlands of Papua New Guinea indicates that a mix of physical and psychological elements accounts for Nekematigi success in treating the chronic infectious diseases that predominate in their environment. This is likely to be true of many previously reported medical systems hitherto interpreted primarily in psychological, social, or symbolic terms.

680. Johnson CK, Gilbert MD, Herdt GH: Implications for adult roles from differential styles of mother-infant bonding: an ethological study. J Nerv Ment Disease 167(1):29–37, 1979.

Ethological observations of maternal and infant behaviors in vervet monkeys indicate that the detachment or separation process of mother-infant interaction is as important a factor during development as the primary maternal bond.

681. Johnson M: An approach to feminist therapy. Psychotherapy: Theory, Research, Practice 13:72–76, 1976.

Feminist therapy invariably requires adoption of new attitudes, not just new techniques. It thus necessitates more introspection and discomfort than many therapists may be willing to undergo.

682. Jonas AD, Jonas DF: A biological basis for the Oedipus complex: an evolutionary and ethological approach. Amer J Psychiatry 132:602–6, 1975.

The Oedipus complex has a strong biological basis in human prehistoric and primate behavior. Understanding the relationship between sex and rank can aid in the therapy of sexual problems.

683. Jonas DF, Jonas AD: Gender differences in mental function: a clue to the origin of language. Current Anthropology 16:626–30, 1975.

The first context in which protolanguage proves adaptive is in the attachment behavior between the hominid mother and her infant. Our human powers of speech and language develop from this matrix.

684. Jones EE, Zoppel CL: Personality differences among blacks in Jamaica and the United States. J Cross-Cultural Psychology 10:435–56, 1979.

Jamaicans see themselves as more spontaneous and excitable than their American counterparts, as well as more orderly and requiring greater certainty and definiteness.

685. Jones IH: Hypochondriacal states and magical acts among tribal Aborigines. In Aboriginal Cognition, edited by GE Kearney and OW McElwain, pp. 324–33. Canberra, Australian Inst. Aboriginal Studies, 1976.

Magic and sorcery, often as the result of group antagonism, may cause or precipitate hypochondriasis.

686. Jones IH: Severe illness followed with anxiety following a reported magical act on an

Australian Aboriginal. Med J Australia 2:93–96, 1977.

Magical sanctions are social conformity mechanisms that had a high survival value in aboriginal society. Ideas of magic may survive even when other ideas are discarded. Magical fright may cause vomiting with consequent fluid imbalance and cardiac arrhythmia.

687. Jones PA: The validity of traditional-modern attitude measures. J Cross-Cultural Psychology 8:207–39, 1977.

It is important to use both the factorial analyses of the interitem correlations and the "predictive validity" coefficients as complementary empirical evidence for moving toward both the refinement of a theoretical conception of modernity and the revision of measures of modern attitudes.

688. Jones R, Jones SK: The Himalayan Woman. Palo Alto, Calif., Mayfield, 1976.

The frequency of divorce and unstable marriage among the Lembu of Nepal is directly linked to economic and social options available to its women.

689. Jones RAK, Belsey EM: Breast feeding in an inner London borough—a study of cultural factors. Social Science Medicine 11:175–79, 1977.

Many women have an irrational distaste for breast feeding. This feeling is strong enough to overcome their belief that it would be better for the baby and their husband's opinion that they should breast feed.

690. Joyce CRB: Cultural variation in the responses to pharmacotherapy and the "nonspecific" factors which may affect this. Transcult Psych Res Review 17:129–48, 1980.

It is unclear whether the lack of studies on cultural or ethnic differences in the response to psychotropic drugs results from inadequate methodology or from the fact that any differences may be small or even nonexistent. Nonspecific influences in individual drug response include constitution (physical make-up, enzyme status, personality, compliance), acquired factors (past disease, induction, expectation, experience), and environment (diseases, nutrition, climate, other therapy, relationship with health professionals, family, friends, and patients). Ten basic methodological research questions are posed, e.g., can samples be reliably drawn from the culturally different populations in an identical fashion?

691. Jules-Rosette B: The veil of objectivity: prophecy, divination, and social inquiry. Amer Anthropologist 80: 549–70, 1978.

The seemingly explicit truths of objective scientific proof are based on beliefs as fantastic and as circular as those carried in a Ndembu divining basket. Central Africans believe that spiritual and social causes are more deeply rooted than any physical explanation of disease.

692. Kaffman M: Kibbutz civilian population under war stress. Brit J Psychiatry 130:489–94, 1977.

During the Arab-Israeli War of 1973 the measures adopted by the kibbutz civilian population and the specific characteristics of an organized cohesive group succeeded in reducing the severity of the reactions of stress and in lowering the incidence of psychiatric casualties among children and adult members of the kibbutzim.

693. Kaffman M: Sexual standards and behavior of the kibbutz adolescent. Amer J Orthopsychiatry 47:207–17, 1977.

The old standards of puritanism and sexual abstinence have almost entirely disappeared among adolescents in the kibbutz. Sexual freedom, governed only by the adolescent's own judgment, in a context of a stable, emotionally meaningful relationship, has become the common and accepted pattern among an increasing number of older high-school students. New sexual standards are tolerated by the adult social system so long as sex involves components of emotional attachment and a love relationship.

694. Kaffman M: Adolescent rebellion in the kibbutz. J Amer Acad Child Psychiatry 17:154–64, 1978.

The increase of adolescent rebellion in the Israeli kibbutz seems to have occurred concurrently with the changes that have taken place in the surrounding environment, making the system of values and norms in the life of the commune less clear and less valid.

695. Kaffman M, Elizur E: Infants who become enuretics: a longitudinal study of 161 kibbutz children. Part 3: Results. Monographs Society Research Child Development 42:14–23, 1977.

Children with early urinary control tend to be self-reliant, have better developmental progress in the areas of autonomy and adaptability to new situations, and have a higher motivational level than children who become enuretics.

696. Kagan J, Klein RE, Finley GE, Rogoff B,

Nolan E: A cross-cultural study of cognitive development. Part 3: Results. Monographs Society Research Child Development 44:29–58, 1979.

In order to solve difficult items in cognitive operations tests, children must first be able to detect the principles used by the examiner manipulating the symbols used on the tests. American children mastered the more difficult operation items which most native Guatemalan Indian children never solved.

697. Kakar S: The Inner World: A Psychoanalytic Study of Childhood and Society in India. Delhi, India, Oxford U. Press, 1978.

Indian traditions such as the cult of Krishna and the mythology of Shiva place a negative value on the ego and replace ego autonomy as a norm of psychic maturity by immersion in social or cosmic totalities.

698. Kalish RA (ed): Death and Dying: Views from Many Cultures. Farmingdale, N.Y., Baywood, 1980.

In traditional societies the dead often play an active role as spirits, ever present and very much a significant part of the events of daily life. Groups studied include the Limbu (Nepal), Anggor (New Guinea), Lebei (Africa), Kaliali (New Britain), Mexican Indians, and Appalachian Kentuckians.

699. Kalish RA, Reynolds DK: Death and Ethnicity. Los Angeles, Andus Gerontology Center, U. of Southern California, 1976.

Mexican-Americans in Los Angeles are expressive at funerals; Japanese-Americans' attitudes toward death are best understood in the context of community cohesion and sensitivity toward others.

700. Kamal S: Observation ethnopsychiatrique des nomads d'Afghanistan. Ethnopsychiatrica 1:163–71, 1978.

When a Pathan family head senses that his death is approaching, he tells his sons of his "fatigue." The family begins to disintegrate if one of the sons is unable to assume leadership following the father's death. The help of a native healer—a monla—may be enlisted.

701. Kamien M: The Dark People of Bourke: A Case Study of Planned Social Change. Canberra, Australian Inst. Aboriginal Studies, 1979.

A psychiatrist describes his partially successful project of directing social change in order to help Aborigines overcome such problems as alcoholism, gambling, discrimination, overcrowded housing, poor sanitation, and malnutrition.

702. Kane SM: Holiness Fire Handling in Southern Appalachia. In Religion in Appalachia, edited by JD Photiadis, 113–24. Morgantown, West Virginia U. Press, 1978.

The immunity to fire of Holiness church members is directly related to peripheral vasoconstriction, to the inhibition of the formation of the vasodilator bradykinin. The entranced fire handler's belief in his invulnerability mobilizes protective nervous-system processes.

703. Kao FF, Kao JJ (eds): Chinese Medicine—New Medicine. New York, Neale Watson, 1977.

Essays on various aspects of Chinese medicine, including psychiatry, are presented.

704. Kao J: Three Millennia of Chinese Psychiatry. New York, Inst. for Advanced Research in Asian Science and Medicine, 1979.

Mental patients in China were often neglected and treated poorly until after the political liberation of 1949. During a visit in 1973 the author discovered that modern and traditional forms of psychiatric care were being combined and that therapy had a political underpinning.

705. Kapferer B: Mind, self, and other in demonic illness: the negation and reconstruction of self. Amer Ethnologist 6(1):110–33, 1979.

Major exorcism rituals in Sri Lanka attempt to transform the identity of a patient from one of illness to one of health. The definition of illness and the exorcisms that follow are settings for the preservation of cultural typifications of the "normal" and of the "abnormal" and are settings in which processes relating to the construction, negation, and reconstruction of self can be identified.

706. Kapferer B (ed): The Power of Ritual. Special Inaugural Issue No. 1, Social Analysis: Journal of Cultural and Social Practice, 1979.

The importance of ritual is presented in studies of folk curing in Sri Lanka and Brazil.

707. Kaplan HB: Self-Attitudes and Deviant Behavior. Pacific Palisades, Calif., Goodyear, 1975.

Deviant behavior results in improved self-attitudes and alleviates subjective distress.

708. Kapur RL: Mental health care in rural India: a study of existing patterns and their implications for future policy. British J Psychiatry 127:286–93, 1975.

A large majority of persons with psychiatric symptoms in rural India consult both traditional and modern healers. Literacy and other sociodemographic factors do not influence the type of consultation. Any scheme for introducing modern psychiatry in rural India should make use of both traditional and modern healers.

709. Kapur RL: The role of traditional healers in mental health care in rural India. Social Science Medicine 13B (1):27–31, 1979.

Healers and patients agree with psychiatrists in the diagnosis and identification of "serious" symptoms of mental illness. The majority of patients in rural India consult more than one kind of healer for their problem.

710. Katakis CD: An exploratory multi-level attempt to investigate intrapersonal and interpersonal patterns of 20 Athenian families. Mental Health Society 3:1–9, 1976.

Relationship patterns in times of social change create conflict and tension in all family members and render cooperation and decisionmaking difficult. Adherence to the dysfunctional patterns serves the function of preserving family stability in a period of transition.

711. Katchadourian H: Human Sexuality. Berkeley, U. of California Press, 1979.

Human sexuality is studied from evolutionary, biological, psychological, sociological, and anthropological perspectives.

712. Katchadourian HA, Sutherland JV: Psychiatric aspects of drug addiction in Lebanon. Intl J Addictions 10:949–62, 1975.

Drug addiction is predominantly a lower-income-class phenomenon in Lebanon. It almost exclusively involves males and Moslems.

713. Kay M: Lexemic change and semantic shift in disease names. Culture Medicine Psychiatry 3:73–94, 1979.

The lexicon of illness terms used by Mexican-American women is affected by the practice of speaking both Spanish and English and by the coexistence of several health systems. When there is changing participation in various health systems, with increasing interference and code switching, linguistic evidence for these changes may be found. In some cases an English disease name is borrowed. In others, a cognate is coined from an English disease name. Some Spanish disease names that do not have equivalents in English or in scientific medical theory may be retained, but there is a shift in the meaning of the words themselves. The direction of the shift is toward semantic correspondence with the concepts of scientific medicine. In these ways the medical lexicon is changed, with the changes reflecting a new medical culture.

714. Kayser-Jones JS: Old, Alone, and Neglected. Berkeley, U. of California Press, 1980.

Elderly persons in the United States and in Scotland describe how it feels to be alone, disabled, and institutionalized. The Scottish healthcare system for the elderly seems to work better than the American system.

715. Keefe SE: Urbanization, acculturation, and extended family ties: Mexican-Americans in cities. Amer Ethnologist 6(2):349–65, 1979.

There is no indication that the traditional Mexican-American extended family breaks down with urbanization, acculturation, or socioeconomic mobility. Discrimination by the Anglo majority reinforces kin ties among Mexican-Americans.

716. Keefe SE, Padilla AM, Carlos LM: The Mexican-American extended family as an emotional support system. Human Organization 38:144–52, 1979.

If the extended family constitutes the primary source of informal support for Mexican-Americans, its absence or malfunction is probably far more distressing than for Anglo-Americans in similar circumstances.

717. Keith J (ed): The Ethnography of Old Age. Anthropological Quarterly (Special Issue), Washington, D.C., Catholic U. of America Press, 1979.

The elderly in new retirement communities are enmeshed in the work of building new communities and new lives and of living in new social, cultural, and spatial environments.

718. Keith-Ross J: Old People, New Lives. Chicago, U. of Chicago Press, 1977.

In a French retirement residence, the members develop a sense of shared fate.

719. Kellam SG, Ensminger ME, Turner J: Family structure and the mental health of children: concurrent and longitudinal community-wide studies. Arch Gen Psychiatry 34:1012–22, 1977.

Fatherless families entail the highest risk in terms of social maladaptation and psychological well-being of the child. However, the absence of the father is less important than the aloneness of the mother.

720. Kelley JH: Yaqui Women. Lincoln, U. of Nebraska Press, 1978.

Biographies of four Yaqui women demonstrate the range and variation of women's roles and emphasize the women's ability to endure stresses, hardship, and violence.

721. Kendell RE: The concept of disease and its implications for psychiatry. Brit J Psychiatry 127:305–15, 1975.

Schizophrenia, manic-depressive illness, some sexual disorders, and some forms of drug dependence can justifiably be regarded as illnesses. Psychiatrists should stick with the tasks that they do best without pretending to be the healers of all the woes of mankind.

722. Kennedy JG, Teague J, Fairbanks L: Qat use in North Yemen and the problem of addiction. Culture Medicine Psychiatry 4:311–44, 1980.

Travelers to North Yemen perceive the Yemeni people as universally addicted to the drug qat and the problems of the country as related to this. The majority of Yemenis claim not only that qat is harmless, but also that it has many virtues. It is necessary to add the social and cultural components to the psychopharmacological theories of drug dependence to achieve any adequate understanding of the widespread or institutionalized use of qat in North Yemen.

723. Kennedy PF: Evaluation of a mental health educational project in Burma. Mental Health Society 4:156–63, 1977.

In attempting to evaluate a brief course on care of the mentally ill given to health personnel in Burma, assessment of clinical knowledge before and after the course and data on treatment prescriptions given to patients by health personnel before and after the course are simple and inexpensive ways of learning about the impact on health care.

724. Kenny MG: Latah: the symbolism of a putative mental disorder. Culture Medicine Psychiatry 2:209–31, 1978.

Latah is intimately related to other aspects of Malay-Indonesian culture and is a well known cultural pattern and not a mental disorder even though it may occur among persons, largely women, in a socially and psychologically marginal situation. Latah is a symbolic representation of marginality and is as appropriate to certain mythological and religious figures as to the socially marginal.

725. Kent I, Nicholls W: The psychodynamics of terrorism. Mental Health Society 4:1–8, 1977.

Terrorism can occur whenever political conditions provide social legitimation for the acting out of deeply repressed hatred. Political terrorism involves the exploitation of mental illness, connived at in turn by the international public through the media.

726. Kenyon FE: Pornography, the law and mental health. Brit J Psychiatry 126:225–33, 1975.

Pornography does little harm to mental health but can be offensive to many people. Instead of further restrictive legislation, a better policy would be increased education, with pornography regarded simply as being in rather poor taste.

727. Kerri JN: Studying voluntary associations as adaptive mechanisms: a review of anthropological perspectives. Current Anthropology 17:23–47, 1976.

Industrialization and urbanization in particular, and social, cultural, and technological change in general, lead to the proliferation of new common-interest associations. Some associations reflect preexisting traditional forms, and others reflect complete innovations or borrowings from other cultures and societies.

728. Kessen W: Childhood in China. New Haven, Conn., Yale U. Press, 1975.

Chinese children are far less restless and less intense in their motor actions and display less crying, whining, fighting, and pushing than American children. Typical school classes include moral lessons and lessons of cooperation rather than competition.

729. Kett JF: Rites of Passage. New York, Basic Books, 1977.

The historical roots of adolescence are traced from 1790 to the present.

730. Khalid MS: Bemerkungen zur symptomatik der schizophrenien in Libyen. Psychiatrie, Neurologie und Medizinische Psychologie 29:46–48, 1977.

The first-rank symptoms of schizophrenic Libyans are similar to those found in Western countries.

731. Khatri AA: Analysis of fiction—a method for intracultural and crosscultural study of family systems. J Marriage Family 42:197–204, 1980.

Analysis of imaginative literature written in the

form of novels can be fruitful in understanding basic values, assumptions, roles, attitudes, intrapersonal processes, and intimate interpersonal relations in the community.

732. Khayyer M, Mojedhi H: Intelligence: Iranian male delinquents compared with nondelinquents on selected WISC scales. Psychological Reports 44:782, 1979.
The results of previous studies on the relationship between intelligence and delinquency are inconsistent.

733. Kiefer CW, Cowan J: State/context dependence and theories of ritual. J Psychol Anthropology 2:53–83, 1979.
The state/context dependence theory proposes relationships between observable ritual acts and measurable physiological and cognitive changes. The function of ritual in the stabilization of state/context is examined, using the Isoma ritual as an example.

734. Kiev A: Cultural perspectives in the range of human behavior. Mental Health Society 3:53–56, 1976.
Traditional societies provide a homogenous world view for everyone and encourage people to work toward specific objectives. In rapidly changing urban settings, unlimited choices create the anxieties that lead people to search for security in unsuitable patterns of beliefs and behavior. In our society a recent reorientation toward a traditional fatalism and a de-emphasis on the puritan work ethic reflects a marked value shift that may stultify many persons, much as it fosters increased individualization among others.

735. Kiev A, Anumonye A: Suicidal behavior in a black ghetto: a comparative study. Intl J Mental Health 5:50–59, 1976.
Ghetto patients tend to be more disoriented, more inclined to drug or alcohol abuse, and more likely to attempt suicide at a greater distance from sources of help than nonghetto patients. Almost as many men as women attempt suicide in the ghetto.

736. Kilbride JE, Kilbride PL: Sitting and smiling behavior of Baganda infants: the influence of culturally constituted experience. J Cross-Cultural Psychology 1:88–107, 1975.
The Baganda of Uganda are comparatively accelerated in the rate of their psychomotor development. Culturally constituted experience is importantly related to the psychomotor development of infants.

737. Kilbride JE, Yarczower M: Recognition of happy and sad facial expressions among Baganda and U.S. children. J Cross-Cultural Psychology 7:181–94, 1976.
American and Baganda children and adults cross-culturally agree on the recognition of happy and sad expressions. Happy expressions are more easily identified by young children than are sad expressions.

738. Killworth PD, Bernard HR: Informant accuracy in social network data. Human Organization 35:269–86, 1976.
Informants' reports of their behavior bear little resemblance to their actual behavior. Due to this low level of informant accuracy, theories of social structure built upon presently available network data are suspect.

739. Kim HA: Transplantation of psychiatrists from foreign cultures. J Amer Acad Psychoanalysis 4:105–12, 1976.
Transplanted psychiatrists are in a special position to understand culturally conflictual problems and to make a definite contribution to our increasingly complicated social structure. In this culturally troubled society, those psychiatrists who have become acculturated and established are urgently needed in the training and consulting of psychiatrists from other cultural communities.

740. Kim K: The Oedipus complex in our changing society: with special reference to Korea. J Korean Neuropsychiat Assn 17:93–103, 1978.
In Korean myths, conflicts between fathers and sons are resolved differently than in Greek myths. In the past, Korean psychiatrists rarely saw Oedipal symptoms but, because of sociocultural changes, such symptoms are now more overt.

741. Kimura B: Transcultural psychiatry and cultural transcendence in the study of psychoses (in German). In Leib, Geist, Geschicte, edited by H Kraus. Heidelberg, Huthig Verlag, 1978.
That guilt is less prevalent in Japanese psychotic, depressed patients than in Western patients can be explained by existential, philosophical concepts.

742. Kinzie JD: Lessons from cross-cultural psychotherapy. Amer J Psychotherapy 32:510–20, 1978.
Effective techniques of cross-cultural psycho-

therapy include the appropriate use of the medical model, recognition of nonverbal communication, and sensitivity to the subjective aspects of the patient's life. When used with self-awareness and flexibility, these techniques can aide the therapist who does not share the cultural background of his patient.

743. Kinzie JD, Tran KA, Breckenridge A, Bloom JD: An Indochinese refugee psychiatric clinic: culturally accepted treatment approaches. Amer J Psychiatry 137:1429–32, 1980.

To be successful with Indochinese refugee patients, the psychiatrist must use a medical approach and work flexibly and broadly with a wide variety of cultural, social, and psychological problems. Mental health workers from each ethnic group should serve as assistants.

744. Kinzie JD, Tseng WS: Cultural aspects of psychiatric clinic utilization: a cross-cultural study in Hawaii. Intl J Social Psychiatry 24:177–88, 1978.

Ethnicity is highly related to utilization of mental health services; however, once entry into the system is made, there is no ethnic difference in the clinic's response to patients.

745. Kitada J: Present status of the psychotherapy of schizophrenia in Japan. Intl J Social Psychiatry 26:151–52, 1980.

In many cases, intensive psychoanalytically oriented psychotherapy in Japan is still in an experimental and exploratory stage.

746. Kitahara M: A cross-cultural test of the Freudian theory of circumcision. Intl J Psychoanal Psychotherapy 5:535–46, 1976.

Freud's theory of circumcision as a symbolic substitute for castration is well supported.

747. Kitzinger S: West Indian adolescents: an anthropological perspective. J Adolescence 1:35–46, 1978.

West Indian adolescents in the United Kingdom have special problems due to their marginal relationship both to adult society and the host culture. The young male may seek his social identity by returning to his African roots through the Rastaman image of masculinity: the adolescent female, by rebelling against the mother through obvious sexual activity and pregnancy. Due to immigration, a mother may leave her children for prolonged periods of time, leading to an unresolved mourning that can cause many difficulties for the adolescent.

748. Klein HE: The taping of both questions and answers as a standardizing technique in transcultural psychiatric research. Transcult Psych Res Review 17:116–20, 1980.

Taping, especially videotaping, of structured interview questions for presentation, with consequent taping of patients' and research subjects' responses, can be advantageous for both research projects and therapy. The technique has been used in comparisons of Turkish and American subjects.

749. Klein HE, Person TM, Cetingok M, Itil TM: Family and community variables in adjustment of Turkish and Missouri schizophrenics. Comp Psychiatry 19:233–40, 1978.

It is not schizophrenic illness alone but also certain variables within the family and community that make for rehospitalization after discharge. If these variables are understood within the context of the patient's culture, there is therapeutic opportunity to help the family and community to keep the patient home. Optimum benefit from psychiatric treatment can be realized only insofar as the social environment can be controlled to meet the patient's needs.

750. Klein JW: Ethnotherapy with Jews. Intl J Mental Health 5:26–38, 1976.

Creating a larger group of healthily identified Jews—not authoritarian chauvinists, on the one extreme, or self-hating disaffiliators, on the other—is crucial to the mental health of the American Jew.

751. Klein J: Susto: the anthropological study of diseases of adaptation. Social Science and Medicine 12(1B):23–28, 1978.

There are large cultural differences in the specific forms of expression of psychophysiological processes. Diseases of adaptation, such as susto, are very much dependent on culture for their genesis, form, content, severity, significance, treatment recognition, and physiological and psychological substrates. Although susto originates in a sudden natural fright, diseases of adaptation can also be associated with any strong emotion or stressful situation, not just fright.

752. Klein MH: Feminist concepts of therapy outcome. Psychotherapy: Theory, Research, Practice 13:89–95, 1976.

Feminist theory, in the best of all possible worlds, converges with humanist and personological theory in its concerns with individual growth; all of the goals articulated as feminist for women should apply equally to men to enhance their personhood.

753. Kleinfeld J, Bloom JD: Boarding schools: effects on the mental health of Eskimo adolescents. Amer J Psychiatry 134:411–17, 1977.

Boarding schools contribute to a high incidence of social and emotional disturbance among Eskimo adolescents. These disturbances are not primarily initial adjustment difficulties that subside later on, but are continuing disturbances. Changes in the boarding school environment can have substantial effects.

754. Kleinman A: Depression, somatization and the "new cross-cultural psychiatry." Social Science Medicine 11:3–10, 1977.

Features of depressive disorders do exhibit cross-cultural differences. These differences are a function of the cultural shaping of normative and deviant behavior.

755. Kleinman A: Clinical relevance of anthropological and cross-cultural research: concepts and strategies. Amer J Psychiatry 135:427–31, 1978.

The clinical social-science approach emphasizes the distinction between disease and illness and cultural influences on the ways "clinical reality" is conflictingly construed in the ethnomedical models of patients and the biomedical models of practitioners. Use of such a model is very useful in the effective understanding and management of patients. Consultation-liaison psychiatry is a particularly appropriate vehicle for introducing clinical social science into medical and psychiatric teaching and practice.

756. Kleinman A: What kind of model for the anthropology of medical systems? Amer Anthropologist 80:661–64, 1978.

Foster's dichotomy of non-Western medical systems into personalistic or naturalistic types is not adequate as a theoretical framework for the kind of cultural analysis that medical anthropology and comparative studies of medical systems require.

757. Kleinman A: Editorial—Major conceptual and research issues for cultural (anthropological) psychiatry. Culture Medicine Psychiatry 4:3–13, 1980.

Major conceptual and research issues for cultural (anthropological) psychiatry are (1) cultural influences on cognitive, affective, communicative, behavioral, and psychophysiological pro-

cess, (2) cultural influences on family and other key social relationships, (3) cultural influences on the perception of and reaction to universal stressors, (4) cultural influences on creation of and coping with culture-specific stressors, (5) cultural influences on psychiatric "disease" and "illness," (6) cultural influences on help seeking, (7) cultural influences on the labeling and societal reaction to social deviance, (8) cultural influences on clinical practice, (9) cultural influences on indigenous and professional therapeutic systems for treating mental illness and the psychosocial concomitants of physical illness, and (10) cultural influences on psychiatric categories.

758. Kleinman A: Patient and Healers in the Context of Culture. Berkeley, U. of California Press, 1980.

As demonstrated by studies in Taiwan, disease and illness problems, therapeutic relationships, and the healing process are affected by systems of cultural meanings and institutionalized social patterns of power. The medical professions' conceptualization of sickness has disappointingly little to contribute to understanding illness as symbolic networks.

759. Kleinman A, Eisenberg L, Good B: Culture, illness, care: clinical lessons from anthropologic and cross-cultural research. Ann Int Medicine 88:251–58, 1978.

Among the primary components of the health-care crisis perceived by the public is the focusing of modern physicians on the diagnosis and treatment of disease—an abnormality in the structure and function of body organs and systems—while ignoring the patient's illness—the experience of devalued changes in states of being and in social function. Folk practitioners usually treat illness effectively, but do not systematically address disease, while modern health professionals are potentially capable of treating both disease and illness. By applying social-science concepts to the patient-doctor encounter in order to formulate and communicate the doctor's explanatory model in terms that the patient can understand, both the disease and illness can be addressed.

760. Kleinman A, Kunstadter P, Alexander ER, Gate JL (eds): Medicine in Chinese Cultures. Washington, D.C., U.S. Govt. Printing Office, 1975.

Health care in China is compared with health care in other countries.

761. Kleinman A, Kunstadter P, Alexander ER,

Gate JL (eds): Culture and Healing in Asian Societies. Cambridge, Mass., Schenkman, 1978.

It is insufficient to study medicine in society solely as a system of beliefs, norms, and values (the cultural system model). Beliefs, norms, and values must be seen as attached not only to distinct cultures but also to particular social structural positions and social roles (the social system model), which are engaged in the processes of modernization, indigenization, and institutional change (the social change model). These changes need to be studied in relation to environmental influences and stress (the adaptive and ecological models). Examples of traditional and modern medical (including psychiatric) systems are described for China, Burma, Thailand, India, and Japan.

762. Kleinman A, Lin TY (eds): Normal and Abnormal Behavior in Chinese Culture. Dordrecht, Netherlands, Reidel, 1980.

Topics discussed include the epidemiology of mental illness in Taiwan, Hong Kong, People's Republic of China, and Chinese-Americans, suicide, deviant marriage patterns, childhood psychopathology, and traditional beliefs about mental illness.

763. Kleinman AK, Mechanic D: Some observations of mental illness and its treatment in the People's Republic of China. J Nerv Ment Disease 167(5):267–74, 1979.

The Chinese report of low rates of mental illness reflects narrow definitions of disorders and somatic expressions of personal and social distress as physical conditions. Acute mental health services are provided at commune and county hospitals, and special psychiatric hospitals are maintained for more intractable patients. Psychiatric practice in teaching hospitals is similar to that in the West.

764. Kleinman A, Sung LH: Why do indigenous practitioners successfully heal? Social Science Medicine 13B(1):7–26, 1979.

Recent research suggests a number of different ways by which indigenous therapies may affect biologically based diseases. Since the epidemiological web causing and sustaining physiological diseases not infrequently includes major psychosocial factors, indigenous healing may at times work to affect such diseases by altering those factors. Thus, to the extent indigenous practitioners provide culturally legitimated treatment of illness, they must heal.

765. Kline F, Acosta FX, Austin W, Johnson RG: The misunderstood Spanish-speaking patients. Amer J Psychiatry 137:1530–33, 1980.

Spanish-speaking patients interviewed with interpreters feel understood, helped, and wish to return. More bilingual and bicultural therapists are needed for direct service.

766. Klineberg O: Historical perspectives: cross-cultural psychology before 1960. In Handbook of Cross-Cultural Psychology, edited by HC Triandis and WW Lambert, 1:31–68. Boston, Allyn and Bacon, 1980.

There has been tremendous recent growth of interest in cross-cultural psychology. Early German studies and contributions by Franz Boas and his students, A. I. Hallowell and Clyde Kluckhohn, are reviewed. Some of the major psychological issues that have been studied and other issues that continue to attract attention are national character, perception, memory, language and thought, psychoanalysis, psychopathology, leadership, acculturation, field dependence, and achievement motive.

767. Klippel MD: Measurement of intelligence among three New Zealand ethnic groups: product versus process approaches. J Cross-Cultural Psychology 6:365–76, 1975.

The education system in New Zealand, which is dedicated to equality of opportunity, in fact is not achieving this aim because educators within the system are not adapting it to meet the particular needs of minority groups such as the Maori, Samoan, and Pakeha.

768. Knight GP, Kagan S: Acculturation of prosocial and competitive behaviors among second- and third-generation Mexican-American children. J Cross-Cultural Psychology 8:273–84, 1977.

Acculturation to the barrio model is not representative of the generational differences in prosocial and competitive behaviors of Mexican-American children, even in a traditional semirural community.

769. Knight GP, Kagan S: Development of prosocial and competitive behaviors in Anglo-American and Mexican-American children. Child Development 48:1385–94, 1977.

With age, Anglo-American children become significantly more competitive while Mexican-American children tend to become slightly more prosocial. In both populations, boys are more rivalrous and less equality oriented than girls.

770. Koentjaraningrat RM: Javanese magic, sorcery and numerology. Masyarakat Indonesia 6:35–52, 1979.

Some Javanese healers diagnose and treat mental illness by utilizing texts on magic as well as Hindu medical texts (usada) written on palm leaves.

771. Kokantzis NA, Ierodiakonou CS: Some considerations on the position of psychotherapy in today's Greek culture. Psychotherapy Psychosomatics 25:254–58, 1975.

Psychotherapy is looked upon as being nonmedical and unscientific by the neurology-oriented psychiatrists of Greece, with only those psychiatrists trained abroad practicing psychoanalytically oriented psychotherapy. Collaboration and systematic contact between psychotherapists in Greece and psychotherapeutic international organizations abroad would aid the cause of psychotherapy in Greece.

772. Kolman PBR: A study of psychiatric patients at the University of Malaya Medical Centre who also consult indigenous healers. Social Psychiatry 11:127–34, 1976.

The advent of modern psychiatry in Malaysia has not replaced more traditional methods of coping with mental illness. Malay patients are more likely than Indians or Chinese to consult healers, but Indian patients are more likely to consult healers of other ethnic origins.

773. Kopp CB, Khoka EW, Sigman M: A comparison of sensorimotor development among infants in India and the United States. J Cross-Cultural Psychology 8:435–52, 1977.

There is greater similarity than difference in the sensorimotor functioning of American and Indian infants.

774. Kopp C, Kirkpatrick M (eds): Becoming Female: Perspectives on Development. New York, Plenum, 1979.

A wide variety of female developmental issues is presented. Included are such topics as problems of the black female, problems in the development of female identity, effects of observed violence on females, cross-cultural perspectives, and biological considerations.

775. Kopteff PJ: A survey of the abuse of medicines and illicit drugs by Finnish students. Intl J Addictions 15:269–75, 1980.

Illicit drugs are less widely abused among Finnish university students than among students in the United States.

776. Korbin JE (ed): Child Abuse and Neglect: Cross-Cultural Perspectives. Berkeley, U. of California Press, 1980.

Examples of child-rearing practices and child maltreatment in America, India, Japan, China, and the Middle East are presented.

777. Kornadt HJ, Eckensberger LH, Emminghaus WB: Cross-cultural research on motivation and its contribution to a general theory of motivation. In Handbook of Cross-Cultural Psychology, edited by HC Triandis and W Lonner, 3:223–321. Boston, Allyn and Bacon, 1980.

The traditional cross-cultural tactic of simply gathering observations or of applying the same tests in different cultures should be abandoned. Cross-cultural research on motivation could and should be devoted to the goal of contributing to the broadening of our knowledge about the universality of human motives or basic motivational patterns and the functional patterns of motive development.

778. Koss JD: Therapeutic aspects of Puerto Rican cult practices. Psychiatry 38:160–71, 1975.

Belief in spirit possession and the ritualized practice of possession trance can create a therapeutic relationship between a cult leader and an adherent committed to spiritism as a means of solving his personal problems. The two important characteristics of this type of relationship are control over the definition of the relationship by an individual directing changes in the behavior of a disturbed person, and mechanisms insuring that the relationship provides a context where change can occur.

779. Koss JD: Social process, healing, and self-defeat among Puerto Rican spiritists. Amer Ethnologist 4(3):453–69, 1977.

Although many studies have shown spirit cults to exert a positive therapeutic influence on their clients, a longitudinal perspective shows that cult socialization may lead to a reverse of the initial benefits. Clients who are diagnosed as seriously disturbed and whose cure depends on their training as healing mediums do initially appear to undergo extensive personal transformations. However, this new personal adjustment can be threatened or even reversed by the dynamics of the cult group itself.

780. Kraft AM, Swift SS: Impressions of Chinese psychiatry. Psychiatric Quarterly 51:83–91, 1979.

The Chinese have a relatively narrow definition of mental illness, excluding such cases as character neuroses, psychosomatic disorders, and borderline states. Treatments combine traditional, folk, and scientific methodologies. The rural and agrarian society has been able to accommodate the mentally retarded without many special programs or facilities, but increasing technology and industrialization may change this.

781. Kramer DA, Kinney WF Jr: The overlapping territories of psychiatry and ethology. J Nerv Ment Disease 167(1):3–22, 1979.

Artifactual differences have been the primary impediment to more interaction between the two rather similar fields of psychiatry and ethology. The area where the most research has occurred and in which the findings of ethology have been the most utilized in psychiatry is that of the attachment systems. A curriculum stressing the writings of Tinbergen, Lorenz, Bowlby, and Hailman can be useful in programs interested in teaching an ethological approach to psychiatry.

782. Kraus RF, Buffler PA: Sociocultural stress and the American native in Alaska: an analysis of changing patterns of psychiatric illness and alcohol abuse among Alaska natives. Culture Medicine Psychiatry 3:111–51, 1979.

The number of Alaska natives treated as inpatients and outpatients for psychiatric illness and alcohol abuse has been rising steadily. Accidental injury and suicidal behavior are common. The treated prevalence rates for psychiatric illness and alcoholism exceed recorded rates for other American native and nonnative groups. For each category of violent death, suicide, homicide, accidents, and alcohol, rates for Alaska natives are higher than rates for Alaska nonnatives, American Indians, and the United States (all rates) and are rising.

783. Krause N, Carr LG: The effects of response bias in the survey assessment of the mental health of Puerto Rican migrants. Social Psychiatry 13:167–73, 1978.

There is no significant relationship between psychiatric symptomatology and the migration status of Puerto Ricans.

784. Kreisman JJ: The curandero's apprentice: a therapeutic integration of folk and medical healing. Amer J Psychiatry 132:81–83, 1975.

Two Mexican-American schizophrenics are successfully treated by a combination of traditional therapy and curanderismo. By working within the patient's cultural reference, the therapist may increase rapport with the patient;

another effect may be to exploit a position of authority in achieving a placebo effect.

785. Krell R: Holocaust families: the survivors and their children. Comp Psychiatry 20:560–68, 1979.

It is the fate of the holocaust family to share the trials and hardships and memories of the parents. Not infrequently, they stand to benefit from the wisdom gained through their parents' intimate encounter with suffering and death.

786. Kris E, Kurz O: Legend, Myth, and Magic in the Image of the Artist. New Haven, Conn., Yale U. Press, 1979.

The artist may be regarded as a hero, a magician, and a contender with divinity. The magic of the visual image is a universal belief and results from the idea that those who possess an image of a person hold some power over that person.

787. Krynicki VE: The double orientation of the ego in the practice of zen. Amer J Psychoanalysis 40:239–48, 1980.

Zen practitioners retain a double orientation of union and separateness and can choose the best of each world, merging during their meditation effort and holding to reality and working at other times. The goal of zen practice is to be able, almost at will, to enter the world of oneness. This ability also relieves separation anxiety.

788. Kuhland D, Feld S: The development of achievement motivation in black and white children. Child Development 48:1362–68, 1977.

Although similar in their respective levels of autonomous achievement motivation, black children display lower levels of social-comparison achievement motivation than white children.

789. Kuhn D, Nash SC, Brucken L: Sex role concepts of two- and three-year-olds. Child Development 49:445–51, 1978.

Girls tend to ascribe positive characteristics to their own sex and negative characteristics to males, while boys do the reverse. There are no differences in the amount of stereotyping as a function of subject's age or sex.

790. Kulhara P, Wig NN: The chronicity of schizophrenia in northwest India: results of a follow-up study. Brit J Psychiatry 132:186–90, 1978.

The course taken by schizophrenia in a newly developed city and its neighborhood in India is similar to the one seen in the Western world.

791. Kumasaka Y, Smith RJ, Aiba H: Crimes in

New York and Tokyo: sociocultural perspectives. Comm Ment Health Journal 11:19–26, 1975.

The rate of infanticides is higher in Tokyo than in New York City. Intruders in New York City seek confrontation with victims more actively than their counterparts in Tokyo.

792. Kunitz SJ: Underdevelopment and social services on the Navajo reservation. Human Organization 36:398–405, 1977.

The fact that unemployment is higher among reservation Indians than in virtually any other segment of the population suggests that labor-intensive areas such as human services will continue to be of relatively more significance there than elsewhere.

793. Kunkas N, Nikelly AG: Group psychotherapy with Greek immigrants. Intl J Group Psychotherapy 25:402–9, 1975.

Group therapy offers a unique solution for psychological problems due to culture stress and conflict among Greek immigrants to the United States. Greek immigrants are exposed to the inadequacies of their defenses and coping mechanisms in a "foreign" culture. Therapy begins with dependency and resentment toward the therapist, who is perceived as authoritarian, but moves toward independence, equality, increased feasibility, and the ability to cope with cultural differences.

794. Kuo W: Theories of migration and mental health: an empirical testing of Chinese-Americans. Social Science Medicine 10:297–306, 1976.

Social isolation indices and cultural shock indices vary positively with the Midtown Psychiatric Impairment Index, CES-D Depression Scale, and Unhappiness Scale, indicating that these theories explain Chinese-Americans' mental health better than those of social change and goal-striving stress.

795. Kuo WH, Gray R, Lin N: Locus of control and symptoms of psychological distress among Chinese-Americans. Intl J Social Psychiatry 25:176–87, 1979.

Chinese-Americans who believe that rewards of life are contingent upon some sort of social force beyond personal control tend to have more psychological distress than do Chinese-Americans who believe that they themselves control their lives.

796. Kuramoto FH: A History of the Shonien 1914–1972: An Account of a Program of Institu-

tional Care of Japanese Children in Los Angeles. San Francisco, R & E Research Associates, 1976.

The ethnically oriented, private social-welfare system (Shonien) developed by the Japanese people in Los Angeles for the out-of-home care of Japanese children is examined historically to better understand the nature of public and private social-welfare institutions in America.

797. Kuroda Y, Suzuki T, Hayashi C: A cross-national analysis of the Japanese character among Japanese-Americans in Honolulu. Ethnicity 5:42–59, 1978.

Japanese-language familiarity is a crucial factor in determining the extent to which Japanese-Americans maintain Japanese culture, although certainly organizational affiliation and contacts with Japanese mass media are important as well.

798. Kutash I, Kutash S, Schlesinger L: Violence: Perspectives on Murder and Aggression. San Francisco, Jossey-Bass, 1978.

Murder and aggression are discussed from multiple viewpoints including ethology, sociobiology, psychoanalysis, and sociology.

799. Kutty IN, Froese AP, Rae-Grant QAF: Hare Krishna movement: what attracts the Western adolescent? Canadian J Psychiatry 24:604–9, 1979.

The Hare Krishna movement may be attractive to some adolescents by providing a sense of belonging as well as answering some questions related to their identity needs.

800. La Barre W: Psychoanalysis and the biology of religion. J Psychol Anthropology 1:57–64, 1978.

All human infants learn ontogenetically the affective stances that are behind both magic and religion. The infant learns that a cry will magically summon the mother to fulfill his needs. As the child develops he learns he must beseech his omnipotent parents to accomplish his needs for him.

801. Lager E, Zwerling I: Time orientation and psychotherapy in the ghetto. Amer J Psychiatry 137:306–9, 1980.

Therapists should understand the present-time orientation of ghetto patients in order to help with understanding precipitating factors, the nature and urgency of patients' communications, and suitability for long-term psychotherapy.

802. Landry B, Jendrek MP: The employment of

wives in middle-class black families. J Marriage Family 40:787–98, 1978.

Black middle-class wives have higher employment rates than both white middle- and black working-class wives because of economic need.

803. Landy D (ed): Culture, Disease, and Healing. New York, Macmillan, 1977.

This collection of well-known articles on medical anthropology covers such areas as theories of disease and healing, divination and diagnosis, emotional states and cultural constraints, statuses and roles of patients and healers, and healers and medical systems in social and cultural change.

804. Langley MS: The Nandi of Kenya. New York, St. Martin's, 1979.

Nandi rituals attached to adolescent initiation, marriage, and divorce persist despite monumental social changes.

805. Laosa LM: Maternal teaching strategies in Chicano families of varied educational and socioeconomic levels. Child Development 49:1129–35, 1978.

The higher the Chicano mother's level of formal education the more she uses inquiry and praise as teaching strategies. The lower the mother's level of formal education the more she uses modeling as a teaching strategy and the more she appears to physically punish and control her boys.

806. Laosa LM: Maternal teaching strategies in Chicano and Anglo-American families: the influence of culture and education on maternal behavior. Child Development 51:759–65, 1980.

Differences in the strategies that Chicano and Anglo-American mothers use when teaching their young children may be the result of differences in the average level of formal education attained by the mothers. The mothers do not differ in their use of negative verbal feedback or disapproval, positive physical control, and physical affection.

807. Laprez LV: Cultural change and psychological stress. Amer J Psychoanalysis 36:171–76, 1976.

As demonstrated by data from the Philippines, the responsibility for recognizing and defining the nature and extent of culture change and identifying the significant encounter points between culture and psyche rests with mental health professionals. In the process of helping the person shift his values and beliefs in the directions that

he himself chooses, the helping person has to recognize his own perceptual and cognitive styles, as well as the parameters of his sociocultural reality.

808. Larraya FP: Ente los ultimos Siriono del ovente de Bolivia. Acta Psiquiatrica y Psicologica de America Latina 23:247–65, 1977.

The Siriono, a rapidly disappearing group of hunters and gatherers from Bolivia, often recreate blissful mythical times through ceremonies. At times they exhibit epidemic group madness, e.g., alternating periods of quiet and frenzy.

809. Larraya FP: El teatro maka del gran chako gualambia. Acta Psiquiatrica y Psicologica de America Latina 24:171–200, 1978.

The Maka of Paraguay have a high incidence of schizophrenia. The tribe's cultural identity is protected from foreign contamination by ritual theatrical performances that preserve traditional practices.

810. Larsen KS: Attitudes toward black and white integration as a function of beliefs about nature versus nurture. Psychological Reports 36:310, 1975.

The nature-nurture question cannot be evaluated on the basis of its scientific tenability alone, for such a belief may also have policy applications as expressed in attitudes toward integration.

811. Lasch C: The Culture of Narcissism. New York, W. W. Norton, 1978.

To live for the moment is the prevailing Western passion, as exemplified by the banality of pseudo-self-awareness. Modern capitalist society not only elevates narcissists to prominence, but also it elects and reinforces narcissistic traits in everyone. By creating so many varieties of bureaucratic dependence, society makes it increasingly difficult for people to lay to rest the terrors of infancy or to enjoy the consolations of adulthood.

812. Lasker GW: Surnames in the study of human biology. Amer Anthropologist 82:525–38, 1980.

Surnames delineate the breeding structure of some human populations over a larger span of time than is usually possible with pedigrees, over a more definite span of time than in genetic studies, and more easily in broad surveys than alternative methods.

813. Lasry JC: Cross-cultural perspective on

mental health and immigration adaptation. Social Psychiatry 12:49–55, 1977.

North African immigrants living in Montreal exhibit a level of mental health similar to that of native French Canadians. Their high level of anxiety seems to be mainly due to the stress of immigration: it diminishes gradually over the years until it reaches the level of the native population.

814. Lasry JM, Sigal JJ: Mental and physical health correlates in an immigrant population. Canadian J Psychiatry 25:391–93, 1980.

High utilization of health services, low level of education, few social contacts, and recent immigration are the simple criteria used by psychiatrists in Canada to consider psychiatric referrals from immigrants. Difficult or infrequent social contacts are predictive of depressive symptomatology, especially for immigrant women.

815. Latorre DL: A Mexican folk interpretation of schizophrenia. J Operational Psychiatry 9(1):37–41, 1978.

This case of a forty-year-old Mexican man illustrates the local folk interpretation of schizophrenia. Mentally disturbed persons receive many rituals aimed at improving their condition or overcoming their illness. These rituals serve to help the outlook of both patient and practitioner, especially if the curer is a relative.

816. Lauterbach W: Current status of Soviet psychotherapy. Comp Psychiatry 19:209–12, 1978.

Although psychotherapy as a psychiatric method of treatment is less important in the Soviet Union than it is in the West, there are many varieties of psychotherapeutic methods in use there.

817. Leach J, Wing JK: The effectiveness of a service for helping destitute men. Brit J Psychiatry 133:481–92, 1978.

The effectiveness of a voluntary organization to help destitute men can be increased by periodic professional assessment and recommendations made to the organization. Setting up a night shelter improves attendance, and appropriate assessment procedures for selection of men who would settle in the house for long periods also improve their length of stay.

818. Leacock E: Women's status in egalitarian society: implications for social evolution. Current Anthropology 19:247–75, 1978.

The structure of egalitarian society has been misunderstood as a result of the failure to recognize women's participation as public and autonomous. Family relations in preclass societies were not merely incipient forms of our own. Social evolution has not been unlineal and quantitative; it has entailed profound qualitative changes in the relations between women and men.

819. Leacock S, Leacock R: Spirits of the Deep. Garden City, N.Y., Anchor, 1975.

The Batuque, an Afro-Brazilian cult, have curing ceremonies that closely resemble the Brazilian pajelanca (shamanism). The cult leaders often accuse each other of sorcery.

820. Lebra J, Paulson J, Powers E: Women In Changing Japan. Boulder, Colo., Westview, 1976.

Although most Japanese women cling to the traditional notion of being a good wife and wise mother, an increasing minority are examining their new legal rights to vote and hold office, to own and to transmit property, and to divorce. The radical feminist movement in Japan is a small underground phenomenon whose deviation is social rather than sexual.

821. Lebra TS: Japanese Patterns of Behavior. Honolulu, U. Press of Hawaii, 1976.

Japanese behavior, mental illness, and therapy are best understood from a psychocultural perspective. The Japanese inclination for compromise, tolerance, and pliability contrasts greatly with the serenity and intolerance of Western emotions. Topics discussed include suicide, Naikan and Morita therapy, delinquency, and the possession behavior of the Salvation cult.

822. Lebra TS: The dilemma and strategies of aging among contemporary Japanese women. Ethnology 18:337–53, 1979.

Most Japanese women, while remaining primarily filiocentric as far as their expressions of fulfillment are concerned, are muted as to their expectations for dependency upon their children. They tend to stress their determination to avoid being a burden upon their children.

823. Lebra WP (ed): Culture-Bound Syndromes, Ethnopsychiatry, and Alternate Therapies. Honolulu, U. Press of Hawaii, 1976.

Studies of Pacific Rim countries include indigenous healing practices, syndromes such as latah, malgri, and shinkeshitu, and Naikan and Morita therapy.

824. Lee RB, DeVore I (eds): Kalahari Hunter-

Gatherers. Cambridge, Mass., Harvard U. Press, 1976.

Data on the !Kung San (Bushmen) are presented in such areas as ecology, social change, health, population, child development, behavior, and the !kia healing dance.

825. Lee RLM, Ackerman SE: The sociocultural dynamics of mass hysteria: a case study of social conflict in West Malaysia. Psychiatry 43:78–88, 1980.

The outbreak of mass hysteria among students in a Malay college in West Malaysia was a result of conflict within the group amplified by illness, intense competition for prestige and leadership, and hostility from the local community. The perception of these objective conditions as extremely stressful was structured by the supernatural world view shared by the group members. This mass hysteria was not cathartic or anxiety relieving as indicated in the published literature.

826. Lee RPL: Perceptions and uses of Chinese medicine among the Chinese in Hong Kong. Culture Medicine Psychiatry 4:345–75, 1980.

The sacred or magical-religious tradition of Chinese medicine is accepted by one-fifth of the ordinary Chinese people in urban Hong Kong and is relatively more popular among women and less-educated people. Both the classical-professional and the local-empirical traditions of secular medicine are resorted to by many Chinese people either for treating diseases or for strengthening their constitution. People are more confident in the Chinese medical tradition than in Chinese-style practitioners in Hong Kong. Chinese medicine is generally perceived to be better than or as good as Western medicine with fewer side effects. Most people follow the pattern of moving from self-medication to Western-style doctors to Chinese-style practitioners and finally to a Western medical hospital.

827. Leff JP, Fischer M, Bertelsen A: A cross-national epidemiological study of mania. Brit J Psychiatry 129:428–42, 1976.

The annual incidence of mania is virtually identical in Aarhus (Denmark) and London. There is a higher proportion of immigrants in the London sample as compared to Aarhus.

828. Lefkowitz M, Eron L, Walder L, Huesmann LR: Growing Up to Be Violent. Elmsford, N.Y., Pergamon, 1977.

A ten-year longitudinal study of children and their parents found that male sex roles and other cultural factors foster aggression.

829. Lefley HP: Female cases of falling-out: a psychological evaluation of a small sample. Social Science Medicine 13B(2):115–16, 1979.

"Falling-out" appears to be a desperate mode of dealing with anxiety in black females with limited coping mechanisms and almost no external support systems.

830. Lefley HP: Prevalence of potential falling-out cases among the black, Latin, and non-Latin white population of the city of Miami. Social Science Medicine 13B(2):113–14, 1979.

Symptoms associated with the falling-out syndrome are more prevalent in the black population than in Latin and non-Latin groups in Miami.

831. Leibowitz L: Females, Males, Families. North Scituate, Mass., Duxbury, 1978.

The ways in which humans organize families are not fixed by biology. Features basic to family arrangements are exemplified by the Irigwe (Africa), the Pahari and the Nayar (India), Marquesan Islanders, and Israelis on kibbutzim. Family forms in Western societies can be contrasted with foragers such as the Tiwi (Australia) and Andaman Islanders.

832. Leiderman PH, Tulkin SR, Rosenfeld A (eds): Culture and Infancy. New York, Academic, 1977.

Topics discussed include child rearing as cultural adaptation, the uses of cross-cultural research in early development, and infancy in various cultures including Ganda, Mayan, Zambian, and Kalahari Desert San.

833. Leininger M: Transcultural Nursing. New York, Wiley, 1978.

The values and beliefs of the patient can act as important variables in determining the success of a nursing situation.

834. Leland J: Firewater Myths: North American Indian Drinking and Alcohol Addiction. New Brunswick, N.J., Rutgers Center of Alcohol Studies, 1976.

Native Americans are not constitutionally predisposed either to develop an inordinate craving for alcohol or to lose control of their behavior when they drink.

835. Leland J: Comment on "Psychocultural barriers to successful alcoholism therapy in an

American Indian patient." J Stud Alcohol 40(7):737–42, 1979.

Popham's contentions regarding Algonquin Indian women demonstrating emotional restraints as described by Hallowell are challenged. The interviews were not conducted appropriately, and there were cross-cultural barriers between the patient and the interviewer.

836. Lemert EM: Koni, kona, kava orange-beer culture of the Cook Islands. J Stud Alcohol 37(5):565–85, 1976.

Orange-beer drinking groups in the Cook Islands have a long history indicating that they served substantial needs and that their significance was neither ephemeral nor marginal. Island drinking customs have cult-like forms, provide for social integration, and control drunken aggression.

837. Lenero-Okro L: Beyond the Nuclear Family Model: Cross-Cultural Perspectives. Beverly Hills, Calif., Sage, 1977.

As evidenced by studies from Poland, the Philippines, India, Japan, Puerto Rico, and Sweden, there are many functional alternatives to the nuclear family model.

838. Lennard SHC, Lennard HL: Architecture: effect of territory, boundary, and orientation on family functioning. Family Process 16:49–66, 1977.

The physical home environment may facilitate or constrain inter- and intrafamily interaction, role relations, values, and identities.

839. Leon CA: "El Duende" and other incubi: suggestive interactions between culture, the devil, and the brain. Arch Gen Psychiatry 32:155–62, 1975.

The belief in persecution or possession by evil spirits is still popular in Latin American countries. Possible psychodynamic mechanisms are involved both in the production of this phenomenon and in the successful "therapeutic" interventions of spiritualist rather than psychiatric or religious healers.

840. Lerner HE: Adaptive and pathogenic aspects of sex-role stereotypes: implications for parenting and psychotherapy. Amer J Psychiatry 135:48–52, 1978.

The degree to which sex-role stereotypes are adaptive and facilitative (as opposed to restrictive and pathogenic) is inversely related to the degree to which an individual has consolidated a comfortable and stable gender identity.

841. Lerner RM, Iwawaki S, Chihara T, Sorell GT: Self-concept, self-esteem, and body attitudes among Japanese male and female adolescents. Child Development 51:847–55, 1980.

Compared to their American counterparts, Japanese adolescents have lower self-esteem and less favorable views of their bodies' attractiveness and effectiveness. Sex differences account for more variance in the self-concepts of Japanese cohorts than they do in comparative American ones.

842. Leung SMR, Miller MH, Leung SW: Chinese approach to mental health service. Canadian Psychiatric Assn J 23:354–60, 1978.

Chinese experiences with mental health raise doubt about the value of professionally oriented emphasis in health programs that are not woven into the social, economic, political, and ethical activities of society. The Chinese maintain that the key to all health and mental health care advances is social and economic reform, grass-roots programs, and a self-reliance strategy with an intense personal motivation to produce change in one's way of life.

843. Levav I, Bilu Y: A transcultural view of Israeli psychiatry. Transcult Psych Res Review 17:7–36, 1980.

A review of the literature indicates that (1) the Israeli public has shown little understanding of mental illness; (2) foreign-born Israelis have higher rates of mental disorder; (3) immigrants from Morocco, Yemen, and other areas maintain folk beliefs about mental illness, e.g., tsira and aslai are disorders caused by demons; (4) these immigrants utilize folk healers; (5) Western medical and psychiatric treatment has attenuated the curing role of traditional healers.

844. Levine EM: Male transsexuals in the homosexual subculture. Amer J Psychiatry 133:1318–21, 1976.

As their gender identity formed, twenty male transsexuals living in a male homosexual subculture were unable to acquire heterosexual partners and sought bisexual partners to confirm their identity as females. Psychiatrists should emphasize the prevention of this futile attempt to be female and help transsexuals shift their gender identity.

845. Le Vine ES, Ruiz RA: An exploration of

multicorrelates of ethnic group choice. J Cross-Cultural Psychology 9:179–90, 1978.

Blacks reveal generally higher own-group preference than Anglos and Chicanos, with Chicanos generally revealing higher own-group preference than Anglos.

846. LeVine S: Mothers and Wives: Gusii Women of East Africa. Chicago, U. of Chicago Press, 1979.

Seven young Gusii mothers relate details about pregnancy, childbirth, anxiety over childbearing capacities, and the hardships of being married to sometimes-absent husbands.

847. LeVine S: Crime or affliction? Rape in an African community. Culture Medicine Psychiatry 4:151–65, 1980.

Among the Gusii of southwestern Kenya, rape is considered a sacrilegious matter to be dealt with in the family, not by the secular authorities. The Gusii are convinced that violent sexual assaults are involuntary and that the criminal is not a criminal but an afflicted person, motivated by the malevolence of the ancestral spirits or of jealous neighbors and kin.

848. Levine SV: Role of psychiatry in the phenomenon of cults. Canadian J Psychiatry 24:593–603, 1979.

It is imperative that psychiatrists have a comprehensive and clear knowledge of the concepts and activities of cults, their effects on young people and their families, and some of the reactions they have caused in society.

849. Levine SV, Salter NE: Youth and contemporary religious movements: psychosocial findings. Canadian Psychiatric Assn J 21:411–20, 1976.

Canadian youths joining contemporary religious movements are young, white, well educated, predominantly middle-class, and from fairly stable backgrounds. Dissatisfaction with life is the main motivating factor for joining, and they feel better with decreased anxiety and depression after joining.

850. Levy JE, Neutra R, Parker D: Life careers of Navajo epileptics and convulsive hysterics. Social Science Medicine 13B(1):53–66, 1979.

Because traditional healers attribute negative social attributes to persons suffering generalized seizures, these practitioners cannot be recommended for treatment of this kind of problem. Instead, acculturated Navajos who are trained as mental health workers are the healer of choice.

851. Levy-Bruhl L: The Notebooks on Primitive Mentality. New York, Harper and Row, 1978.

Primitive man is capable of analytical and logical thought. An emotional, vested interest in certain forms of behavior, however, appears to show his perceptual orientation in a prelogical, intuitive direction.

852. Lewis DO, Shanote SS, Cohen RJ, Kligfeld M, Frisone G: Race bias in the diagnosis and disposition of violent adolescents. Amer J Psychiatry 137:1211–16, 1980.

Violence and severe psychiatric symptomatology are equally prominent in adolescents sent to correctional schools or psychiatric hospitals. Black adolescents from the lower socioeconomic class, girls, and those with head injury are more often in correctional institutions.

853. Lewis G: Knowledge of Illness in a Sepik Society. Atlantic Highlands, N.Y., Humanities, 1975.

The recognition and explanation of illness among the Gnau of New Guinea are linked with their world view and culture.

854. Lewis HB: Sex differences in superego mode as related to sex differences in psychiatric illness. Social Science Medicine 12(3B):199–205, 1978.

Men and women differ in their prevailing mode of superego functions. This difference in superego mode may be one determinant of sex differences in "choice" of psychiatric illness. There is evidence for a connection between patients' perceptual style and their proneness to shame or guilt.

855. Lewis J (ed): Symbols and Sentiments. New York, Academic, 1977.

Among the topics discussed are symbolic behavior in a Sudanese healing cult, the meaning of Africa in Haitian voodoo, symbolism in psychoanalysis, moral order and mental derangement, Hindu asceticism, and the roots of violence and symbolism in childhood and adolescence.

856. Lewis TH: A culturally patterned depression in a mother after loss of a child. Psychiatry 38:92–95, 1975.

The phenomenology of clinical psychiatric syndromes, like grief, is conditioned by the cultural ambience of the patient.

857. Lewis TH: A syndrome of depression and

mutism in the Oglala Sioux. Amer J Psychiatry 132:753–55, 1975.

The wacinko syndrome of the Oglala Sioux, not previously recognized by non-Indian practitioners, varies from mild response to disappointment to severe psychosis and suicide. Most cases are recognizable as reactive depressive illnesses.

858. Leyton E: Dying Hard: The Ravages of Industrial Carnage. Toronto, McClelland and Stewart, 1975.

Miners of Newfoundland dying from silicosis and lung cancer describe their bitterness.

859. Lichtman AJ, Challinor JR (eds): Kin and Communities: Families in America. Washington, D.C., Smithsonian Institution Press, 1979.

Roles in the American family have changed as a response to environmental, economic, and social settings. Topics include the women's roles, the adaptation of sick or alcoholic roles as a response to economic insecurity, social isolation among older blacks, and the changing roles of the family in the care of the mentally ill.

860. Lidz RW, Lidz T: Male menstruation: a ritual alternative to the oedipal transition. Intl J Psychoanalysis 58:17–31, 1977.

Initiation rituals serve to separate young males from their mothers' influence and to establish an intense bond with the male group. Among several primitive societies, nose bleeding—male menstruation—and vomiting are used to cleanse the boy of the mother's womb blood and serve to mark the beginning of his maturation.

861. Lieban RW: Traditional medical beliefs and the choice of practitioners in a Philippine city. Social Science Medicine 10:289–96, 1976.

Traditional medical systems in developing areas complement modern medicine and serve different purposes or functions than modern medicine does.

862. Lieblich A, Kuglemass S, Ehrlich C: Patterns of intellectual ability in Jewish and Arab children in Israel. Part 2: Urban matched samples. J Cross-Cultural Psychology 6:218–26, 1975.

The intellectual pattern difference found in previous studies is not likely to be related to the Arab-Jewish ethnic difference per se, but probably reflects an interaction of ethnicity and subcultural environment.

863. Lifshitz M, Ramot L: Toward a framework for developing children's locus-of-control orientation: implications from the kibbutz system. Child Development 49:85–95, 1978.

Children (girls more so than boys) raised in kibbutzim characterized by a greater degree of authoritarian educational methods combined with intimate early contacts with parents are less internal in their locus of control than those raised under an ideology espousing more peer-group autonomy and lesser contacts with parents.

864. Lifton RJ, Kato S, Reich M: Six Lives/Six Deaths: Portraits from Modern Japan. New Haven, Conn., Yale U. Press, 1978.

The life and death of six Japanese elite men are presented. All the subjects had written about their attitudes to their own death.

865. Light D, Spiegel J: The Dynamics of University Protest. Chicago, Nelson-Hall, 1977.

Student unrest and protest are examined in context, as are the tactics of student, faculty, and administrative responses, and the psychology of university protest.

866. Lilly JC: Simulations of God. New York, Simon and Schuster, 1975.

The Christian-Jewish God, like other gods such as sex, money, and drugs, is a projection of individuals and of a culture.

867. Lin TY, Lin MC: Service delivery issues in Asian–North American communities. Amer J Psychiatry 135:454–56, 1978.

A traditional Chinese view of mental illness is prevalent among Chinese-Canadians. Sociocultural factors such as moralistic, religious, psychological, and familial characteristics influence the help-seeking behavior of Chinese psychiatric patients in North America.

868. Lin TY, Tardiff K, Donetz G, Goresky W: Ethnicity and patterns of help-seeking. Culture Medicine Psychiatry 2:3–13, 1978.

Ethnicity is a prime factor in differentiating patterns of help-seeking. Chinese patients are kept for prolonged periods of time within their families, while Anglo-Saxons and Middle Europeans are referred by their families or themselves to multiple social and mental health agencies. Native Indians are referred by persons other than family members or themselves between social and legal agencies in the community.

869. Lincoln JR: Household structure and social stratification: evidence from a Latin American city. J Marriage Family 40:601–12, 1978.

Data on household structure and the educational and occupational patterns of male household heads in Santiago, Chile, reveal no relationship between status and household composition. Ascriptive factors (father's occupation and father's education) are more influential determinants of the statuses attained by men from extended family households, whereas achievement factors (education and early job status) are more influential with regard to men from nuclear households.

870. Lindenbaum S: Kuru Sorcery. Palo Alto, Calif., Mayfield, 1979.
Kuru, a fatal, slow virus disease devastated the Fore of Papua New Guinea, who blamed the disease on sorcery.

871. Linn MW, Shane R, Webb NL, Pratt TC: Cultural factors and attrition in drug abuse treatment. Intl J Addictions 14:259–80, 1979.
Even though black and white drug patients are very different on many cultural variables, most of these variables have no effect on their staying in treatment.

872. Lippman D: Psychiatry in Ethiopia. Canadian Psychiatric Assn J 21:383–88, 1976.
Ethiopia has a mental health system involving psychiatrists and two psychiatric hospitals. There is a high frequency of some neurological syndromes; depression is rare.

873. Littlewood R: Anthropology and psychiatry—an alternative approach. Transcult Psych Res Review 17:238–41, 1980.
Transcultural psychiatry is determined primarily by its method, which is based on the assumption that symbolism is crucial to humans. Transcultural psychiatry is to social psychiatry as anthropology is to sociology.

874. Littlewood R, Lipsedge M: Acute psychotic reactions in Caribbean-born patients. Transcult Psych Res Review 17:194–97, 1980.
Caribbean and West African blacks in London are being overdiagnosed as suffering from schizophrenia. These patients may be actually demonstrating an acute psychotic reaction of the type previously described in Africa and the Caribbean.

875. Liu X: Mental work in Sichuan. Brit J Psychiatry 137:371–76, 1980.
In Sichuan, China, psychiatric patients are mostly treated in large mental hospitals with a blend of traditional Chinese and Western therapies. Most of the inpatients are schizophrenics.

Affective disorders and substance abuse disorders are less prevalent. Most of the outpatients in teaching hospitals are neurotics. ECT without anesthesia is widely used.

876. Lloyd BB, Easton B: The intellectual development of Yoruba children: additional evidence and a serendipitous finding. J Cross-Cultural Psychology 8:3–16, 1977.
Yoruba children growing up in a privileged environment show increasingly superior mental ability.

877. Lo WH, Lo T: A ten year follow-up study of Chinese schizophrenics in Hong Kong. Brit J Psychiatry 131:63–66, 1977.
Sixty-five percent of an evaluated group of Chinese schizophrenics in Hong Kong have full and lasting remission or show no or mild deterioration after some relapses in a ten-year follow-up. Females with shorter duration of illness, with acute onset, and with no symptoms affecting emotions or volition, have a better prognosis.

878. Lock MM: Scars of experience: the act of moxibustion in Japanese medicine and society. Culture Medicine Psychiatry 2:151–75, 1978.
Beliefs and practices surrounding moxibustion, a cautery technique used in Japan, demonstrate that the concept of holism is culture-bound and that the practice of East Asian medicine is often reductionistic. Socialization practices concerning attitudes toward illness reflect pluralistic values derived from traditional medical systems. One dominant set of values encourages patient and family responsibility during the healing process, adaptation to psychosocial relationships regarded as causal in disease occurrence, and avoidance of verbal analysis of problems. These concepts cannot be readily adapted in the West as part of a holistic approach to health care.

879. Lock MM: East Asian Medicine in Urban Japan: Varieties of Medical Experience. Berkeley, U. of California Press, 1980.
East Asian medicine based on classical Chinese theories is practiced widely in Japan and is generally regarded favorably by cosmopolitan physicians. Therapies such as herbal medicine, acupuncture, moxibustion, and massage often contain symbolic components that ameliorate some social and psychological aspects of illness.

880. Locke BC: Being black is detrimental to one's mental health: myth or reality? Phylon 38(4):408–28, 1977.
Stressful social conditions that come about as a

result of blackness, such as experiences of loss or failure, denial of respect, ordinary dignity, and courtesy, and being viewed as inferior, along with other effects of racism, are what contributes to the high prevalence of mental disorders among blacks rather than the amount of melanin in their skin.

881. Loehlin JC, Lindzey G, Spuhler JN: Race Differences in Intelligence. San Francisco, W. H. Freeman, 1975.

Racial differences in intelligence may in great part be nutritional in origin. The problem could best be approached by improving nutrition and education and by deemphasizing IQ test performance.

882. Loflin MD, Winogrond IR: A culture as a set of beliefs. Current Anthropology 17:723–25, 1976.

Culture is the sum of the acts and experiences represented by the shared beliefs of individuals in a social grouping. Enculturation is both the process of coming to share beliefs and the process of evolving new propositions that have the potential of being shared. Belief acquisition is the result of inferential processes involving acts and experiences or generalizations from them.

883. Logan MH: Variations regarding susto causality among the Cakchiquel of Guatemala. Culture Medicine Psychiatry 3:153–66, 1979.

As with other folk syndromes common among traditional peoples, susto (fright-sickness) is largely a socially based phenomenon. Ethnographic data from two villages in Guatemala suggest that patterning exists in reference to explanations of susto causality. This patterning centers on the relative significance Cakchiquel villagers attach to sorcery in their interpretations of fright-sickness. Susto is not simply a belief buried in peasant traditionalism, but rather is a syndrome of cultural trait having diverse functions of alleviating individual anxiety, controlling antisocial behavior, and providing a sense of ethnic identity for those who move from rural areas to large, culturally pluralistic urban centers.

884. Logan MH, Hunt EE: Health and the Human Condition: Perspectives on Medical Anthropology. North Scituate, Mass., Duxbury, 1978.

Anthropology is valuable to the medical sciences because it combines in one discipline the approaches of the biological sciences, the social sciences, and the humanities.

885. Lomas HD: Graffiti: some clinical observations. Psychoanalytic Review 63:451–57, 1976.

Graffiti are both a portrayal of an intrapsychic crisis and an attempt to actively ward off and master a passive experience that was no doubt previously very traumatic.

886. Lomnity LA: Networks and Marginality. New York, Academic, 1977.

Social networks contribute to economic survival for residents of a Mexico City shanty town.

887. Longabaugh R: The systematic observation of behavior in naturalistic settings. In Handbook of Cross-Cultural Psychology, edited by HC Triandis and JW Berry, 2:57–126. Boston, Allyn and Bacon, 1980.

Direct measurement of human behavior in settings of its natural occurrence must be a high priority of a transcultural science of human behavior. However, this is a very difficult methodology to use. In fact, its most difficult application is probably in cross-cultural field studies, exactly the point where it is most needed.

888. Longclaws L, Barnes GE, Grieve L, Deemoff R: Alcohol and drug use among the Brokenhead Ojibwa. J Stud Alcohol 41:21–36, 1980.

Most of the drinking in the Brokenhead community occurs on weekends in group settings. The three major predictors of alcohol and drug use among students are age, family relationships, and participation in hobbies. Teenagers view drinking and drug use as confirmation of their adult status. Native American children use alcohol and drugs in response to the same conditions that lead to drug use in the non-Native community. Cultural factors, such as level of acculturation and traditional upbringing, do not prove to be important predictors of drug use. In an adult sample, people who have a more traditional upbringing use more cannabis.

889. Longhofer J, Floersch JE: Dying or living? The double bind. Culture Medicine Psychiatry 4:119–36, 1980.

Kubler-Ross's five-stage theory describing the behaviors of terminally ill patients is meaningful only when used to describe behaviors occurring among patients, families, or medical practitioners. A plausible explanation of these behaviors is accomplished by examination of communication patterns containing the structure of paradox or double bind. Patients are forced to perceive realities about their physical conditions not as they appear to them but as they are defined by those in their environment. By exploring communication patterns in relation to the structure of social relationships and the specific contents of messages being transmitted and received, a "plausible" explanation for certain behaviors can be obtained.

890. Lonner WJ: The search for psychological universals. In Handbook of Cross-Cultural Psychology, edited by HC Triandis and WW Lambert, 1:143–204. Boston, Allyn and Bacon, 1980.

Behavioral universals are summarized from the perspectives of anthropology, biology, language and linguistics, and psychology. A taxonomy, summary, and analysis of possible universals in interpersonal structure are presented. Anthropological field work such as the six-cultures project is summarized. Also presented are societal and ecological bases upon which comparisons can be attempted with an assumed substantial degree of universality. It is concluded that conceptions of basic interpersonal structures converge with psychocultural models, the latter having better explanatory power.

891. Lorion RP: Ethnicity and mental health: an empirical obstacle course. Intl J Mental Health 5:16–25, 1976.

The community mental health movement remains surprisingly distant from the people it aims to serve. Recognition of ethnic influences on adaptation and on the acceptance and impact of therapeutic interventions can help to reduce this distance.

892. Lotstein LM: Human territoriality in group psychotherapy. Intl J Group Psychotherapy 28:55–71, 1978.

There is a great need for obtaining empirical data on human territoriality in group therapy. Such a data base would enhance the growing body of anecdotal literature about the importance of spatial variables in the group psychotherapy setting.

893. Loudon JB (ed): Social Anthropology and Medicine. New York, Academic, 1976.

Examples from African societies demonstrate the social contextualization of illness.

894. Luckert KW: Coyoteway. Tucson, U. of Arizona Press, 1979.

A Navajo Holyway Healing Ceremony is presented in detail.

895. Lumsden DP: On transcultural psychiatry, Africans, and academic racism. Amer Anthropologist 78:101–4, 1976.

Many psychiatric studies in general, and Ari Kiev's textbook *Transcultural Psychiatry* in particular, present ethnocentric, distorted views on Africans.

896. Lyketsos G: Emigration: psychopathologic reaction in the families left behind. Mental Health Society 4:263–69, 1977.

Family members who were left behind following the emigration of their head show a significantly higher rate of psychopathology related to the stress of emigration as compared with family members of the family whose head is a candidate for emigration. Wives and children are mainly affected.

897. Lynn R: The social ecology of intelligence in the British Isles. Brit J Social Clinical Psychology 18:1–12, 1979.

Mean population IQ in the British Isles is highest in London and southeast England and tends to drop with distance from this region. Mean population IQs are highly correlated with measures of intellectual achievement, per capita income, unemployment, infant mortality, and urbanization.

898. Lynn R: The social ecology of intelligence in France. Brit J Social Clinical Psychology 19:325–31, 1980.

The social ecology of intelligence is concerned with the relationship between a population's mean IQ and a variety of social and economic phenomena. Internal migration in France has created regional differences in mean population IQ, which are in turn responsible for some of the regional variation in intellectual achievement, earnings, and infant mortality.

899. Lynn R, Hampson SL: National differences in extraversion and neuroticism. Brit J Social Clinical Psychology 14:223–40, 1975.

Among a group of nations the most extraverted is the United States, and the most introverted is Japan. The most neurotic is Austria, and the least neurotic is Ireland.

900. Lynn R, Hampson SL: The fluctuations in national levels of neuroticism and extraversion, 1935–1970. Brit J Social Clinical Psychology 16:131–37, 1977.

Levels of neuroticism rose significantly in the nations that suffered military defeat and occupation in the Second World War and then declined during the 1950s to prewar levels. National levels of extraversion have been generally rising over this period.

901. Lyons HA: Civil violence—the psychological aspects. J Psychosomatic Research 23:373–93, 1979.

In situations of civil disturbance such as in Northern Ireland, there is no increase in psychiatric illness in the general population. Those immediately exposed to acute danger or who have been victims of terrorist activity tend to show an anxiety reaction. Normal children have learned that violence is an acceptable and successful way of life, and this will have a disturbing effect on their personality development in the future.

902. McAdoo H: Family therapy in the black community. Amer J Orthopsychiatry 47:75–79, 1977.

Black, upwardly mobile families face all the stresses experienced by other families dealing with developmental crises and economic changes, but are subject to the additional strain of discrimination. Support, often unavailable from the community, is received instead from the family and others involved in the kinship network.

903. McAdoo HP: Factors related to stability in upwardly mobile black families. J Marriage Family 40:761–78, 1978.

Examination of the impact of upward mobility over three generations on the extended kin network of black parents in the mid-Atlantic area indicates that extended help patterns are culturally, rather than solely economically, based.

904. McBride DC, Page JB: Adolescent Indian substance abuse. Youth and Society 2:475–92, 1980.

Alcohol and other substance abuse is common among Native American adolescents. The high prevalence can be explained by sociocultural factors. Treatment intervention services are enumerated.

905. McCarthy FE: Bengali village women as mediators of social change. Human Organization 36:363–70, 1977.

Any attempt to involve Bengali village women in change programs is far more complicated and culturally related than is indicated by the present concept of mobilization. Exposure to machines, urban life, consumer goods, and changing agricultural occupations is a relevant dimension perhaps for men in a developing nation, but not for women.

906. McCarthy PD, Walsh D: Suicide and the consequences for national statistics. Brit J Psychiatry 126:301–8, 1975.

There are real differences in national suicide rates, at least between Ireland, England and Wales, and Scotland. The discrepancy between official and "true" suicide rates in Ireland is greater than in England, Wales, and Scotland.

907. McCreery JL: Potential and effective meaning in therapeutic ritual. Culture Medicine Psychiatry 3:53–72, 1979.

Rituals are "symbolic constructions" analogous to works of art or literature. Rituals, like plays, appeal to audiences in different ways, sometimes by providing profound reflections on the human condition or some recurrent situation in human life, sometimes by sheer spectacle. The presentation of ritual is also important. Rituals do not heal by physical action or human bodies; their power lies in making illness meaningful to human beings. What is crucial is not simply potential meaning but effective meaning. Chinese healing rituals are examined to support the proposed arguments.

908. McDermott JF, Tseng WS, Maretzki TW: People and Cultures of Hawaii. Honolulu, U. Press of Hawaii, 1980.

The problems of Hawaiian ethnic groups (Chinese, Japanese, Portuguese, Okinawan, Korean, Filipino, Samoan, Vietnamese, and Hmong) are best understood by relating psychological to cultural factors.

909. McDonald T: Group psychotherapy with Native-American women. Intl J Group Psychotherapy 25:410–20, 1975.

Group therapy with Native American women relocated from the reservations to major urban centers provides a welcome addition to their lives in helping them to cope with a new and confusing world. In therapy sessions they learn to share each other's difficulties, thus increasing their self-esteem and confidence.

910. McDonald WS, Oden CW: Aumakua: behavior direction visions in Hawaiians. J Abnormal Psychology 80:189–94, 1977.

Disturbing visions of an Aumakua—the spirit of a dead relative—often appear to Hawaiian adolescents who have behaviorally deviated from cultural norms. Compliance with the spirit's wishes allows the person to change his behavior to conform to authority while allowing him to maintain that these changes were made of his own free will.

911. McGill JC: MMPI score differences among Anglo, Black and Mexican-American welfare recipients. J Clin Psychology 36:147–51, 1980.

Differences on several MMPI scales are only present between Mexican-Americans and Anglos, and not between Blacks and Anglos. MMPI scores may tend to vary as a function of education and economic considerations in addition to any racial differences.

912. McGoodwin JR: Ethnosemantic analysis of cognition in the alcoholic patient. Intl J Addictions 11:619–28, 1976.

Ethnosemantic analysis is a research method developed by structural anthropologists and linguists to provide a more objective understanding of the cognitions and internal symbology of persons whose social situations are "alien" from those of the researcher.

913. Mack DE: Husbands and wives in Lagos: the effects of socioeconomic status on the patterns of family living. J Marriage Family 40:807–16, 1978.

In most areas of family life in Lagos, Nigeria, middle-income couples have different attitudes and behavior patterns than do urban and rural low-income couples. Husbands and wives seldom agree in either their marital attitudes or reported behavior.

914. Mack DE, Tosan-Imade G: The effects of ethnicity and education on attitudes toward mental illness in southern Nigeria. Intl J Social Psychiatry 26:101–7, 1978.

Education influences one's attitudes toward mental illness. There are no differences between Nigeria's three ethnic groups with respect to their attitudes about mental illness.

915. Mack DE, Tosan-Imade G: The effects of ethnicity and education on attitudes toward mental illness in southern Nigeria. Transcult Psych Res Review 15:191–92, 1978.

There is no difference in attitudes toward mental illness among the Ibo, Yoruba, and Bim in Nigeria. Market traders differ significantly in attitudes from University of Lagos undergraduate students, however, in regard to beliefs that mental illness could be caused by the machinations or ill wishes of people, that Indian hemp causes mental illness, and that mental illness runs in families. There is also a difference between students and traders in attitudes toward native doctors.

916. McKernan J, Russell JL: Differences of religion and sex in the value systems of Northern Ireland adolescents. Brit J Social Clinical Psychology 19:115–18, 1980.

Protestants and Catholics in Northern Ireland differ in the ranking of "Protestant ethic" values, i.e., a sense of accomplishment, salvation, ambition, independence, and responsibility. Female pupils may be socialized into adopting a subservient role in Irish society. Catholics place a higher value on political values than do Protestants.

917. Mackey WC, Day RD: Some indicators of fathering behaviors in the United States: a cross-cultural examination of adult male-child interaction. J Marriage Family 41:287–99, 1979.

American men (compared to American women) do not associate or interact with children much differently than men in other countries (Ireland, Spain, Japan, Mexico). American men do associate with children in large numbers when the societal norms allow them access to the children, and American men interact with children at levels consonant with adult female-child dyads.

918. McLean AA: Work Stress. Reading, Mass., Addison-Wesley, 1979.

The relationships among individual vulnerability, particular stresses, and the broader social context are major factors in occupational stress.

919. MacNutt F: The Power to Heal. Notre Dame, Ind., Ave Maria, 1977.

The healing of illness is central to Christianity. The basic types of sicknesses are those of the spirit, of the emotions, and of the body. Spiritual healing commonly works by speeding up the recuperative forces of the body through prayer. A long-term program for persons with severe mental illness should include a regular schedule of prayer (including the reading of Scripture and the receiving of sacraments) and participation in a supportive Christian community.

920. MacWhinney B: The acquisition of morphophonology. Part 5: The acquisition of German morphophonology. Monographs Society Research Child Development 43:53–69, 1978.

The order of acquisition of strategies in plural formation is determined by the interaction of applicability and correctness.

921. Madanes C, Dukes J, Harbin H: Family ties of heroin addicts. Arch Gen Psychiatry 37:889–94, 1980.

Contrary to the conventional assumption that

addicts are basically peer-oriented sociopaths, there is accumulating evidence that they are enmeshed in dependent relationships with their families of origin or parental surrogates.

922. Madge NJH: Context and the expressed ethnic preferences of infant school children. J Child Psychol Psychiat Allied Disciplines 17:337–44, 1976.

Children are aware of ethnic differences. The extent and direction of their expressed ethnic preferences are strongly influenced by the situational context and by the competing variables upon which their choices of figures can be alternatively based.

923. Magaro P, Gripp R, McDowell D: The Mental Health Industry: A Cultural Phenomenon. New York, Wiley-Interscience, 1978.

Social expectations and demands define the deviant as mad. Treatment systems are created by cultural structures and have become solidified in order to perpetuate their own beliefs.

924. Magusson G, Aurelius G: Illness behavior and nationality: a study of hospital care utilization by immigrants and natives in a Stockholm district. Social Science Medicine 14A: 357–62, 1980.

In Swedish health-care planning, too little attention has been paid so far to the special problems of immigrants. Because of communication problems, immigrants experience difficulties in getting across institutional barriers. For the same reason they lack information about the organization of medical care, a prerequisite for intelligent use of health services.

925. Mahania KM: La psychotherapie dans le systeme medical traditionnel et le prophetisme chez les Kongo du Zaire. Psychopathologie Africaine 13:149–96, 1977.

The Kongo of Zaire recognize brief illnesses as natural and treat them with herbs and plants, while long-lasting or intermittent diseases are felt to be supernatural and are attributed to group social tensions. Healers include herbalists, priests who organize healing rites and practice psychotherapy, and charismatic leaders, who have ecstatic visions and dreams.

926. Mail PD: American Indian drinking behavior. J Alcohol Drug Education 26:28–39, 1980.

Teaching the American Indian how to drink rather than not to drink may provide the best solution to the myth of Indian alcoholism.

927. Mala TA: Status of mental health for Alaskan natives. Alaska Medicine 21:1–3, 1979.

The numerous social and economic changes faced by the native Alaskans have resulted in an increase in suicide, alcoholism, and alcohol-related deaths. A breakdown of intimate, traditional human associations leads to loneliness, anxiety, frustration, continuing stress, and despair, especially among the young. The community mental health center and cross-cultural workshops and seminars to educate mental health workers about the personal backgrounds and experiences of their patients can fulfill a much needed role.

928. Maloney C (ed): The Evil Eye. New York, Columbia U. Press, 1976.

The evil-eye belief is found in many cultural groups in Italy, Greece, Tunisia, Iran, Ethiopia, India, the Philippines, Guatemala, Mexico, and the United States (Italian-Americans and Slovak-Americans).

929. Mann L: Cross-cultural studies of small groups. In Handbook of Cross-Cultural Psychology, edited by HC Triandis and RW Brislin, 5:155–209. Boston, Allyn and Bacon, 1980.

Most work on cross-cultural aspects of small-group behavior has sought to test differences between cultures in the scope and intensity of conformity and cooperative behavior. In all societies the group exerts pressures toward conformity and cooperation. The exact nature and strength of the relationship between the two processes is a problem that awaits investigation.

930. Manning FE: The salvation of a drunk. Amer Ethnologist 4(3):397–412, 1977.

The religious conversion of a drunken man at a Pentecostal worship service in Bermuda gives understanding of how modes of thought based on empirical fact are phenomenologically related to nonempirical forms of consciousness in a ritual context and also throws light on the current appeal of Pentecostalism, both within its own churches and in many other denominations where aspects of Pentecostal ritual have been introduced along with the search to rediscover transcendence.

931. Manning PK: The Sociology of Mental Health and Illness. Indianapolis, Ind., Bobbs-Merrill, 1976.

Since concepts of mental illness are vague, it would be better to focus on concepts of mental health that avoid the mind/body dichotomy.

932. Manschreck TC, Petri M: The atypical psychoses. Culture Medicine Psychiatry 2:233–68, 1978.

Studies of the atypical psychoses with more rigorous methodology in descriptive and cross-cultural psychiatry indicate several methodologic problems such as inadequate assessment and certain naive notions about psychopathology in different cultures. Upon the present evidence, it is possible that atypical psychoses may represent variants of traditional psychiatric disorders, may represent independent disorders, or may be a variety of behavioral sequences found worldwide that have multiple determinants but are particularly shaped by sociocultural influences.

933. Maoz B, Tyano S, Wijsenbeck H, Erez R, Rav-Or M: Community psychiatry in border settlements in Israel. Social Psychiatry 11:163–69, 1976.

Israel, like most countries throughout the world, is struggling with the problem of how to supply adequate psychiatric services to medical centers. The success of this clinic's operation can be explained by appropriate initial classification of referrals, concentration on short-term therapy, close cooperation between the team members, and effective interaction with the relevant agencies in the community.

934. Marcos LR: Bilinguals in psychotherapy: language as an emotional barrier. Amer J Psychotherapy 30:552–60, 1976.

The bilingual patient, while faced with a language barrier that can cause the misinterpretation and distortions of his problems, may be better able to verbalize emotionally charged material through the linguistic detachment afforded by the second language.

935. Marcos LR, Alpert M: Strategies and risks in psychotherapy and bilingual patients: the phenomenon of language independence. Amer J Psychiatry 133:1275–78, 1976.

Two separate languages can complicate psychotherapy with bilingual patients; language switching may be used by them to block treatment. Therapists should carefully assess the degree of language independence in bilingual patients in order to minimize its impact on therapy and to insure that all aspects of the patient's emotional experience are available to treatment.

936. Marcus DE, Overton WF: The development of cognitive gender constancy and sex role preferences. Child Development 49:434–44, 1978.

Gender constancy is related to cognitive level with most children conforming to a developmental sequence in which conservation precedes gender constancy. Gender constancy performance is better when the concept is applied to the self versus another child and when applied to pictorial representations versus live forms. Gender constancy is not related to sex-role preferences.

937. Maretzki TW: What difference does anthropological knowledge make to mental health? Australian New Zealand J Psychiatry 10:83–88, 1976.

Most anthropologists believe that the greatest value of their work lies in their comparative and contrastive studies, where they increse understanding of how other cultures function. For the psychiatrists who must treat a specific member of a culture group, however, the anthropologist who is not psychologically oriented cannot supply a useful perspective. The anthropologist, by supplying systems analysis in a mental health context, must strive to bridge the communication gap.

938. Maretzki TW: Anthropology and mental health: reflections on interdisciplinary growth. Culture Medicine Psychiatry 3:95–110, 1979.

Westermeyer's *Anthropology and Mental Health: Setting a New Course* is the departure point for taking stock of past and present links between anthropology and psychiatry. This article reviews some of the critical links mentioned in Westermeyer's book and suggests other recent or current works that are representative of some of the promising results of anthropological contributions to psychiatric interests. Questions are raised but left unanswered that might be further examined in attempts to continue long-established interdisciplinary collaboration.

939. Maretzki TW, McDermott JF: Viewpoint of interdisciplinary team of educators: a project illustrating sensitivity to cross-cultural perspectives. Psychiatric Opinion 13(4):31–36, 1976.

A specially designed project involving an intensive year of training in the subspecialty of child psychiatry at a medical school in Hawaii for psychiatrists from Indonesia (who had completed three years of basic psychiatry residency training in their home country) indicates that learning about the training process cross-culturally is a rather elusive enterprise in which criteria for having reached the goal seem to shift as the experience progresses.

940. Mar'i SK, Levi AM: Modernization or

minority status: the coping style of Israel's Arabs. J Cross-Cultural Psychology 10:375–89, 1979.

Israeli Arabs, influenced by the majority, have advanced more than their West Bank neighbors.

941. Marin G: Social-psychological correlates of drug use among Colombian university students. Intl J Addictions 2:199–207, 1976.

Among Colombian university students the factors that differentiate the users from the nonusers are related to their attitudes and the presence of models and social reinforcers that together interact to help initiate and continue their behavior. Parents' attitudes and disapproval do not influence their behavior, but the modeling situations presented do serve to validate the use of drugs in the subjects' minds. Friends are more important in modeling and granting of social approval than "pushers."

942. Marin-Foucher M: Psychiatry in Mexico: past and present. Psychiatric Opinion 12:27–30, 1975.

In spite of the great impetus that Mexican psychiatry has received in the last ten years, it still lacks a great deal. Health centers have opened, psychiatric services have been incorporated into general hospitals, forming a liaison with the other specialities, meritorious efforts have been made to improve psychiatric education, and there are better perspectives for research. Uncontrollable demographic explosion is a reason for the slow progress.

943. Marjoribanks K: Ethnicity, family environment and cognitive performance. Psychological Reports 42:1277–78, 1978.

After accounting for joint effects and the unique influence of the environment, ethnicity generally continues to make small, but significant, unique contributions to variation in cognitive performance.

944. Marks AF: Male and Female and the Afro-Curacaoan Household. The Hague, Martinus Nijhoff, 1976.

Patterns of domestic organization among Afro-Curacaoans constitute a unique variant within the broader Afro-American spectrum.

945. Marrett CB, Leggon C (eds): Research in Race and Ethnic Relations. Greenwich, Conn., JAI, 1979.

Studies presented include ethnicity and class in Nigeria and black perspectives on race relations.

946. Mars L: The Crisis of Possession in Voodoo. San Francisco, Barbary Coast, 1980.

Voodoo in Haiti is a form of possession by the loa spirit.

947. Marsella AJ: Thoughts on cross-cultural studies on the epidemiology of depression. Culture Medicine Psychiatry 2(4):343–57, 1978.

Present cross-cultural depression studies are faced with the problems of poor diagnostic reliability for depressive disorders and profound differences in manifestation and experience of depression among different ethnocultural groups. Many ethnocultural groups do not demonstrate any of the psychological components of depression associated with its presence among Western groups. An entirely new approach to the cross-cultural study of depression is warranted.

948. Marsella AJ: Depressive experience and disorder across cultures. In Handbook of Cross-Cultural Psychology, edited by HC Triandis and JG Draguns, 6:237–87. Boston, Allyn and Bacon, 1980.

Depressive experience and disorder vary considerably as a function of sociocultural factors. Depression assessment methods are highly ethnocentric and need to emphasize greater attention to somatic and interpersonal processes in non-Western cultural settings. Existing sociocultural theories of depression are lacking in explanatory and predictive power and require more comprehensive views of the mechanisms by which sociocultural factors influence the various parameters of depression.

949. Marshall M: The politics of prohibition on Namoluk Atoll. J Stud Alcohol 36(5):597–610, 1975.

The attempts to institute prohibition during 1969–1971 on Namoluk Atoll, in the eastern Caroline Islands, became a symbol of intergenerational struggle for political power, which was eventually won by the younger antiprohibitionists.

950. Marshall M: Weekend Warriors. Palo Alto, Calif., Mayfield, 1979.

Young Trukese men are under tremendous social pressure to use alcohol and tobacco, while young women are under pressure to avoid using them. Young men are considered irresponsible, whether drunk or sober, and public displays of drunken bravado are endorsed.

951. Marshall M (ed): Beliefs, Behaviors, and

Alcoholic Beverages. Ann Arbor, U. of Michigan Press, 1979.

Cultural factors influence both the use and abuse of alcoholic beverages in important ways, including ways relevant to the treatment of alcohol problems, as exemplified by multiple cross-cultural studies.

952. Martin JP (ed): Violence and the Family. New York, Wiley, 1978.

Criminological data, clinical vignettes, and historical perspectives on family violence and on women refugees in England are presented.

953. Martin K, Voorhies B: Female of the Species. New York, Columbia U. Press, 1975.

The nature of human sex roles has an adaptive advantage for society. Physical aggression may be sex linked, but intelligence, dependency, ambition, and nurturance are not. Learning is the primary factor in most behavioral difference.

954. Martinez C: Curanderos: clinical aspects. J Operational Psychiatry 8(2):35–38, 1977.

Curanderos—Mexican-American folk healers —have a role in the mental health system of the Southwest, and in certain conditions such as evil eye (mal ojo), susto, and mal puesto, can be used as consultants or auxiliary therapists. Some case reports in clinical practice are presented.

955. Martinez C: Group process and the Chicano: clinical issues. Intl J Group Psychotherapy 27:225–31, 1977.

Chicano patients in groups differ from others by a certain reticence to deal with feelings toward the therapist, by the various manifestations of a second language, and by a unique ethnic background. In other areas, Chicano patients do not differ from others as long as language, economic, and cultural factors are dealt with actively and sensitively.

956. Martinez JL, Martinez SR, Olmedo EL, Goldman RD: The semantic differential technique: a comparison of Chicano and Anglo high school students. J Cross-Cultural Psychology 7:325–34, 1976.

The concepts *self, male, female, mother,* and *father,* all basic to the traditional Mexican family structure, have different affective meanings for Chicanos and Anglos.

957. Martinez ME, Hays JR, Solway KS: Comparative study of delinquent and non-delinquent Mexican-American youths. Psychological Reports 44:215–21, 1979.

Nondelinquent Mexican-Americans score higher on self-concept, school attitude, and level of aspiration than delinquents. Cultural and social-class biases must be considered in evaluating the self-concepts of minority delinquent youth.

958. Martino M: Emergence: A Transsexual Autobiography. New York, Crown, 1977.

An Italian-American describes personal struggles with transsexuality.

959. Matanda H: The role of paramedical workers in the mental health care of children in developing countries. Intl J Mental Health 7:106–11, 1978.

Paramedical workers should be taught to recognize signs of mental problems in children and be cognizant of the environmental factors that may be at the root of the difficulties.

960. Matejcek Z: Mental health services for children in Czechoslovakia. Intl J Mental Health 7:90–95, 1978.

Mental health care of children in Czechoslovakia is, in some ways, representative of such care in the socialist countries; in other respects, it rather anticipates developments in some of those countries.

961. Mathis A: Contrasting approaches to the study of black families. J Marriage Family 40:667–76, 1978.

Studies of black families have been influenced by two competing perspectives. The first perspective assumes that black families are patterned after the dominant culture, while the other perspective holds that at least part of black family life is linked to African forms of culture. Future research would be most useful in developing a cohesive view of the nature of black families.

962. May R: Values, myths and symbols. Amer J Psychiatry 132:703–6, 1975.

Symbol draws together and unites experience; myth is a cluster of symbols set in dramatic form. Modern society lacks symbol and myth, prompting the need for psychotherapy for the individual to define his own values.

963. Mazer M: People and Predicaments. Cambridge, Mass., Harvard U. Press, 1976.

Psychiatric services provided to residents of Martha's Vineyard were established in a cultural context that stresses the values of the islanders, many of whom are Portuguese-Americans.

964. Mechanic D (ed): Readings in Medical Sociology. New York, Free Press, 1980.

The delivery of health services is discussed, as are the social factors that influence psychiatric diagnosis, the interaction between patients and health professions, and stress.

965. Meer F: Race and Suicide in South Africa. London, Routledge and Kegan Paul, 1976.

White suicides stem largely from emotional deprivation, while black suicides stem largely from economic deprivation.

966. Mehryar AH: Mental retardation in developing countries. Intl J Mental Health 7:112–28, 1978.

Mental retardation among both children and adults will pose a serious health and social problem in developing countries in years to come.

967. Mehryar A, Khajavi F: Some implications of a community mental health model for developing countries. Intl J Social Psychiatry 21:45–52, 1974/1975.

Development of an efficient and effective mental health service will go a long way toward facilitating the social and economic progress of developing nations, while also helping to prevent some of the undesirable side effects of rapid industrialization and urbanization suffered by Western society.

968. Mehryar AH, Tashakkori GA: Sex and parental education as determinants of marital aspirations and attitudes of a group of Iranian youth. J Marriage Family 40:629–37, 1978.

Despite the trends toward modernization of marriage with a view to safeguarding the young people's rights and freedom of choice, there is much consistency between the expressed attitudes and preferences of Iranian youth and the established values and traditions of Iranian culture. A presumed generation gap is much less evident in the youth segment of Iranian society.

969. Meigs AS: Male pregnancy and the reduction of sexual opposition in a New Guinea Highlands society. Ethnology 15:393–407, 1976.

All New Guinea Highlands ethnographies describe societies in which an extreme opposition is made between male and female. This opposition is made with tremendous force among the Hua as well. The more dramatically or rigidly a category distinction is drawn, the more we can expect to find alternatives through which the tensions and dissatisfactions set up by the original distinctions are refuted.

970. Mernissi F: Beyond the Veil: Male-Female Dynamics in a Modern Muslim Society. Cambridge, Schenkman, 1975.

Women are equal to men in Islamic ideology but are subordinate to men in Islamic law and institutions. The heterosexual family unit is a threat to Islam, and Muslim women's liberation will take the form of generational rather than sexual conflict.

971. Messing SD: Health care, ethnic outcasting, and the problem of overcoming the syndrome of encapsulation in a peasant society. Human Organization 34:395–97, 1975.

Ethnic outcasting of craftsmen among Ethiopians discourages their young people from entering skilled trades. Encapsulation not only cultivates attitudes of fear, witch-hunting, and scapegoating, but also reinforces nonscientific beliefs in the causation of disease.

972. Meyer B: The development of girls' sex-role attitudes. Child Development 51:508–14, 1980.

The sex-role attitudes and aspirations of eleven-year-olds are more varied and flexible than those of seven-year-old girls. Most younger girls seem to identify primarily with a common sex-role model, while olders girls are apparently able to transcend the simplified analysis of behavior presented by societal stereotypes.

973. Meyer GC: The professional in the Chicano community.Psychiatric Annals 7(12):9–19, 1977.

Many Chicanos have a fear of institutions and a reluctance to separate themselves from their families. An active interest in the patient and the community can help ensure that the therapist does not overdiagnose psychoses because of a lack of communication and that family psychotherapy is appropriately utilized in addition to medication and hospitalization.

974. Mezzich JE, Raab ES: Depressive symptomatology across the Americas. Arch Gen Psychiatry 37:818–23, 1980.

A basic commonality of core depressive symptoms and signs exists between adult depressive patients in Peru and the United States. However, more complaints and higher scores on somatic symptoms and daily fluctuation of depression are found among the Peruvians, while the United States group has higher scores on suicidal manifestations.

975. Micklin M, Leon CA: Colombian views on causes and treatments for mental disorder: a comparative analysis of health workers and the public. Social Psychiatry 12:133–48, 1977.

In Colombia, mental disorder is interpreted in physical terms by a sizable segment of the population. However, this belief appears to be less firmly held with regard to etiological factors than to methods of treatment. Beliefs regarding causes and treatments for mental disorder vary between health workers and the public according to social position.

976. Micklin M, Leon CA: Cultural bases of images of causation in psychological disorder: a Colombian survey. Intl J Social Psychiatry 24:79–94, 1978.

Human beings generally seem to attribute their psychological problems to a limited set of etiological factors.

977. Migamoto T: Some characteristics of schizophrenic delusions in Japan. Seishin Igaku 21:152–63, 1979.

The schizophrenic delusions of Japanese patients differ from those of German patients. Germans tend to hear voices that come from outside themselves, while Japanese are more likely to believe that they are possessed by or transformed into spirits of living or dead persons, gods, or even the sun or the moon.

978. Miles A: Staff relations in psychiatric hospitals. Brit J Psychiatry 130:84–88, 1977.

In studying the roles of doctors, nurses, occupational therapists, and social workers, most respondents regard the occupational importance of psychiatrists as being higher than various groups regarding their specific roles and areas of occupational competence. Existing intergroup contacts are evaluated as much less satisfactory by nonmedical staff than by psychiatrists.

979. Miller DB: A partial test of Oscar Lewis's culture of poverty in rural America. Current Anthropology 17:720–23, 1976.

To identify the impoverished, most analysts simply determine an annual income below which they believe an individual or family will inevitably be deprived of what are considered basic necessities in life. A more definitive examination of the rural poor in the United States would compare their degree of social participation with the number of negative values they possess.

980. Miller JB: Toward a New Psychology of Women. Boston, Beacon, 1976.

Topics discussed include sex-role relationships, women's self-concept, and historical, interpersonal, and intrapersonal perspectives of women.

981. Miller RA, Miller MG: The golden chain: a study of the structure, function, and patterning of comparatico in a south Italian village. Amer Ethnologist 5:116–36, 1978.

Comparatico (Italian ritual kinship complex) is the best of all potentially integrative devices in the Italian community as it not only reinforces other bonds, but also complements them by actually linking domestic units that are not linked by other bonds.

982. Minde KK: Psychological problems in Ugandan school children: a controlled evaluation. J Child Psychol Psychiat Allied Disciplines 16:49–59, 1975.

The incidence of psychological disturbances is significantly related to place of residence, with urban children showing the highest rate. Children from multinuclear homes who have changed living places are not only seen as being disturbed more often than those who have not changed living places, but also do worse academically and have a much more unrealistic concept of their futures.

983. Minde K: Child psychiatry in developing countries. J Child Psychol Psychiat Allied Disciplines 17:79–83, 1976.

While the available literature gives a fair estimate of the problems child psychiatrists face in Africa and Southeast Asia, the delivery of services to the patients and the teaching of child psychiatry have received very little scrutiny.

984. Minde KK: Children in Uganda: rates of behavioral deviations and psychiatric disorders in various school and clinical populations. J Child Psychol Psychiat Allied Disciplines 18:23–37, 1977.

A number of African children suffer from psychological disorders and are given diagnostic labels originally created to describe European children. The majority of symptom-screening test items seem to possess transcultural relevance.

985. Minde K, Minde R: Children of immigrants: the adjustment of Ugandan Asian primary school children in Canada. Canadian Psychiatric Assn J 26:371–81, 1976.

There are increased psychological and academic adjustment problems in Ugandan Asian immigrant children in Canada. The psychopathology of the children significantly correlates with the family's drop in income and professional prestige.

986. Mindel CH, Habenstein RW: Ethnic Families in America. New York, Elsevier, 1976.

Areas discussed include the demographic characteristics of the ethnic family, family structure, cultural patterns that define family roles and statuses, cultural family values that affect life style, achievement, and economic aspirations, and stages of the family life cycle. The ethnic families examined are Polish-American, Japanese-American, Italian-American, American Catholic Irish, Chinese-American, Arab-American, Greek-American, Puerto Rican, Black American, North American Indian, Mexican-American, Amish, Franco-American, Jewish-American, and Mormon. Ethnic families are adaptive; new foci of attention arise first as problems, then change to adaptations, then become folkways. These followings, as community, neighborhood, and group preoccupations, then may become central to family belief and behavior.

987. Minor JH: Interrole conflict, coping strategies, and satisfaction among black working wives. J Marriage Family 40:799–806, 1978.

In black employed wives with children, type of conflict influences the choice of coping strategy, but choice of coping strategy is not related to satisfaction with role performance. Professional and nonprofessional subjects differ in degree of work satisfaction. The husband's approval does not affect satisfaction with worker role.

988. Miranda MR, Kitano H: Mental health services in third world communities. Intl J Mental Health 5:39–49, 1976.

When third-world communities encounter the dominant society in urban settings, the conflict in cultural values frequently presents monumental problems for those attempting to provide the full continuum of social services as well as for those in need of such services.

989. Mitchell IS, Cawte JE: The Aboriginal family voluntary resettlement scheme: an approach to Aboriginal adaptation. Australian New Zealand J Psychiatry 11:29–35, 1977.

A governmental program successfully offers assistance to Aboriginal families who themselves seek help in migrating and adjusting to a new environment. Counseling is provided, housing and employment are prearranged, a sense of identity is encouraged, psychological stress is minimized, and migrants who are unable to cope are assisted to return home without prejudice.

990. Mitchell RE, Trickett EJ: Task force report: Social networks as mediators of social support: an analysis of the effects and determinants of social networks. Comm Mental Health J 16:27–44, 1980.

The study of social networks has significant implications both for an understanding of community life and for the design of intervention programs. When viewed as a way of thinking about persons and programs, social network analysis can heuristically inform a number of the assessment, program development, and program evaluation functions of community mental health centers. The specific translation of such concepts into intervention activities, however, is still mediated by various social forces and value choices in the immediate situation.

991. Moerman D: Anthropology of symbolic healing. Current Anthropology 20:59–80, 1979.

A patient's construction of symbolic image need not be reconstructed in another order or dimension to effect his physiological, specifically healing, process. The construction of healing symbols *is* healing.

992. Moffic HS, Cheney CC, Barrios FX, Adams GL, Tristan MP, Gonzalez ID: Culture, primary care, and community mental health. Intl J Mental Health 8:89–107, 1979.

In spite of an enhanced general awareness of the importance of sociocultural variables in the provision of effective health and mental health services, problems involving the incongruence of the care rendered to subcultural groups continue to exist.

993. Mojdehi H: Change and stability of self-concepts of Iranian psychiatric patients and normals. Psychological Reports 43:403–6, 1978.

While the self-concept and discrepancy of self-concept/ideal-self of normals remained stable over a four-week period, those of mental patients significantly improved but were still lower than those of normals.

994. Mollica RF, Blum JD, Redlick F: Equity and the psychiatric care of the black patient, 1950–1975. J Nerv Ment Disease 168:279–86, 1980.

Black patients in 1975, as compared to 1950, continued to utilize almost exclusively the state hospital for inpatient care. In addition, black patients in 1975 received previously nonexistent outpatient services at regional community mental health centers in units characterized by low intervention treatment by semi- and nonprofessional staff.

995. Monfouga-Brousta J: Phenomene de possession et plant hallucinogene. Psychopathologie Africaine 12:317–48, 1976.

The Bori cult (Niger) is run by women who have been cured of sickness by joining the cult. The datura plant, a hallucinogen, is used by cult members in many different situations, e.g., to be in a trance, to demonstrate happiness, to secretly drive a person mad, and to enhance the performance of actresses during spirit possession sessions as a form of theatrical drama.

996. Montagu A: The Nature of Human Aggression. Oxford and New York, Oxford U. Press, 1976.

Aggression is a result of both nature and nurture. Too great an emphasis on biological influences could easily be exploited by a nationalistic racist identity, as could social programs aimed at equalizing the conditions of life.

997. Moore SF, Meyerhoff BG (eds): Secular Ritual. Atlantic Highlands, N.J., Humanities, 1978.

Analyses of ritual forms blend ethnographic scrutiny with questions of social dynamics, as exemplified by studies of Sinhalese healing rituals and rituals in old-age homes.

998. Moos RH: The Human Context. New York, Wiley Interscience, 1976.

Social ecology is the multidisciplinary study of the impact of physical and social environments on human beings.

999. Morgan R: Three weeks in isolation with two chronic schizophrenic patients. Brit J Psychiatry 131:504–13, 1977.

Living for three weeks in isolation with chronic schizophrenic patients gives the observer an unusually close view of schizophrenic and institutional behavior and some insight into the natural outcome of staff-patient interaction.

1000. Morley P, Wallis R: Culture and Curing. Pittsburgh, U. of Pittsburgh Press, 1978.

Folk medical beliefs and practices in Mexico, Serbia, the Philippines, Melanesia, Africa, and Vermont are examined anthropologically.

1001. Morris RJ, Hood RW: Religious and unity criteria of Baptists and Nones in reports of mystical experience. Psychological Reports 46:728–30, 1980.

An experience of unity may be a major characteristic of both religious and nonreligious mysticism.

1002. Morrison JK, Nevid JS: Attitudes of mental patients and mental health professionals about mental illness. Psychological Reports 38:565–66, 1976.

A variety of attitudes toward mental illness, such as from staff in hospital settings and from the popular media, may often lead to divergent staff-client expectations for service.

1003. Morsy S: Sex roles, power, and illness in an Egyptian village. Amer Ethnologist 5:137–50, 1978.

The incidence of Uzr illness and perceived stress are linked to power relations associated with subservient status and deviation from culturally stipulated role behavior. Reference to individual manipulations and individual cases of wielding power is incomplete without parallel attempts to isolate structural regularities associated with the availability and exercise of power. Theoretical statements about power relations cannot be abstracted from individual choices, manipulations, or influences but should go beyond the enumeration of choices and the exercise of power toward isolating their determinants, not in terms of alleged universals but by reference to specific social formations.

1004. Mosse GL: Toward the Final Solution. New York, Howard Fertig, 1978.

European racists appropriated legitimate scientific findings and occasionally enlisted reputable scientists for their own ends. "Racial thinking" led to the destruction of the Jews by the Nazis.

1005. Mostwin D: Uprootment and anxiety. Intl J Mental Health 5:103–16, 1976.

Uprootment can produce attitudes, fears, priorities, values, and related anxieties in the attempt to adjust to a new culture.

1006. Moulton R: Some effects of the new feminism. Amer J Psychiatry 134:1–6, 1977.

The new freedom for women has brought both expanded opportunities and problems in work, sexual, and family settings. A stable equilibrium will be achieved only after the effects of rapid cultural change have been dealt with individually and socially.

1007. Mounier B, Dubuis J: The North African immigrant in France. Intl J Mental Health 5:96–102, 1976.

North Africans seem dominated by an agonizing and crippling ambivalence and a search for identity. Making use of values derived from native traditions is very uncertain. The nature of these problems determines how well the immigrants adapt in France and, especially, their reaction to the physical and psychological impact the host country makes on them.

1008. Moy CS: Determining ethnic origins in an interview survey: problems and recommendations. Public Health Reports 92:414–20, 1977.

The acquisition of accurate data of ethnic origin is a great concern of many United States programs providing financial assistance. Several steps are recommended for identifying minorities, including a listing and definition of the desired groups, a system of classifying persons within these groups, wording of questions for self-identification that are easily understood and inoffensive, and the use of flashcards that are unambiguous and inoffensive.

1009. Muecke MA: An explication of "wind illness" in northern Thailand. Culture Medicine Psychiatry 3:267–300, 1979.

"Wind illness" is a very common complaint among the northern Thai, yet is rarely recognized by physicians trained in biomedics. Adult women who have ever borne a child are most susceptible. "Wind illness" has no consistent pattern of organic pathology and is a cover-all term of sundry disorders that are particularly circumscribed by cultural traditions. Neither biomedicine nor indigenous medicine in northern Thailand is oriented to treat disturbances of interpersonal relationships. "Wind illness" is a residual category that includes emotional disturbances when they are not all alleviated by indirect treatment of their somaticized or displaced symptomatology.

1010. Mueller DP: Social networks: a promising direction for research on the relationship of the social environment to psychiatric disorder. Social Science Medicine 14A: 147–61, 1980.

There is a need for systematic investigations of the relationship of social network characteristics to specific psychiatric disorders, particularly depression.

1011. Muensterberger W (ed): The Psychoanalytic Study of Society, Vol. 7. New Haven, Conn., Yale U. Press, 1976.

Both northern and southern Athabascans demonstrate a pattern of delayed maturation. Ghost sickness—cannabalistic fantasies with concomitant gastrointestinal psychophysiological reactions and overt ghost fears—is experienced by a majority of Kiowa Apache adults at times of mourning. The case history of a Filipino faith healer is presented, as is a psychoanalytic interpretation of a Siberian shaman.

1012. Muensterberger W, Boyer LB (eds): The Psychoanalytic Study of Society, Vol. 8. New Haven, Conn., Yale U. Press, 1979.

Articles include studies of fear in Zambian natives, Arctic hysteria in an Eskimo, dreams of Brazilian Indians, and a Siberian myth of death and reincarnation.

1013. Muensterberger W, Esman AH (eds): The Psychoanalytic Study of Society, Vol. 6. New York, Intl. Universities Press, 1975.

Areas covered include aggression in two Canadian Eskimo groups, the psychocultural significance of the Alaska Athabascan potlatch ceremony, and an Apache myth.

1014. Muhlin GL: Mental hospitalization of the foreign-born and the role of cultural isolation. Intl J Social Psychiatry 25:258–66, 1979.

Cultural isolation is highly related to the psychiatric hospitalization rates of the foreign-born in small areas in New York City.

1015. Munoz L: Exile as bereavement: socio-psychological manifestations of Chilean exiles in Great Britain. Brit J Med Psychology 53:227–32, 1980.

The psychodynamics of exile are akin to those of bereavement and must be understood in terms of loss followed by stress caused by adaptation to the new environment.

1016. Munro D: Locus-of-control attribution factors among blacks and whites in Africa. J Cross-Cultural Psychology 10:157–72, 1979.

In attributing causality in familiar events, both blacks and whites take independent account of (a) the participant's efforts and abilities and (b) the intervention of chance and supernatural forces.

1017. Munroe RL, Munroe RH: Perspective suggested by anthropological data. In Handbook of Cross-Cultural Psychology, edited by HC Triandis and WW Lamberts, 1:253–317. Boston, Allyn and Bacon, 1980.

Anthropology has consistently employed two complementary approaches that are of value to cross-cultural psychology: a comparative orientation and an emphasis on context. The definite limits to cross-cultural variability indicate that possible adaptive solutions to the problems of existence are finite. The concept of limiting factors can be applied to the analysis of sociocultural change pervasive in the modern world. Psychology and anthropology can join together to achieve understanding of the process of change.

1018. Murdock GP, Wilson SF, Frederick V: World distribution of theories of illness. Ethnology 17:449–70, 1978.

Theories of natural causation of illness include infection, stress, organic deterioration, accident, and overt human aggression. Theories of supernatural causation fall into three groups: mystical causation (fate, ominous sensations, contagion, mystical restitution), animistic causation (soul loss, spirit aggression—the most common and widespread of all types of supernatural causation), and magical causation (witchcraft, sorcery). A disproportionate number of societies emphasizing witchcraft theories are found in Africa and the circum-Mediterranean, of those stressing spirit aggression in East Asia and the insular Pacific, and of those showing sorcery in North and South America.

1019. Murillo-Rhode I: Family life among mainland Puerto Ricans in New York City slums. Perspectives Psychiatric Care 14:174–79, 1976.

Puerto Rican families see their personal relationships and values being replaced by a system of impersonal relationships and norms that threatens the very core of their being. As their children assimilate American values, they challenge their parents' values, reject their ways, and rebel against parental authority and control.

1020. Murphy HBM: Migration, culture and mental health. Psychological Medicine 7:677–84, 1977.

The mental health of a migrant group is determined by factors relating to the society of origin, factors relating to the migration itself, and factors operating in the society of resettlement.

1021. Murphy HBM: Transcultural psychiatry should begin at home. Psychological Medicine 7:369–71, 1977.

The time is overdue for the relationship among cultural backgrounds, psychopathology, and forms of therapy in developed countries to be more formally examined.

1022. Murphy HBM: European cultural offshoots in the New World: differences in their mental hospitalization patterns. Part 1: British, French and Italian influences. Social Psychiatry 13:1–9, 1978.

While there are significant differences in the mental hospitalization patterns of Canadians with British, French, Italian, and Irish origins, such epidemiological features offer only pointers to the existence of deeper, more significant differences.

1023. Murphy HBM: Historic changes in the sex ratios for different disorders. Social Science and Medicine 12(3B): 143–49, 1978.

The imagination may have more relevance for pathology than real-life roles that one plays. Societies may markedly affect the risk of pathology by dominating the imaginations of their members. Regarding changing sex ratios for disorders, it is often the ideal self-image of one or the other sex that appears to lead to an excess vulnerability to a disease.

1024. Murphy HBM: Depression, witchcraft and super-ego development in pre-literate societies. Canadian J Psychiatry 24:437–49, 1979.

Guilt feelings and self-accusations first appeared as symptoms of depression in Europe and Africa following a period of witchcraft beliefs. Heightened witchcraft beliefs were a defense against an individualizing change that would eventually lead to symptoms of depression.

1025. Murphy HBM, Taumoepeau BM: Traditionalism and mental health in the South Pacific: a re-examination of an old hypothesis. Psychological Medicine 10:471–82, 1980.

Mental disorders are rare in the stable, traditionally rural society of Tonga.

1026. Myerhoff B: Number Our Days. New York, E. P. Dutton, 1979.

Residents of a center for elderly Jews in California deal with old age, isolation, and poverty by developing survival techniques that were instrumental in their Eastern European countries of origin.

1027. Myerhoff B, Simic A: Life's Career—Aging: Cultural Variations on Growing Old. Beverly Hills, Calif., Sage, 1977.

Essays on aging among the Chagga (Africa), Yugoslavs, Mexican-Americans, and Jews demonstrate that the rewards possible in old age depend on individual ability, resourcefulness, good judgment, and luck at every point during the life cycle.

1028. Nadler A, Romek E, Shapira-Friedman A: Giving in the kibbutz: pro-social behavior of city and kibbutz children as affected by social responsibility and social pressure. J Cross-Cultural Psychology 10:57–72, 1979.

Kibbutz children are more socially responsible and generous than city children.

1029. Nagera H: Female Sexuality and the Oedipus Complex. New York, Jason Aronson, 1975.

Femininity contains elements of passivity and masochism. Since clitoral masturbation is phallic, the clitoris has to be renounced if femininity is to be established.

1030. Nahas GG, Zeidenborg P, Lefebure C: Kif in Morocco. Intl J Addictions 10:977–93, 1975.

Chronic cannabis intoxication of a significant fraction of the male population still prevails in Morocco.

1031. Nahemou N: Residence, kinship, and social isolation among the aged Baganda. J Marriage Family 41:171–84, 1979.

Values of individualism, self-reliance, and independence of aged Baganda people in Uganda parallel those of the United States. The majority of Baganda people do not view old age as a period of loneliness or isolation. Loneliness is found to be associated with widowhood, residential separation from kin, and poor health.

1032. Nakagawa T, Nakano S, Mori S, Sugita M: Psychosomatic studies of Japanese youth under social changes: an overview. Psychotherapy Psychosomatics 30:216–28, 1978.

A study of psychosomatic disorders in adolescent patients at Kyushu University Hospital reveals that the incidence of irritable colon syndrome ranks first. Through matched-pair studies with high-school students, significant interrelationships are proved to exist between the occurrence of diarrhea and constipation and the awareness of illness and psychological factors, with diarrhea and constipation increasing rapidly from junior to senior high school.

1033. Nandi DN, Mukherjie SP, Boral GC, Banerjie G, Ghosh A, Sarkar S, Ajamany S: Socio-economic status and mental morbidity in certain tribes and castes in India: a cross-cultural study. Brit J Psychiatry 136:73–85, 1978.

In caste groups residing in a cluster of villages

in West Bengal, India, the higher socioeconomic classes have higher rates of mental morbidity. Different groups with a similar cultural pattern show no difference in their rates of morbidity whereas groups with different cultural patterns differ significantly in their rates of morbidity. In lower-caste tribes anxiety states and obsessive disorders are absent.

1034. Nandy A: Woman versus womanliness in India: an essay in social and political psychology. Psychoanalytic Review 63:301–15, 1976.

Redefinition of womanhood in present-day India has required a redefinition of the concept of man and of public functioning. To make the issues of emancipation of woman and equality of sexes primary, one needs a culture in which conjugality is central to male-female relationships.

1035. Nardi TJ, Di Sipio WJ: The Ganser syndrome in an adolescent Hispanic-black female. Amer J Psychiatry 134:453–54, 1977.

Closer examination of children who are sometimes considered "flippant" in their responses may lead to the finding of Ganser syndrome. The validity of the Ganser states is questionable because many of the signs and symptoms may appear in children as well as in adults with limited coping mechanisms.

1036. Naroll R, Levinson D: Human Relations Area Files: resources for social psychiatry. J Operational Psychiatry 10(2):141–44, 1979.

The Human Relations Area Files pertain mainly to the behavior of individuals in societies without cities and serve as a cost-effective tool for worldwide testing of theories of human behavior.

1037. Naroll R, Michik GL, Naroll F: Worldwide Theory Testing. New Haven, Conn., Human Relations Area Files, 1976.

The step-by-step details of procedures for completing an adequate holocultural study are illustrated by two hypotheses regarding the relationships between drunken brawling and suicide frequency, and between witchcraft and suicide frequency.

1038. Naroll R, Michik GL, Naroll F: Holocultural research methods. In Handbook of Cross-Cultural Psychology, edited by HC Triandis and JW Berry, 2:479–521. Boston, Allyn and Bacon, 1980.

Worldwide cross-cultural surveys, although neither as sensitive nor as accurate as other kinds of cross-cultural theory tests, must be used before a general theory of cultural variation can be scientifically established. The computer program and holocultural manual library of the Human Relations Area Files are especially intended to make the solution to many survey problems easier.

1039. Neki JS: Psychotherapy in India: past, present, and future. Am J Psychotherapy 29:92–100, 1975.

The future of psychotherapy in India lies in discovering the strengths and weaknesses of traditional techniques and developing them into clinically serviceable therapeutic systems that make use of the native metapsychologic concepts and idioms.

1040. Neki JS: Sahaja: an Indian ideal of mental health. Psychiatry 38:1–10, 1975.

Sahaja is an Indian ideal of mental and spiritual health that has received special emphasis in the Sikh scriptures. It is possible to divest Sahaja of its esoteric, mystic connotations and to define it as a mental health ideal in the context of contemporary conditions.

1041. Neki JS: An examination of the cultural relativism of dependence as a dynamic of social and therapeutic relationships. Part 1: Socio-development. Brit J Med Psychology 49:1–10, 1976.

Western and the Indian cultures, though considerably distant from one another, are not essentially irreconcilable polarities. Nonetheless, despite great social changes, the two cultures still retain their distinctive ideals for child development.

1042. Neki JS: An examination of the cultural relativism of dependence as a dynamic of social and therapeutic relationships. Part 2: Therapeutic. Brit J Med Psychology 49:11–22, 1976.

Most of the methodological strategies as well as conceptual formulations of various psychotherapeutic systems revolve round the phenomenon of dependence. Any system that neglects cross-cultural factors and makes ethnocentric assumptions its basis lacks universal validity.

1043. Neki JS: Culture-conflict and psychotherapeutic approach. Mental Health Society 4:245–54, 1977.

Both the psychodynamic conceptualization and the operational technique of psychotherapy are rooted in culture. Psychodynamics have to be

viewed against the background of ethnodynamics and sociodynamics, and the techniques chosen for therapy have to be syntactic with cultural practices and expectations. Cultural distance between the therapist and the patient can make the possibility of successful therapy rather remote.

1044. Neki JS: An examination of the extent of responsibility of mental health services from the standpoint of developing communities. Intl J Social Psychiatry 25:203–8, 1979.

The delineation of the extent of responsibility of mental health services in any given community ought to be made very carefully and realistically by planners. It should be based on estimation of projected community needs and resource availability, as well as the priority of demands on these resources.

1045. Nekipelov V: Institute of Fools. New York, Farrar, Straus and Giroux, 1980.

The Serbsky Forensic Psychiatry Institute in the Soviet Union is notorious for detaining political dissidents for nonmedical purposes.

1046. Nelson MC: The Narcissistic Condition. New York, Human Sciences, 1977.

Narcissistic pathology is present in current politics, cults, and character disorders in children and adolescents.

1047. Ness RC: The old hag phenomenon as sleep paralysis: a biocultural interpretation. Culture Medicine Psychiatry 2:15–39, 1978.

The body paralysis and hallucinations characteristic of the "old hag" syndrome of Newfoundland may be likened to the clinical condition termed sleep paralysis. "Old hag" may simply be a local explanation for a cross-cultural phenomenon.

1048. Ness RC: The impact of indigenous healing activity: an empirical study of two fundamentalist churches. Social Science Medicine 14(B):167–80, 1980.

Study of a Pentecostal church in Canada reveals that it has an "assumptive system" of the causes and treatment of illness, a charismatic preacher who is considered a healer, a belief that healing or insight into personal problems can come through church participation, and formal healing rituals. The community's Protestant church has none of these. Dissociative states, such as glossolalia and possession, occur in the men but not the women. While the amount of time spent in church activity is positively correlated with symptoms relief, the perceived obligation to perform specific ritual is stressful.

1049. Nettleship MH, Givens RD, Nettleship A (eds): War, Its Causes and Correlates. Chicago, Aldine, 1975.

War is studied from varied perspectives such as anthropology, sociology, political science, economics, psychiatry, psychology, ethology, zoology, and medicine.

1050. Neutra R, Levy JE, Parker D: Cultural expectations versus reality in Navajo seizure patterns and sick roles. Culture Medicine Psychiatry 1:255–75, 1977.

Three distinct seizure conditions are recognized among the Navajo: ichaa, characterized by generalized convulsions and stigmatized as resulting from incestuous relations; frenzy witchcraft, resembling fugue states and viewed as the result of witchcraft and deserving help; and hand-trembling, considered a sign of shamanistic ability and rewarded as an asset. Hysterics demonstrate more frenzy witchcraft and hand-trembling seizures than do epileptics, who were often physically abused. While social reward did not abolish a sick role, social stigmatization aggravated it.

1051. Newman GR: Toward a transitional classification of crime and deviance. J Cross-Cultural Psychology 6:297–315, 1975.

Deviance protest and moral indignation operate on different levels across all countries.

1052. Newman R: Comparative Deviance. New York, Elsevier, 1976.

There is a consistent and similar structure in perceptions of deviance across all countries surveyed.

1053. Ney P, Lieh-Mak F, Cheng R, Collins W: Chinese autistic children. Social Psychiatry 14:147–50, 1979.

In tightly structured family situations where there is overcrowding, Chinese autistic children have many more opportunities for tactile contact and nonverbal communication. Thus they are more social and socialized although still inept at verbal expression.

1054. Ngubane H: Body and Mind in Zulu Medicine. New York, Academic, 1977.

Zulu disease causation has three elements: natural processes, morality, and mystical processes. Curing is a rite of passage. Zulu medicines have color symbolism.

1055. Nielsen J, Nielsen JA: Eighteen years of community psychiatric service in the island of Samso. Brit J Psychiatry 131:41–48, 1977.

In the Danish island of Samso a majority of patients are referred to the community psychiatric clinic by the general practitioners. Close cooperation between the psychiatrists and the local physicians is essential. Fifty percent of all patients referred can be treated by the local physicians after examination and advice from the psychiatrist. The local population benefits from the clinic by much easier access to psychiatric treatment, earlier intervention, and shorter periods of mental illness.

1056. Nobles WW: Toward an empirical and theoretical framework for defining black families. J Marriage Family 40:679–88, 1978.

The importance of a culturally consistent theoretical and empirical framework lies in its ability to clarify and amplify the phenomena associated with a group of people like the black family. It is only with a culturally sensitive empirical and theoretical framework that such an amplification and clarification can be obtained.

1057. Noesjirwan J: A laboratory study of proxemic patterns of Indonesians and Australians. Brit J Social Clinical Psychology 17:333–34, 1978.

Indonesians use a smaller interpersonal distance and more touching and smiling than Australians.

1058. Notman M: Midlife concerns of women: implications of the menopause. Amer J Psychiatry 136:1270–74, 1979.

Menopause is not the central event of women's middle age nor is it responsible for most of the symptoms. Midlife stresses are the result of a combination of personal, family, social, and biological variables, with post-menopausal development an important phase.

1059. Nowak M, Durrant S: The Tale of the Nisan Shamaness: A Manchu Folk Epic. Seattle, U. of Washington Press, 1978.

A Nisan shamaness goes on an ecstatic trance journey to the netherworld to retrieve a soul.

1060. Nudelman AE: Christian Scientists' beliefs about the role of suggestion in illness and healing. Psychological Reports 47:358, 1980.

Most Christian Scientists contend that suggestion is not only a necessary, but also a sufficient, cause of illness.

1061. Nurbakhsh D: Sufism and psychoanalysis: what is Sufism? Intl J Social Psychiatry 24:204–12, 1978.

Sufism is the school of inward illumination and not of discussion. Hence, everything that has been said by eminent Sufis concerning Sufism is only an attempt to express in words their own inward states. The goal of Sufism is knowledge of absolute reality, not as learned men explain it to us through logic and demonstration, but as it is in itself.

1062. Nurbakhsh D: Sufism and psychoanalysis: a comparison between Sufism and psychoanalysis. Intl J Social Psychiatry 24:213–19, 1978.

Transference is the establishment of the appropriate relationship between patient and the analyst, and it may result in curing the patient and bringing him to the state of a "normal" person. Iradah (the motive force of the heart), on the other hand, is the spiritual relationship between the murid (disciple) and the murad (master) established in order to elevate the state of the normal person to that of the perfect man.

1063. Nyiti RM: The development of conservation in the Meru children of Tanzania. Child Development 47:1122–29, 1976.

Defects in methodological procedures rather than the child's education and cultural milieu seem to be largely responsible for the time lag so often reported among children from non-European cultures.

1064. Obeyesekere G: Sorcery, premeditated murder, and the canalization of aggression in Sri Lanka. Ethnology 14:1–23, 1975.

The low frequency of premeditation in homicide and violence in Sri Lanka implies that the motives for such acts are canalized through functional alternatives such as sorcery.

1065. Oboler RS: Is the female husband a man? Woman/woman marriage among the Nandi of Kenya. Ethnology 19:69–88, 1980.

Among the Nandi of Kenya, only men can hold and manage the means of production. Thus, a woman who marries another woman is culturally recoded as a man to reduce the contradiction implicit in her role with regard to property.

1066. O'Bryant SL, Corder-Bolz CR: Black children's learning of work roles from television commercials. Psychological Reports 42:227–30, 1978.

Although black children's knowledge of occupations increases after television exposure, their views of stereotypic roles do not change.

1067. Obudho CE: Black-White Racial Attitudes. Westport, Conn., Greenwood, 1976.

An annotated bibliography of 475 items dealing with racial attitudes.

1068. Ochberg FM, Gunn J: The psychiatrist and the policeman. Psychiatric Annals 10(5):30–45, 1980.

Psychiatrists and policemen will be working together more often in the future because of such disparate factors as changes in the laws, the evolution of specialty clinics for aggressive and antisocial persons, specialization within psychiatry, and such catastrophic events as the recent terrorist sieges.

1069. Odejide AO: Cross-cultural psychiatry: a myth or reality. Comp Psychiatry 20:103–9, 1979.

It is evident that cross-cultural psychiatry is real, but there is little evidence in support of the theory of cultural relativity in the diagnosis of psychiatric disorders.

1070. Odejide AO: A study of the inpatient service of a Nigerian psychiatric hospital. Comp Psychiatry 21:302–7, 1980.

The three most common diagnoses in psychiatric inpatients in Abeobuto, Nigeria, are schizophrenia, affective disorders, and psychosis associated with other cerebral conditions. Polypharmacy is commonly practiced with psychiatric patients in Nigeria.

1071. Oetting ER, Edwards R, Goldstein GS, Garcia-Mason V: Drug use among adolescents of five southwestern Native American tribes. Intl J Addictions 15:439–45, 1980.

Native Americans show a higher use of alcohol, marijuana, and inhalants from the seventh through twelfth grades than does the nation as a whole.

1072. Ogbu JU: African bridewealth and women's status. Amer Ethnologist 5(2):241–62, 1978.

There is little evidence to support previous conclusions about the functions of bridewealth and women's status in Africa. Recent studies suggest that the one function of bridewealth common to African societies is the legitimation of marriage, a function that enhances rather than diminishes the status of women in the African context.

1073. Ogunremi OO, Okonofua FE: Abuse of drugs among Nigerian youth. African J Psychiatry 3:107–12, 1977.

Results of an anonymous questionnaire given to Nigerian university students indicate that most drug abusers came from urban areas and that drugs were used in a social setting, often during exam times.

1074. Ohnuki-Tierney E: Ainu illness and healing: a symbolic interpretation. Amer Ethnologist 7(1):132–51, 1980.

Ainu "metaphysical illnesses" are characterized by the presence of spiritual beings, such as demons or deities, in illness causation or aggravation or as a source of curing power. A symbolic interpretation of Ainu metaphysical illnesses by reference to the basic cognitive structure of Ainu medical epistemology, which is founded upon sacred-profane dyads within a "social network" of cosmic organization, is possible.

1075. Ohnuki-Tierney E: Illness and Healing Among the Sakhalin Ainu. Cambridge and New York, Cambridge U. Press, 1980.

The Ainu, a small hunting and gathering group, relate their illness to their view of the universe; their medical system is interwoven with their moral cosmology and social networks.

1076. Okasha A: Psychiatric symptomatology in Egypt. Mental Health Society 4:121–25, 1977.

The main clinical symptomatology of schizophrenia, affective disorders, hysteria, and obsessional disorders as presented in Egypt are described. The differences in the presentation of symptoms in Egypt as compared to Western conditions are discussed.

1077. Okasha A, Bishery Z, Osman NM, Kamel M: A psychosocial study of accidental poisoning in Egyptian children. Brit J Psychiatry 129:539–43, 1976.

The highest age incidence for both sexes in accidentally poisoned children in Egypt (Cairo) is thirty-six months. Behavioral problems occur more often in poisoned children than in controls. The families of poisoned children differ significantly from the controls in their large size, low level of education, disturbed home atmosphere, and the accessiblity to the child of the poisonous substance.

1078. Okasha A, Demerdash A: Arabic study of cases of functional sexual inadequacy. Brit J Psychiatry 126:446–48, 1975.

Kuwaitis are more active sexually before puberty than Egyptians or Palestinians. Impotent patients are less inclined to indulge in cigarette smoking as compared to normal healthy controls recruited from each ethnic group. The somatic complaints most frequently reported by patients as an accompaniment of their sexual complaint are backache, orchalgia, shoulderache, and headache.

1079. Okasha A, Sadek A, Moneim A: Psychosocial and electroencephalographic studies of Egyptian murderers. Brit J Psychiatry 126:34–40, 1975.

In Egypt clearly motivated murders are committed by a group of men among whom the incidence of EEG abnormality is about the same as in the neurotic population. Prisoners with motiveless crimes have a higher incidence of abnormal EEGs than a group of psychopaths.

1080. Okonogi K: Japanese psychoanalysis and the Ajase complex (Kosawa). Psychotherapy Psychosomatics 31:350–56, 1979.

The Ajase complex, rooted in Buddhist thought, views the psychological peculiarity of the Japanese as being evidenced in the acceptance of oral dependency toward the mother and the repression of resentment at the mother, with guilt about being forgiven and a need to make restitution for harboring this resentment. This guilt feeling is different from traditional Freudian guilt feeling as fear of punishment.

1081. Olatawura MO: Psychotherapy for the Nigerian patient: some aspects of the problems involved. Psychotherapy Psychosomatics 25:259–66, 1975.

Conventional Western psychotherapy needs substantial modification when dealing with the traditional Nigerian. Various cultural factors —such as belief in witchcraft—as well as common psychotherapeutic processes—such as resistance and transference phenomenon—must be appreciated by the therapist during treatment.

1082. Olatawura MO: Mental health services for children in the African region. Intl J Mental Health 7:34–38, 1978.

There is an urgent need to overhaul the health education policy at all levels of training of the health-delivery teams serving in Africa.

1083. Olatunbosum DA, Akindele MO, Adadevoh BK, Asuni T: Serum copper in schizophrenia in Nigerians. Brit J Psychiatry 127:119–21, 1975.

Serum copper concentrations are significantly

higher in schizophrenic patients than in normal subjects in Nigeria. The average serum copper in schizophrenic females is higher than in schizophrenic males.

1084. O'Lears JF, Hanson J: Sexual duality, religion and the mythic imagination. J Psychol Anthropology 3:1–15, 1980.

Mythic imagination expresses the fundamental duality of identities and is conditioned by sexual differentiation. Thus, mythic imagination and its religious and political expressions are based on the erotic metaphors that serve both fantasy and dream.

1085. Olson DR (ed): The Social Foundations of Language and Thought. New York, W. W. Norton, 1980.

The major areas discussed are the interactions between social contexts, language and cognition, the learning of communication by children, and the relationship between cultural values and cognitive processes.

1086. Omark D, Strayer F, Leedman D (eds): Dominance Relations. New York, Garland STPM, 1980.

In a variety of cultural settings, relationships between children conform to the definition of dominance as predictable interaction based on force or a threat of force.

1087. Onat T, Koptagel-Ilal G, Enbiyaoglu G, Mahmutoglu M, Uctum N: The relationship between somatic growth and psychological development in Turkish adolescents. Psychotherapy Psychosomatics 32:313–21, 1979.

The results of a study of 148 Turkish adolescents and preadolescents from a middle-level school in Istanbul reveal no relationship between rate of somatic growth and psychological development. Parental cultural environment has some influence on the degree of intellectual capacity. The variations of psychological characteristics in adolescents may not only be due to internal factors—the tempo and degree of somatic development independent of cultural and environmental effects—but also due to external, social-environmental factors.

1088. O'Nell CW: Dreams, Culture, and the Individual. San Francisco, Chandler and Sharp, 1976.

Dreams differ with age, sex, and culture, and they function physiologically, psychologically, and sociologically to shape the dreamer and his society.

1089. O'Nell CW: Nonviolence and personality dispositions among the Zapotec: paradox and enigma. J Psychol Anthropology 2:301–22, 1979.

The nonviolent Zapotec community of La Paz differs from its more violent neighbors in that its child-rearing methods instill a high degree of social dependency that serve as the primary factor governing interpersonal behavior and bonding.

1090. O'Nell CW, O'Nell ND: A cross-cultural comparison of aggression in dreams: Zapotecs and Americans. Intl J Social Psychiatry 23:35–41, 1977.

Not only is there less sex and age variation in the dreamed aggression of Zapotecs, but this dreamed aggression is far more physical and less verbal for Zapotecs than it is for Americans.

1091. Orley J, Wing JK: Psychiatric disorders in two African villages. Arch Gen Psychiatry 36:513–20, 1979.

Depressive disorders are more common and more severe in rural Ugandan female populations than in the female population in London.

1092. Orubuloye IO: Sexual abstinence patterns in rural western Nigeria: evidence from a survey of Yoruba women. Social Science Medicine 13A(6):667–72, 1979.

Traditional sexual abstinence has been the main method of child-spacing for the Yoruba of Nigeria and is likely to remain so for some years to come.

1093. Osborne OH, Nakagawa H, Hartmann K: Social processes and psychiatric symptom pattern change: Wallace revisited. Human Organization 35:287–93, 1976.

Concepts of deviance and psychopathology must be reexamined and used with extreme caution. The images prevailing in the community and its institutions mold the images of appropriate behavior held by agents of socialization and social control as well as by their patients, clients, and students.

1094. Osgood CE, May WH, Miron MS: Cross-Cultural Universals of Affective Meaning. Champaign, U. of Illinois Press, 1975.

The principles and methodology of cross-cultural research using the semantic differential can be used to test hypotheses, e.g., cross-cultural similarities in the affective meaning attributed to color names.

1095. Osmond MW: Cross societal family research: a macrosociological overview of the seventies. J Marriage Family 42:995–1016, 1980.

The decade of the 1970s saw a revival of interest in cross-societal family research. Macrosociological comparative research focused particularly on the interrelationship of marital, family, and stratification systems with other societal elements. A substantive emphasis was on comparative analyses of changing sex roles.

1096. Ostendorf D, Hammerschlag CA: An Indian-controlled mental health program. Hosp Community Psychiatry 28:682–85, 1977.

The control of health-care programs for American Indians is shifting slowly from the federal government to the tribes. Agencies run by Indians can be successful.

1097. Ostwald PF (ed): Communication and Social Interaction. New York, Grune and Stratton, 1977.

Areas discussed are basic elements of human communication, disturbed patterns of communication, communication as a therapeutic tool, and communication adapted to space, time, and social realities.

1098. O'Sullivan K: Observations on vaginismus in Irish women. Arch Gen Psychiatry 36:824–26, 1979.

Although vaginismus is a relatively common gynecological complaint, vaginismus manifesting as a psychological source of sexual dysfunction is less common.

1099. Ottenberg P: Terrorism. Psychiatric Annals 10(5):10–22, 1980.

When psychiatric consultants are used in negotiations with terrorists for the sake of the hostages, there is a danger that they may become identified with the official viewpoint of their government. Psychiatry, to remain professional, requires independence; its members must not be co-opted consultants to covert agencies, courts, the military, prisons, industry, and government.

1100. Oyebola DDO: The method of training traditional healers and midwives among the Yoruba of Nigeria. Social Science Medicine 14(A):31–37, 1980.

No formal tests of competence are used by Yoruba healers in determining whether the training received by an apprentice has been sufficient. However, trainees are assessed by their performance on the job and are subjected to constant oral interviews to assess the body of knowledge they have acquired.

1101. Oyebola DDO: Traditional medicine and its practitioners among the Yoruba of Nigeria: a classification. Social Science Medicine 14(A):23–29, 1980.

If traditional healers are to be used in providing primary health care in Nigeria, it is important that all qualified traditional healers should be registered first.

1102. Ozbek A, Volkan VD: Psychiatric problems within the satellite-extended families of Turkey. Amer J Psychotherapy 30:576–82, 1976.

Emigration of Turkish villagers to urban centers in Turkey and Europe creates satellites of families left behind. Circumstances stimulate the members of satellite families to become more psychically independent of parental authority, often leading to anxiety and the formation of psychiatric symptoms.

1103. Ozturk OM: Psychotherapy under limited options: psychotherapeutic work with a Turkish youth. Amer J Psychotherapy 32:307–19, 1978.

Standard psychotherapy proved unsuitable for a severely and chronically disturbed rural Turkish male due to his personality traits and sociocultural background. Unusual treatment maneuvers had to be employed, beginning with an anamnestic evaluation followed by shocking confrontation and demanding recommendations. Then an intensive relationship formed between the therapist and patient through the mail, and finally face-to-face psychotherapy was used.

1104. Padilla AM (ed): Acculturation: Theory, Models and Some New Findings. Boulder, Colo., Westview, 1980.

Theoretical perspectives on acculturation are presented, as are case examples involving Cuban-Americans, Mexican-Americans, and Puerto Ricans.

1105. Paine HJ: Attitudes and patterns of alcohol use among Mexican-Americans: implications for service delivery. J Stud Alcohol 38:544–53, 1977.

In delivering alcoholism services to Mexican-Americans, specific cultural characteristics directly affect the impact of outreach and treatment efforts. A finding of real significance is the family structure and its system of maintenance. Most important from the standpoint of those involved in delivering services to Mexican-Americans is biculturalism, which recognizes and affirms the cultural identity of the group.

1106. Palazzoli MS, Boscolo L, Cecchin GF, Prata G: Family rituals a powerful tool in family therapy. Family Process 16:445–53, 1977.

The prescribing of a family ritual can be an extremely effective therapeutic task in family therapy.

1107. Palmore E: The Honorable Elders. Durham, N.C., Duke U. Press, 1975.

Modernization does not inevitably decrease the status of the elderly, as is evident in Japan.

1108. Papenfus SC: Witchcraft, faith-healing and psychiatry—an exploration of the grounds of therapeutic praxis. Transcult Psych Res Review 15:92–96, 1978.

Practices at a mental hospital in Swaziland are unaligned to tribal-traditional power bases and their accompanying mystical traditional legitimations; yet they are required to rehabilitate patients who come from tribal-traditional settings. Psychiatric personnel should couch their therapeutic efforts in formats that are culturally meaningful and appropriate to their patients' prior experiences and expectations.

1109. Paredes A: Social control of drinking among the Aztec Indians of Mesoamerica. J Stud Alcohol 36:1139–53, 1975.

In the Aztec culture of pre-Columbian Mexico, the rules for the use of alcoholic beverages were clearly defined and strictly enforced. Drinking was permitted only on religious occasions and the amount drunk was restricted.

1110. Paredes A, Hepburn MJ: The split brain and the culture-and-cognition paradox. Current Anthropology 17:121–27, 1976.

There are discrete modes of thought that have at best only indirect and weak connections with language. An effort must be made to develop a vocabulary for discussing the visual, "nonverbal" modes of thought characteristic of the right hemisphere, difficult and paradoxical-seeming as that effort may be.

1111. Parikh B: Development of moral judgement and its relation to family environmental factors in Indian and American families. Child Development 51:1030–39, 1980.

For both Indian and American children, twelve and thirteen year olds score at a lower level in their development of moral judgment than older children do. When a child from either culture is

fifteen to sixteen years old, the chances of his being at the conventional stage of morality are significantly greater when his parents use high as opposed to low encouragement.

1112. Parin P: The microscope of comparative psychoanalysis and the macrosociety. J Psychol Anthropology 1:141–64, 1978.

Every culture establishes a self-perpetuating model through its child-rearing methods that can only be altered by outside forces, as is shown in the anal fixations and ego components of the Dogon and Anyi of West Africa and of lower-middle-class Swiss.

1113. Parin P, Parin-Matthey G: The Swiss and southern German lower-middle class: an ethno-psychoanalytic study. J Psychol Anthropology 1:101–19, 1978.

The ethnopsychoanalytical method is applied to Swiss and German lower-middle-class patients who underwent psychoanalytical treatment in Switzerland during the fifties and sixties. The method serves to define the relationships among a small number of typical ego functions and to reconstruct their psychogenesis.

1114. Parin P, Morgenthaler F, Parin-Matthey G: Fear Thy Neighbor As Thyself: Psychoanalysis and Society Among the Anyi of West Africa. Chicago, U. of Chicago Press, 1980.

Data gathered from psychoanalytically based interviews indicate that the Anyi are distrustful of each other and that they have an obsessive concern with discharge of feces (daily enemas are an important health rite). Anyi mothers almost never play with, praise, scold, or talk to a child until it is about nine months old; this behavior may stem from a high infant-mortality rate, i.e., by being detached from an infant the mother will be relatively unaffected if it dies.

1115. Paris J: The symbolic return: psychodynamic aspects of immigration and exile. J Amer Acad Psychoanalysis 6:51–58, 1978.

The need for continued rapprochement between young adults and their parents and the conflicts arising from this need are a reflection of the still insecure identity formation of young adults.

1116. Parker G, Lipscombe P: Parental characteristics of Jews and Greeks in Australia. Australian New Zealand J Psychiatry 13:225–29, 1979.

In the assessment of parental characteristics, Jewish subjects saw their mothers as being less caring than did those in the non-Jewish control group, while the Greek subjects viewed both parents as being more protective. Further investigation found that the parents were overprotective of their daughters only and that this characteristic is resistant to acculturation and may be selectively disadvantageous to the Greek girls.

1117. Parker S: The precultural basis of the incest taboo. Amer Anthropologist 78:285–305, 1976.

Incest avoidance is widespread among the vertebrata. For humans, it and its later elaboration into a cultural taboo serve to motivate exploration of and attachment to a wider social nexus than the family.

1118. Parker S, Parker H: The myth of male superiority. Amer Anthropologist 81:289–309, 1979.

The male's agonistic propensities are becoming irrelevant, and females no longer need be confined to reproductive and domestic activities. Women will increasingly enter traditionally "masculine" occupations, and men will enter "feminine" ones.

1119. Parr L: Alcohol in Colonial Africa. Helsinki, Finnish Foundation for Alcohol Studies, 1975.

The great evils of Colonial Africa—the slave trade and liquor traffic—became close partners when colonials used alcohol as payment for slaves.

1120. Parres R: The first American psychiatrists. Psychiatric Annals 10(6):25–35, 1980.

The Nahuas of pre-Columbian Mexico could be considered the first American psychiatrists. The elucidative element of their psychotherapy included psychological analysis leading to the removal of symptoms by discovering their causes.

1121. Pataki-Schweizer KJ: Transcultural coping: psychiatric aspects in squatter settlements. Papua New Guinea Medical Journal 21:270–75, 1978.

While the squatter settlement in Papua New Guinea is a community surviving under pressure, there is a pervasive indifference and lack of enthusiasm among some of the younger, childless couples and single males, reminiscent of incipient clinical depression. Thus, the effects of extensive change on the populace deserve closer monitoring.

1122. Pattison EM: The fatal myth of death in the family. Amer J Psychiatry 133:674–78, 1976.

The observed pathogenic effects on a child of a parent's death result from the family's culture-bound inability to integrate death into the process of living. Dealing with death by the avoidance mechanisms of myth and family mystification is pathogenic as illustrated by a case report.

1123. Pattison EM: Psychosocial interpretations of exorcism. J Operational Psychiatry 8(2):5–21, 1977.

Widespread belief in exorcism and demonology occurs only when there is social aggression and loss of social integration. Modern demonology is part of the social repudiation of the scientific determinism of rational man. In terms of symbolic actions, psychoanalytic psychotherapy is also a practice of exorcism. Western psychotherapy is just as much a part of its culture as other healing systems.

1124. Pattison EM, Defrancisco D, Wood P, Frazier H, Crowder J: A psychosocial kinship model for family therapy. Amer J Psychiatry 132:1246–51, 1975.

The basic family system may not be the traditional nuclear family, but the extended psychosocial kinship system of family relatives, neighbors, friends, and associates. A formal theoretical framework and model for family theory encompassing this extended kinship system is presented.

1125. Pattison EM, Llamos R, Hund G: Social network mediation. Psychiatric Annals 9(9):56–67, 1979.

Arousal of anxiety, the modulation of anxiety, and the resolution of anxiety are critically related to the social environment—and expressly to the social unit termed the "personal psychosocial network." Anxiety is generated out of the person's inability to cope with ambient internal or external stress.

1126. Pattison EM, Pattison ML: "Ex gays": religiously mediated change in homosexuals. Amer J Psychiatry 137:1553–62, 1980.

Profound behavioral and intrapsychic change in sexual orientation is possible with religious mediation.

1127. Paul RA: Instinctive aggression in man: the Semai case. J Psychol Anthropology 1:64–79, 1978.

The range of human behavior, especially in cultures with nonviolent ethical rules, is best understood by postulating that one of man's primary instincts is the desire to cause pain and death, and that this desire is a cause of the Oedipus complex. The Semai, a hunting and gathering people of Malaysia, are examined with this premise in mind.

1128. Peach C: Segregation of black immigrants in Britain: spatial pattern and social process. Current Anthropology 19:612–13, 1978.

While only a small part of the West Indians' segregation pattern could be expected from their class structure, there is evidence to suggest that significant parts of the observed segregation levels are due to voluntary self-segregation rather than externally imposed sanctions.

1129. Peacock JL: Muslim Puritans: Reformist Psychology in Southeast Asia. Berkeley, U. of California Press, 1978.

Javanese Muslim reformists experience more depression and less latah than nonreformists and feel guilty and sinful. Singapore Muslim reformists are more apt to hold patrist domestic values and concern themselves more with pleasing father than mother. Traditionally reared, agrarian Malaysians are more reformist and psychologically rationalist than the cosmopolitan, urban reformists of Java and Singapore.

1130. Peal E: "Normal" sex roles: an historical analysis. Family Process 14:389–409, 1975.

Social role performance is an unsatisfactory criterion for identifying pathogenic families.

1131. Pebley AR, Dilgado H, Brineman E: Family sex composition preferences among Guatemalan men and women. J Marriage Family 42:437–47, 1980.

The predominant preference of men and women in rural and semiurban locations in Ladino communities in Guatemala is for equal numbers of sons and daughters. Yet agreement between husbands and wives is low. Motivations for preferring equal numbers of children differ between rural and semiurban areas.

1132. Pedersen PP, Draguns JG, Lonner WJ, Trimble JE: Counseling Across Cultures. Honolulu, U. Press of Hawaii, 1976 (rev. ed. 1981).

Topics include racial and ethnic barriers in counseling; counseling specific groups such as Asian Americans, Chicano college students, Native Americans, and foreign students; behavioral approaches to counseling across cultures; and psychological tests and intercultural counseling.

1133. Peele R, Luisada PV, Lucas MJ, Rudisell D, Taylor D: Asylums revisited. Amer J Psychiatry 134:1077–81, 1977.

Institutionalization and secondary adjustment phenomena still exist in asylums. Institutionalization may be the approach of choice for some patients.

1134. Pellow D: Women in Accra. Algonac, Mich., Reference, 1977.

Women in Accra remain subservient because they lack the fundamental consciousness of liberation to conceive of alternatives to their situation.

1135. Pellow D: Work and autonomy: women in Accra. Amer Ethnologist 5:770–85, 1978.

Autonomy is inoperative in the choices of urban work roles of nonelite Ghanaian women. The association of education and employment and the exclusion of women, traditional notions about "the woman's place" and female occupations, the influence of others, and financial considerations are all influential in the lack of autonomy.

1136. Penk WE, Robinowitz R, Woodward WS, Hess JL: Differences in MMPI scores of black and white compulsive heroin users. J Abnormal Psychology 87(5):505–13, 1978.

MMPI responses by black and white compulsive heroin users refute the assumption of personality trait communality among compulsive heroin users and suggest that ethnicity is an influential subject background characteristic by which subgroups of heroin users might be identified.

1137. Penningroth PE, Penningroth BA: Cross cultural mental health practice in Guam. Social Psychiatry 12:43–48, 1977.

Cultural beliefs about the cause of illness largely determine methods of treatment. For Guamanians, "crazy" behaviors simply happen and are accepted as facts of life. Persons with symptoms of "craziness" are often taken to a native healer for treatment.

1138. Peristiany JG: Mediterranean Family Structures. Cambridge and New York, Cambridge U. Press, 1976.

The differing types of family structures found in most of the circum-Mediterranean countries are described in terms of British social anthropology.

1139. Perlin S (ed): A Handbook for the Study of

Suicide. Oxford and New York, Oxford U. Press, 1975.

Anthropology is concerned with the social elements common to the acts of self-destruction that occur in a community, how these relate to roles, structures, and related development, and resolution of conflicts in that community. Yet these studies do not reveal which particular individuals are potential suicides.

1140. Perlman C, Givelber F: "Women's issues" in couples treatment—the view of the therapist. Psychiatric Opinion 13(1):6–12, 1976.

With the changing status of women, "women's issues" emerge in marriage therapy. A female therapist may experience opportunities and countertransference problems when working with these issues. The work can stir up women therapists' own conflicts and threaten their personal solutions.

1141. Perry JW: Roots of Renewal in Myth and Madness. San Francisco, Jossey-Bass, 1976.

Psychosis is a visionary state that recapitulates the evolution of consciousness in American history. The renewal process of healing attempts to evolve a new level of consciousness in the individual by inducing an identification first with the mythology of social kingship, then with that of messianic democratization. Finally, it reaches a vision of the potential spiritual consciousness for life in today's world society.

1142. Peters G: Psychotherapy in Tamang shamanism. Ethos 6:63–91, 1978.

Tamang (Nepal) culture is male dominated. Most healing rituals are done for women. Shamanistic healing may involve reciting a mantra or a major ritual (puja). A case study describes a woman with symptoms of headache, backache, blurred vision, and apathy who is cured when she speaks with the voice of a spirit, which is then exorcised.

1143. Peters LG: Concepts of mental deficiency among the Tamang of Nepal. Amer J Mental Deficiency 34:352–56, 1980.

Mental retardation is thought by the Tamang to be caused by a curse either on the victim, his father, or his patrilinear ancestors, or by karma, i.e., the effects of deleterious acts performed in former lives. Verbal incompetence is a major factor in the Tamang folk diagnosis of mental retardation. Although retarded persons are treated kindly, their disorder is considered incurable.

1144. Peters LG, Price-Williams D: Towards an experimental analysis of shamanism. Amer Ethnologist 7:397–413, 1980.

Shamanic ecstasy is a specific class of altered states of consciousness involving voluntary control of entrance and duration of trance, posttrance memory, and transic communicative interplay with spectators.

1145. Pfeiffer WM, Schoene W (eds): Psychopathology in Cultural Comparison (in German). Stuttgart, Ferdinand Enke, 1980.

This collection of cultural psychiatric papers covers such areas as epidemiology, psychosomatic disorders, emics and etics, delusions, altered states of consciousness, attitudes toward the mentally ill, epilepsy, mental retardation, aging, culture-bound syndromes, and psychotherapy.

1146. Philbrick JL, Opolot JA: Love style: comparison of African and American attitudes. Psychological Reports 46:286, 1980.

Subjects from an African culture who have been free from the influence of Western notions of romantic love tend to endorse many of the attitudes essential to this phenomenon.

1147. Philippe J, Romain JB: Indisposition in Haiti. Social Science Medicine 13B(2):129–33, 1979.

Indisposition is a Haitian syndrome that falls between psychic and somatic ailments. It is said to be caused by conditions and actions of the blood and by magic.

1148. Phillips RE: Impact of Nazi holocaust on children of survivors. Amer J Psychotherapy 32:370–78, 1978.

Within families of survivors of the holocaust, the child is regarded as the family's savior and is forced to adhere to an orthodox lifestyle. Being so overprotected and burdened, the child becomes fearful of real or imagined dangers, and his own personal development is frustrated.

1149. Phillips S, King S, DuBois L: Spontaneous activities of female versus male newborns. Child Development 49:590–97, 1978.

High-intensity activity increases in the evenings and over an interfeeding period, and low-intensity oral activity increases over days, with both types of activity being independent of sex. Males may be slightly more irritable than females.

1150. Pick AD: Cognition: psychological perspectives. In Handbook of Cross-Cultural Psychology, edited by HC Triandis and WJ Lonner, 3:117–53. Boston, Allyn and Bacon, 1980.

Three culture-related factors potentially relevant for understanding variations in general intelligence are early social and cognitive stimulation, early nutrition, and education. Clear interpretation of apparent cultural differences in general intellectual functioning is virtually impossible because of the culture-specific nature of tests of intelligence and because of the difficulty of ensuring the representativeness of samples of subjects' tests.

1151. Pilowsky I (ed): Cultures in Collision. Adelaide, Australian Natl. Assn. for Mental Health, 1975.

Papers from the 1973 World Federation for Mental Health meeting in Australia are presented. Topics include migration, cognitive development in Aboriginal children, criminal guilt and moral fault in Papua New Guinea, and epidemic hysteria in Malaysia.

1152. Pilowsky I, Spence ND: Ethnicity and illness behavior. Psychological Medicine 7:447–52, 1977.

Relationships observed between ethnicity and illness behavior among Greeks and Anglos are to some extent dependent upon age and sex.

1153. Piotrkowski CS: Work and the Family System. New York, Free Press, 1979.

The travails of working-class and lower-middle-class families are studied naturalistically.

1154. Pitta P, Marcos LR, Alpert M: Language switching as a treatment strategy with bilingual patients. Amer J Psychoanalysis 38:255–58, 1978.

In bilingual patients the dominant language has a richer emotional structure that can capture greater richness of experience but may at the same time inhibit the patient's ability to gain distance and profit from intellectual coping mechanisms. Language switching during the course of therapy with a bilingual patient can be very helpful if used appropriately by a bilingual therapist.

1155. Piuck CL: Child rearing patterns of poverty. Am J Psychotherapy 29:485–502, 1975.

Harsh and repressive child-rearing methods among the chronically poor create a class of socially disabled, emotionally and intellectually stunted individuals. To reverse this trend, the therapist must foster verbal self-expression and

support the individual as he seeks role models other than his parents.

1156. Plemons G: A comparison of MMPI scores of Anglo- and Mexican-American psychiatric patients. J Consulting Clin Psychology 45:149–50, 1977.

Mexican-American psychiatric patients respond differently than Anglo-Americans on the MMPI. Mexican-Americans may experience comparable distress to Anglo-Americans, but they may be less apt to report it.

1157. Pollack D, Shore JH: Validity of the MMPI with Native Americans. Amer J Psychiatry 137:946–50, 1980.

MMPI profiles of American Indian patients from Pacific Northwestern tribes are influenced by culture and result in similar profiles for different diagnostic groups.

1158. Pollnac RB, Jahn G: Culture and memory revisited: an example from Buganda. J Cross-Cultural Psychology 7:73–86, 1976.

Quantitative and qualitative differences in free recall within a specific age-education group suggest that there is interschool variability in some component of the educational process related to memory skills. Years of education must be more carefully defined in cross-cultural studies of cognition.

1159. Polsky RH, Chance MRH: An ethological perspective on social behavior in long stay hospitalized psychiatric patients. J Nerv Ment Disease 167:658–74, 1979.

Research dealing with the behavior of psychiatric patients in ward settings from an ethological perspective indicates that there is individual variability in the amount of social interaction, there are differences in the modes of interaction between individuals who interact relatively frequently as opposed to infrequently, and correlative relationships distinguish high interactions from low interactions.

1160. Polsky R, McGuire MT: An ethological analysis of manic-depressive disorder. J Nerv Ment Disease 167:56–65, 1979.

Ethological techniques used to identify behavioral characteristics of hospitalized manic-depressive patients show distinctive patterns of behavior characteristics of manic and depressed patients. There are also characteristic patterns of behavior for patients who improve as compared to patients who show no improvement.

1161. Ponce DE, Lee V: Intraethnic violence in a Hawaii school: a mental health consultation experience. Amer J Orthopsychiatry 47:451–55, 1977.

Mental health intervention during school crises involving local-born and immigrant Filipino students in an Hawaiian high school has been very helpful in solving the crises and preventing future violence in the school.

1162. Poortinga YH: Basic Problems in Cross-Cultural Psychology. Amsterdam, Swets and Zeitlinger, 1977.

Problem areas in cross-cultural psychology include the semantic differential technique, the concept of psychological differentiation, and lack of cultural knowledge by psychologists.

1163. Popham RE: Psychocultural barriers to successful alcoholism therapy in an American Indian patient: the relevance of Hallowell's analysis. J Stud Alcohol 40:656–76, 1979.

The patterns of emotional restraint described by A. I. Hallowell as characteristic of northeastern Indians are consistent with the response of the Algonquin Indian women during clinical interview.

1164. Press I: Urban folk medicine. Amer Anthropologist 80:71–84, 1978.

Folk illness and cure in cities minimize the trauma of acculturation. Under severe competition from modern medical and welfare systems, folk illness will decline in importance, but folk medicine may shift toward adjunct functions of health.

1165. Price J, Karim I: An evaluation of psychiatric after-care in a developing country (Fiji). Brit J Psychiatry 129:155–57, 1976.

Very little expertise is available in Fiji for the development of an effective community mental health program.

1166. Price J, Karim I: Matiruku, a Fijian madness: an initial assessment. Brit J Psychiatry 133:228–30, 1978.

Matiruku is a recurrent mental illness in Fiji corresponding to hypomania with special features, e.g., short duration, frequent recurrence, and an intensification of symptoms in the morning.

1167. Price-Williams DR: Anthropological approaches to cognition and their relevance to psychology. In Handbook of Cross-Cultural Psy-

chology, edited by HC Triandis and W Lonner, 3:155–84. Boston, Allyn and Bacon, 1980.

There is a tendency in anthropology to treat cognition more as a matter of product than process and to be more group and institutionally oriented than individually oriented. Cognitive psychologists tend to work on the basis of a theory, and their findings have reference to a general theory of cognition. Cognitive anthropologists have no theory of mind, no general theory of cognition; their concern is how different people organize their cultures.

1168. Priest RG: The homeless person and psychiatric services: an Edinburgh survey. Brit J Psychiatry 128:128–36, 1976.

Those persons presenting to psychiatric services from common lodging houses in Edinburgh are a highly selected group, quite unrepresentative of homeless single persons in general.

1169. Prince R: Some Yoruba views of the causes and modes of treatment of anti-social behavior. African J Psychiatry 1,2:133–37, 1975.

The Yoruba hold contradictory beliefs about antisocial behavior related to contradictions between free will and determinism and between individual responsibility and lack of it. One view holds that untreatable antisocial behavior results from the often unwitting choice of a person's double in the spirit world to be a thief or to engage in antisocial behavior. A second view holds that a curse or sorcery is etiological and may lead to amok behavior including multiple murders or suicide. Treatment consists of ritual cleansing and of sacrifices to the victim's spiritual double.

1170. Prince R: Symbols and psychotherapy: example of Yoruba sacrificial ritual. J Amer Acad Psychoanalysis 3:321–38, 1975.

Symbolism has much more to do with conscious wishes than with unconscious conflicts. In the more detailed example of Yoruba sacrifice, the verbal, symbolic, and motor activities all represent expressions of consciously desired ends in varying degrees of concreteness.

1171. Prince R: Variations in psychotherapeutic procedures. In Handbook of Cross-Cultural Psychology, edited by HC Triandis and JG Draguns, 6:291–349. Boston, Allyn and Bacon, 1980.

Examination of the relationship between psychoanalysis and other psychotherapeutic techniques suggests that psychoanalysis is a unique and probably superior system for the understanding of psychopathology. As a form of therapy, however, there are severe limitations on its applicability and, indeed, a lack of convincing evidence for its superior therapeutic power where it can be applied. Altered states of consciousness, mystical states, dreams, meditation, and shamanism are also discussed.

1172. Pritchard DA, Rosenblatt A: Racial bias in the MMPI: a methodological review. J Consulting Clin Psychology 48:263–67, 1980.

Testing the accuracy of predictions or inferences made within racial subgroups on the basis of the MMPI is the most adequate method of examining racial bias in the MMPI, since it provides clear and unequivocal evidence of test bias whenever such bias actually exists.

1173. Proskauer S: Oedipal equivalents in a clan culture: reflections on Navajo ways. Psychiatry 43:43–50, 1980.

Key determinants of the way in which oedipal elements manifest themselves in various cultures include matrilineality versus patrilineality and unclear family structure versus clan-extended family structures.

1174. Puthenkalam FJ: Marriage and Family in Kerala. New Dehli, Printaid, 1977.

Social and economic stresses have led to the breakdown of the major matrilineal joint family, as well as to changes in such ceremonies as tali-tying and sambandham.

1175. Rabinowitz S: The Ulpan as a model for effective integration of new immigrants: a psychological overview of an Israeli absorption center. Israel Ann Psychiatry 15:397–402, 1977.

Psychological adjustment of new immigrants is by no means a haphazard sequence of events but a clear and often difficult process of change and acculturation.

1176. Rabkin JG: Ethnic density and psychiatric hospitalization: hazards of minority status. Amer J Psychiatry 136:1562–66, 1979.

In New York City the smaller the ethnic group, the higher its psychiatric hospitalization rate in comparison to both the rate of other residents in the same area and that of members of the same ethnic group living in areas where they constitute a numerical majority. The effect of ethnic density on risk of psychiatric hospitalization cannot be accounted for by the differences in poverty, family cohesiveness, or population mobility.

1177. Rabkin LY: Superego processes in a collective study: the Israeli kibbutz. Intl J Social Psychiatry 21:79–86, 1975.

In a collective society such as the Israeli kibbutz, there exists a superego based on internalized values rather than introjected specific figures—a collective superego. The result is a shame-oriented, as opposed to a guilt-oriented, conscience, with resulting emphasis on the need for the presence of others as controlling forces.

1178. Racy J: Somatization in Saudi women: a therapeutic challenge. Brit J Psychiatry 137:212–16, 1980.

In Saudi women somatic complaints express emotional problems that have no other outlets. The women are passive, and for therapy to succeed an alliance with a male relative is necessary. Measures to combat passivity can be of great benefit.

1179. Rahe RH, Looney JG, Ward HW, Tung TM, Liu WT: Psychiatric consultation in a Vietnamese refugee camp. Amer J Psychiatry 135:185–90, 1978.

Psychiatric consultation in a Vietnamese refugee camp can help with the adaptation of refugees to the camp setting. A psychiatric crisis clinic and a mental health survey of a random sample of refugees may give an understanding to the camp organizers about the refugees' response to camp experience.

1180. Ramon S, Shanin T, Stimpel J: The peasant connection: social background and mental health of migrant workers in Western Europe. Mental Health Society 4:270–90, 1977.

In Western Europe rates of mental illness among migrants are lower than would be predicted on the basis of the severity of the stress they face. Coming mainly from peasant origins and perceiving themselves as peasants-in-town are central aspects in understanding their capacity to cope with the stress due to migration.

1181. Rao AV: Some aspects of psychiatry in India. Transcult Psych Res Review 15:7–27, 1978.

Syndromes that occur particularly in India include spirit possession, sexual neurosis (ascetic syndrome and Indian Dhat syndrome), obsessional neurosis (suchi-bai), and malignant anxiety. Depression is characterized by somatic symptoms and by a rarity of depressed mood and of guilt feelings. Psychotherapists often refer to stories from epics such as Ramayana and Mahabharata in explanations to their patients.

1182. Rao AV: Geropsychiatry in Indian culture. Canadian J Psychiatry 24:431–36, 1979.

Geriatric psychiatry will be increasingly important in years to come as the care of the elderly becomes a health problem in India. Improved health care promises longevity, but social and economic conditions like poverty, breakup of the joint family system, and poor services pose a psychiatric threat to the aged in India.

1183. Rao AV, Nammalvar N: The course and outcome in depressive illness: a follow-up study of 122 cases in Madurai, India. Brit J Psychiatry 130:392–96, 1977.

In South India affective disorders do not carry a uniformly favorable prognosis. The occurrence of chronic symptoms in the depressives is likely to be underestimated, but these chronic symptoms do not preclude the diagnosis of endogenous depression.

1184. Rappaport H: The tenacity of folk psychotherapy: a functional interpretation. Social Psychiatry 12:127–32, 1977.

Prescientific psychotherapy in Tanzania is not simply a comfortable habit but represents a dynamic approach to psychosocial disorders that must be considered in conjunction with Western practices in future mental health planning.

1185. Rappaport H, Dent PL: An analysis of contemporary East African folk psychotherapy. Brit J Med Psychology 52:49–54, 1979.

Patients with emotional problems make use of both folk and Western therapists. A clear conceptual distinction between the two services is made by the patients.

1186. Raskin A, Crook TH, Herman KD: Psychiatric history and symptoms differences in black and white depressed inpatients. J Consulting Clin Psychology 43:73–80, 1975.

Blacks have a greater tendency toward negativism and the introjection of anger than whites. Depressed black males indicate that they are more likely to strike back, either verbally or physically, when they feel their rights are being violated than are their white counterparts.

1187. Reed J: From Private Vice to Public Virtue. New York, Basic Books, 1978.

The history of the birth control movement in American society from 1830 to the present is described.

1188. Regev E, Beit-Hallahmi B, Sharabany R: Affective expression in kibbutz-communal, kibbutz-familial, and city-raised children in Israel. Child Development 51:232–37, 1980.

Kibbutz-communal children, to a greater degree than kibbutz-familial and city-raised children, avoid the expression of both positive and negative feelings when dealing with significant others.

1189. Reich W: The case of General Grigorenko: a psychiatric reexamination of a Soviet dissident. Psychiatry 43:303–23, 1980.

A psychiatric reexamination of General Grigorenko of Russia by American psychiatrists indicates that he did not suffer from a diagnosable mental illness. Soviet description of Grigorenko's mental condition was skewed. The Soviets characterized perseverance as obsessions, rationality as delusions, and committed devotion as psychotic recklessness.

1190. Reichel-Dolmatoff G: The Shaman and the Jaguar. Philadelphia, Pa., Temple U. Press, 1975.

The use of hallucinogenic drugs such as ayahuasca and yaje is interwoven with religious belief and shamanism among the Tukamo and other tribes in Colombia, Peru, and Ecuador.

1191. Reid FT: Space, territory, and psychiatry. Mental Health Society 3:77–91, 1976.

Space and territory are the hidden dimensions of human and other animal life. Mastering the unwritten rules of space and territory, which differ with individual cultures in relation to the behavioral aberrations possibly resulting from the disrupted territoriality of modern urban life, is important.

1192. Reid J: A time to live, a time to grieve: patterns and processes of mourning among the Yolngu of Australia. Culture Medicine Psychiatry 3:319–46, 1979.

The elaborate and extended mortuary rites ("Murngin") of the people of Northeastern Arnhem Land, Australia, have several characteristics that promote and structure the mourning process and facilitate the full reintegration of the bereaved into the social life of the community.

1193. Reiser MF: Psychosomatic medicine: a meeting ground for oriental and occidental medical theory and practice. Psychotherapy Psychosomatics 31:315–23, 1979.

Psychosomatic medicine is a common meeting ground for East-West medical theory and practice. Eastern physicians can more easily accept the importance of spiritual relationships. Advances in neurobiology over the past two decades implicate the central nervous system mechanisms in the pathogenesis of medical illness. Central nervous system mechanisms linking the psychosocial and physiologic realms are vital to the maintenance of health.

1194. Reiss D, Costell R: The multiple family group as a small society: family regulation of interaction with nonmembers. Amer J Psychiatry 134:21–24, 1977.

In family groups, changes in either parents' or the adolescents' group participation levels are quickly matched by comparable changes in the other generation, suggesting a continuously operating family-control mechanism governing participation of members in interaction with nonmembers.

1195. Reminick RA: The symbolic significance of ceremonial defloration among the Amhara of Ethiopia. Amer Ethnologist 3:751–63, 1976.

The principles of the Amhara social order and world view, as well as the oppositions of masculinity and femininity contained within them, are dramatically reflected in ceremonial defloration. This symbolic pattern of behavior appears well suited to the maintenance of traditional Amhara peasant life because the relationships conceived between honor and virginity, on the one hand, and land and legitimate access to it, on the other, are the most important attributes of such peasant social structures.

1196. Remschmidt H: Mental health services for children and adolescents in the European region. Intl J Mental Health 7:65–74, 1978.

If most European countries could gain some cooperation between their education officials and social welfare departments, they would diminish costs and increase the effectiveness of the work of all concerned.

1197. Renik O: Some observations on "sisterhood" in the feminist movement. Bull Menninger Clinic 39:345–56, 1975.

"Sisterhood" is not only a means of gaining strength against sexism but is also an end in itself. Female chauvinism operates at the expense of real sisterhood.

1198. Reschly DJ: WISC-R factor structures among anglos, blacks, chicanos, and native-American Papagos. J Consult Clinical Psychology 46:417–22, 1978.

The use of the Full Scale IQ as an index of general intelligence appears to be appropriate for all groups, as is the Verbal-Performance scale distinction.

1199. Reynolds DK: Naikan therapy—an experimental view. Intl J Social Psychiatry 23:252–63, 1977.

Naikan therapy is a form of directed meditation practiced in Japan that aims at reconstructing the client's view of his past in order to reshape his attitudes and behaviors in the present.

1200. Reynolds DK: The Quiet Therapies. Honolulu, U. Press of Hawaii, 1980.

Japanese psychotherapy (Morita, Naikan, Shadan, Seiza, Zen) teaches ways to accept the discomforts of life. Behaviors, not feelings, are determinative of fulfillment. Understanding the dynamics of symptoms is irrelevant.

1201. Reynolds DK, Farberow N: Endangered Hope: Experiences in Psychiatric Aftercare Facilities. Berkeley, U. of California Press, 1977.

By posing as a patient, an anthropologist entered four psychiatric aftercare settings to define their supportive and destructive elements.

1202. Reynolds FE, Waugh EH (eds): Religious Encounters with Death: Insights from the History and Anthropology of Religions. University Park, Pennsylvania State U. Press, 1977.

The meanings of death in various religions and cultures are discussed.

1203. Rhoades ER, Marshall M, Attneave C, Echohawk M, Bjork J, Beiser M: Impact of mental disorders upon elderly American Indians as reflected in visits to ambulatory care facilities. J Amer Geriatric Society 23:33–39, 1980.

Data from the Indian Health Service show that in comparison with younger age groups, elderly Indians utilize the mental health ambulatory care less, with rates of one visit for every ten persons in the 0–44 age group, one for every five persons in the 45–54 age group, and only one visit for every twenty-five persons in the 65 + age group. Most visits by the older Indians are for "social" problems rather than "mental" disorders. Following the treatment rates of the younger groups may yield information helpful in designing social and health programs for elderly Indians.

1204. Rich GW: The domestic cycle in modern Iceland. J Marriage Family 40:173–83, 1978.

Traditional Icelandic patterns of domestic organization have not changed significantly with industrialization and economic growth. The majority of Icelanders go through a transitional phase after marriage, during which they establish an engaged family in the context of an extended family household. The association of engagement with procreational rights accounts for a large portion of Iceland's traditionally high premarital birth rate.

1205. Rieber RW (ed): Applied Psycholinguistics and Mental Health. New York, Plenum, 1980.

Linguistics is important for psychiatry in such areas as schizophrenic language (as documented in American and Russian studies) and communication with children, adolescents, and bilingual patients.

1206. Riley JN: Western medicine's attempt to become more scientific: examples from the United States and Thailand. Social Science Medicine 11:549–60, 1977.

As compelling and productive as the enterprise of science has been for modern Western medicine, the commitment to science has not produced an altogether consistent trend in the historical struggle of acculturation. The costs of attempting to make medicine extremely scientific can have negative effects on health as well as positive ones.

1207. Riley MW (ed): Aging From Birth to Death. Boulder, Colo., Westview, 1979.

Life-span developmental psychology is linked with social factors that affect and are affected by the aging process.

1208. Ritchie K: The patient's primary group. Brit J Psychiatry 132:74–86, 1978.

Patients spend the same amount of time as normals with their primary group, but proportionately more of that time is affectively unpleasant. They have fewer good friends and fewer contacts with persons outside the household.

1209. Ritter PL: Social organization, incest, and fertility in a Kosraen village. Amer Ethnologist 7(4):759–73, 1980.

An examination of Yewan (Kosrae Island) social organization in light of past historical and demographic events shows that fertility reduction can be understood as resulting from the bilateral extension of the incest taboo during a past period of depopulation and the rapid growth of the current population from a few individuals. There is a complex interrelationship between population and social organization, and an understanding of this relationship is needed to interpret aggregate demographic data in the context of the history and social system of the people involved.

1210. Rizzuto AM: The Birth of the Living God: A Psychoanalytic Study. Chicago, U. of Chicago Press, 1979.

God is an object representation of a special type. The process of creating and finding god never ceases in the course of human life.

1211. Robarchek CA: Frustration, aggression, and the nonviolent Semai. Amer Ethnologist 4(4):762–79, 1977.

Emotional behavior can be viewed as the product of the complex interaction of hierarchically organized systems with circular rather than linear causality. This model can be employed to understand better the genesis of and the relationships between the subjectively perceived emotions of fear and anger and their behavioral concomitants in a specific ethnographic context.

1212. Roberts A, Mosley KY, Chamberlain MW: Age differences in racial self-identity of young black girls. Psychological Reports 37:1263–66, 1975.

Racial self-identity is formulated during the preschool years for most black children, and for most it is more firmly established by the beginning school years.

1213. Robertson A, Cochrane R: Deviance and cultural change. Intl J Social Psychiatry 22:79–85, 1976.

During the past decade there has been a dramatic increase in the incidence of all forms of deviant behavior. More important is the fact that within this overall increase there has been a relatively greater increase in deviance among the young than among the old.

1214. Robins LN, West PA, Hernaic BL: Arrests and delinquency in two generations: a study of black urban families and their children. J Psychol Psychiat Allied Disciplines 16:125–40, 1975.

Juvenile records of parents and their children show similar rates and types of offenses. Parental arrest histories are powerful predictors of their children's delinquency.

1215. Rochester S, Martin JR: Crazy Talk: A Study of the Discourse of Schizophrenic Speakers. New York, Plenum, 1979.

The cognition and language of schizophrenics make deviations in "crazy" discourse more understandable. Two important linguistic methods of study are cohesion analysis and the network system of reference and retrieval categories.

1216. Rock PH: Some practical problems in providing a psychiatric service for immigrants. Mental Health Society 4:144–51, 1977.

Immigrant minority groups in a multicultural society create certain problems for psychiatric-service providers because of differences in language and in treatment expectations. Some of the problems encountered by a clinical team that has been established at an English psychiatric hospital for Asian patients are discussed.

1217. Rohner RP: They Love Me, They Love Me Not: A Worldwide Study of the Effects of Parental Acceptance and Rejection. New Haven, Conn., Human Relations Area Files, 1975.

There is a phylogenetic proclivity to form warm affective attachments at critical periods. Parental rejection is associated with a cluster of traits for both children and for adults who were rejected as children.

1218. Rohrbaugh J: Women: Psychology's Puzzle. New York, Basic Books, 1979.

Mental health professionals should consider women's own opinions and experiences especially in such areas as sexuality, birth control, pregnancy, rape, the battered woman, and participation in sports. Hysteria may be a form of superfemininity.

1219. Rohrl VJ: Culture, cognition, and intellect: towards a cross-cultural view of "intelligence." J Psychol Anthropology 2:337–64, 1979.

Intelligence is affected by such cultural factors as language, values, cognitive modes, environment, abstraction, and space conceptualization. By systematizing new knowledge gained about these factors, a new culturally pluralistic model of learning can be applied in the classroom.

1220. Rohrl V: A trace on Freud's "mystic writing-pad"? J Psychol Anthropology 2:465–78, 1979.

The structure of the mind as presented by Freud is comparable to the traditional Jewish structuring of the soul and shows the influence of Jewish tradition on the mind and works of Freud.

1221. Rohrlich-Leavitt R (ed): Women Cross-Culturally. Chicago, Aldine, 1975.

Woman's biologically invariant role as reproducer is less important than her social and productive activities. Feminism is revolutionary.

1222. Rolle A: The Italian Americans. New York, Free Press, 1980.

The experience of immigration from Italy to the United States can be better understood by using psychiatric and psychoanalytic insights. The first phase involved cultural shock, and survival was the immigrants' central concern. Then came an emerging self-consciousness. Still later came more self-affirmation. Not until the second and third generations could most of the immigrants afford to become disillusioned. This disguised form of repression helped them to move out across America and determined the places they would live in and the kinds of lives they would lead.

1223. Roman PM, Gebert PJ: Alcohol abuse in the U.S. and the U.S.S.R.: divergence and convergence in policy and ideology. Social Psychiatry 14:207–16, 1979.

There are several forces that will likely increase the similarity between the United States and the Soviet Union in the definition and management of alcohol abuse and alcoholism. Participation of Soviet physicians in international bodies such as the W.H.O. is likely a support for institutionalization of the medical model and might serve to reduce some of the punitive practices that are currently evident.

1224. Roosens E: Des Fous dans la Ville? Paris, Presses Universitaires de France, 1979.

Mental patients in Gheel, Belgium, often live with lower-class foster families. Most are indistinguishable from other citizens in public life.

1225. Rosen DH, Voorhees-Rosen D: The Shetland Islands: the effects of social and ecological change on mental health. Culture Medicine Psychiatry 2:41–67, 1978.

A longitudinal, epidemiological study is necessary to examine the impact that industrialization and urbanization have on the mental health and social order of the people living not only on the Shetland Islands, but in other regions as well.

1226. Rosen S: Sibling and in-law relationships in Hong Kong: the emergent role of Chinese wives. J Marriage Family 40:621–28, 1978.

Role reorganization within the nuclear family, and specifically the changing role of Chinese wives, has created a new family structure that reinforces rather than rejects traditional norms of shared residence and reciprocal aid among kin. Life-cycle variation, inclusion of uxorial relatives, emergence of "extended family households" encompassing several separate residences, and strengthening of intergenerational ties along with attitudinal changes have contributed to the new style of extended family interaction.

1227. Rosenbaum MT: Gender-specific problems in the treatment of young women. Amer J Psychoanalysis 37:215–21, 1977.

In the changing roles facing young women there are few guidelines, much open space, much ambiguity, and few positive role models. Women tend to be more aware of the negatives to which they do not aspire rather than choosing and working toward some positive goal. Therapists should explore options with female patients, look for new combinations of old ingredients, and allow and encourage the complexities involved in becoming mature women and freely accepting, expecting, and respecting a multitude of different routes to autonomous adulthood.

1228. Rosenberg ML: Patients: The Experience of Illness. Philadelphia, Pa., Saunders, 1980.

A physician describes the differing responses to medical illness of six patients from their perspectives.

1229. Rosenblatt PC, Walsh P, Jackson DA: Grief and Mourning in Cross-Cultural Perspective. New Haven, Conn., HRAF, 1976.

Results of a holocultural study of seventy-eight cultures indicate that grief and mourning are universal responses to bereavement. Grief in American culture may be prolonged or complicated by a relative lack of institutionalized practices that support bereaved persons.

1230. Roskies E: Sex, culture and illness—an overview. Social Science Medicine 12(3B):139–41, 1978.

In spite of its importance and complexity, the problem of sex differences in illness has until recently aroused little interest in the scientific community. Even the few researchers who have sought to explore the issues have been hampered by the lack of communication between the biological and social sciences.

1231. Ross JK: Social borders: definitions of diversity. Current Anthropology 16:53–72, 1975.

The diversity of ways to distinguish individuals

from one another is the result of a universal human activity, the definition of social borders. The past successes of anthropology in seeing through diversity to structural universality suggest that the definition of social borders is not only a problem anthropology needs to face, but one it is particularly well equipped to resolve.

1232. Ross MH, Weisner TS: The rural-urban migrant network in Kenya: some general implications. Amer Ethnologist 4:359–75, 1977.

Rural-urban bonds in Kenya are characterized by high levels of two-way interaction between the city and the countryside. Social behavior must be conceptualized as taking place in two locations within a single social field.

1233. Rotenberg M, Nachshon I: Impulsiveness and aggression among Israeli delinquents. Brit J Social Clinical Psychology 18:59–63, 1979.

Israeli delinquents are impulsive in the sense of hastiness, and impatient rather than aggressive against others.

1234. Rowlands R: The psychopathology of Haitian females. Intl J Social Psychiatry 25:217–23, 1979.

Valuable ethnopsychological and sociopsychological studies of the Haitian population in the future will be those that are limited to either the African-oriented segment of the society or to the Western-oriented segment.

1235. Roy M: Bengali Women. Chicago, U. of Chicago Press, 1976.

Bengali women experience the dichotomies of eroticism, romantic expectation, unrequited love, and resigned functionality.

1236. Roy M (ed): Battered Women. New York, Van Nostrand Reinhold, 1977.

The historical, sociological, psychological, and legal aspects of domestic violence are reviewed.

1237. Rozynko V, Ferguson LC: Admission characteristics of Indian and white alcoholic patients in a rural mental hospital. Intl J Addictions 13:591–604, 1978.

Indian-white patient differences may not be the result of excessive drinking but instead may be the result of relative economic status of the two populations in American society. Indian-white patient differences in drinking patterns, arrest record, and age, however, show configurations not accounted for by population differences alone. There is need for the education of police and Native Americans in the area concerning treatment resources available to Native-American problem drinkers.

1238. Rubin JC, Jones J: Falling-out: a clinical study. Social Science Medicine 13B(2):117–27, 1979.

The problems of a patient with "falling-out" overlapped two health-care systems (orthodox and traditional), and he improved because of appropriate interaction between the two.

1239. Rubin V, Comitas L: Ganja in Jamaica. The Hague, Mouton, 1975.

Study of thirty ganja (cannabis) smokers and thirty controls, all of whom are working-class native men, reveals no significant differences. There is little correlation between ganja use and crime. The incidence of alcoholism is low among ganja smokers.

1240. Rubins JL: The relationship between the individual, the culture, and psychopathology. Amer J Psychoanalysis 35:231–49, 1975.

Individual development and personality, extending along a continuum from the healthy or normal to the definitely psychopathological, can be initiated, exacerbated, or modified by sociocultural influences and changes. But rarely, if ever, can mental and emotional illness be created by sociocultural factors alone, especially by simply labeling it abnormal.

1241. Rubinstein D: Beyond the cultural barriers: observations on emotional disorders among Cuban immigrants. Intl J Mental Health 5:69–79, 1976.

Therapists who are versed in the various cultural expressions of Cuban immigrants are able to understand the nature and meanings of apparently dissimilar syndromes.

1242. Rueveni U: Network intervention with a family in crisis. Family Process 14:193–203, 1975.

Network intervention can provide the opportunity for a troubled family to mobilize its own resources by assembling family members, relatives, friends, and neighbors to serve as a network of concerned and active people.

1243. Ruffin JE: The relevance of racism to the goals of psychotherapy. Perspectives Psychiatric Care 14:160–64, 1976.

The psychosocial phenomenon of racism demands serious study by all institutions if its insidious and pervasive effects are to be eliminated.

The therapist's use of his or her position of power to influence positive, nonracist attitudes is crucial to therapeutic conduct, whether or not he or she is aware of it.

1244. Ruhland D, Feld S: The development of achievement motivation in black and white children. Child Development 48:1362–68, 1977.

Although similar in their respective levels of autonomous achievement motivation, black children display lower levels of social comparison achievement motivation than white children display.

1245. Ruiz EJ: Influence of bilingualism and communication in groups. Intl J Group Psychotherapy 25:391–95, 1975.

In bilingual groups, feelings and thought processes that are basic to the development of the personality are strongly tied into the first language learned by the group members.

1246. Ruiz P: Spiritism, mental health, and the Puerto Ricans. Transcult Pysch Res Review 16:28–43, 1979.

Puerto Rican immigrants to the United States believe in and practice spiritism, a religious system that contains beliefs in reincarnation, contact with spirits, the pathological influence of some spirits, and healing mediums. An understanding of spiritism is a necessity for mental health practitioners who treat Puerto Ricans.

1247. Ruiz P, Langrod J: Psychiatry and folk healing: a dichotomy? Amer J Psychiatry 133:95–97, 1976.

The experience of a Bronx mental health center with folk healers reveals a Hispanic belief system that helps its members to cope with distress. Folk healers can be valuable members of the mental health team.

1248. Ruiz P, Langrod J: The role of folk healers in community mental health services. Comm Ment Health Journal 12:392–98, 1976.

If people are uncertain about their chances of achieving socially valued goals, they are likely to seek and accept alternative paths to these goals, magic included.

1249. Rumbaut R: John of God: His Place in the History of Psychiatry and Medicine. Miami, Ediciones Universal, 1978.

Juan Duarte founded a religious order that cared for the mentally ill.

1250. Rumbaut RD, Rumbaut RG: The family in

exile: Cuban expatriates in the United States. Amer J Psychiatry 133:395–99, 1976.

The ordeal of expatriation for Cuban exiles has meant anguish, uprootedness, challenge, and accomplishment. The success of their struggle, due to their high educational and occupational levels, positive ethnic communities, and organized reception by the United States, shows that the influx of refugees could be a creative and enriching process for both the host country and the individual refugee.

1251. Runions JE: The mystic experience: a psychiatric reflection. Canadian J Psychiatry 24:147–51, 1979.

Mystical experiences may occur in the contexts of epilepsy, toxicity, organic brain syndromes, major psychosis, and hysterical dissociative states as well as in apparently normal persons. There are two fallacies that await the unwary psychiatrist: the fallacy of reductionalism, which defines the mystical experience in pathological terms only; and the fallacy of speculations without adequate philosophical or theological tools.

1252. Russell G: The father role and its relation to masculinity, femininity, and androgyny. Child Development 49:1174–81.

Androgynous fathers carry out more childcare tasks and interact more with their children than masculine fathers do. Fathers high on femininity participate more than fathers low on femininity.

1253. Rutter M: Changing Youth in a Changing Society. Cambridge, Mass., Harvard U. Press, 1980.

Patterns of adolescent development and disorder such as depression, delinquency, drug abuse, sexual activity, and stress events are described.

1254. Rutter M, Yule B, Morton J, Bagley C: Children of West Indian immigrants: home circumstances and family patterns. J Child Psychol Psychiat 16:105–23, 1975.

West Indian immigrant families have many more children than and differ somewhat in their patterns of childrearing from nonimmigrants. Parents of immigrant families living in England are more likely to hold semiskilled or unskilled manual jobs and to live in poor-quality, overcrowded housing.

1255. Rwegellera GGC: Psychiatric morbidity among West Africans and West Indians living in London. Psychological Medicine 7:317–29, 1977.

Migrant populations have higher rates of psychiatric morbidity than nonmigrants.

1256. Rwegellera GGC: Suicide rates in Lusaka, Zambia: preliminary observations. Psychological Medicine 8:423–32, 1978.

Differences in suicide rates between African and European residents are not statistically significant. There is no definite seasonal variation in suicide rate. Hanging is by far the most commonly used method of suicide in Africa. Domestic quarrels, mental illness, and physical disease are some of the important precipitating factors of suicide in Lusaka.

1257. Rwegellera GGC: Differential use of psychiatric services by West Indians, West Africans and English in London. Brit J Psychiatry 137:428–32, 1980.

Migrant and nonmigrant patients differ in their use of psychiatric agencies in London. Migrant patients refer themselves or are referred by agencies. More migrant than nonmigrant patients show disturbed behavior prior to psychiatric contact. There is no association between length of stay in England prior to developing mental illness and disturbed behavior.

1258. Sabatier E: Astride the Equator. Melbourne, Oxford U. Press, 1977.

A summary of the history and culture of the Gilbert Islands includes data on spirit possession and exorcism.

1259. Sabeau-Jouannet L: Essai de psychologie transculturelle appliquee au groupe ethnique Merina. Supplement aux Confrontations Psychiatriques 14:5–54, 1976.

The Merina ethnic group are a type of ruling "caste" of a section of Malagasy. The group members differ from the lower classes by an extremely reserved behavior, by marked suppression of expressive affects, by obedience to ancestors, and by respect for numerous taboos. Using Kardiner's theories it is possible to demonstrate how the Merina's secondary institutions derive from basic personality traits. Some secondary institutions such as possession by ancestor spirits, male transvestism, and special days of collective transgressions are safety valves for frustrations.

1260. Sacks K: Sisters and Wives. Westport, Conn., Greenwood, 1979.

A social-Darwinistic view of women's roles is

countered by a feminist-Marxist analysis of women in preclass societies such as Mbuti, Lovedu, Mpondo, Buganda, Dahomey, and Onitsha.

1261. Sadler PO: The "crisis cult" as a voluntary association: an international approach to Alcoholics Anonymous. Human Organization 36:207–10, 1977.

The understanding of currently proliferating self-help groups will be more reflective of members' perceptions if investigators scrutinize on-the-ground interaction of members rather than the literature of the groups.

1262. Sagan E: The Lust to Annihilate. New York, Psychohistory, 1979.

The widespread violence in ancient Greek culture is examined from a psychoanalytic perspective. Homer's epic poems, Thucydides' history, and Greek tragedies are analyzed.

1263. Sagarin E: Deviance and Social Change. Beverly Hills, Calif., Sage, 1977.

Deviance may be destructive or creatively adaptive.

1264. Sahlins M: The Use and Abuse of Biology. Ann Arbor, U. of Michigan Press, 1976.

An anthropological critique reveals that kin selection—the central dogma of sociobiology—is important in human mating groups because such groups are culturally rather than biologically constituted.

1265. Sainsbury P, Wood E: Measuring gesture: its cultural and clinical correlates. Psychological Medicine 7:63–72, 1977.

The ultrasonic system provides a reliable and sensitive method for measuring gesture activity and can be applied clinically to the study of psychomotor behavior.

1266. Sakamoto Y: Some experiences through family-psychotherapy for psychotics in Japan. Intl J Social Psychiatry 22: 265–71, 1976/1977.

Although the history of family psychotherapy spans over a decade, there is still no definite method established in Japan.

1267. Saklofske DH, Eysenck SBG: Cross-cultural comparison of personality: New Zealand children and English children. Psychological Reports 42:1111–16, 1978.

The Eysenck scales measure substantially similar or identical factors in England and New Zealand. However, all cross-cultural compari-

sons suffer from the difficulty of discovering whether measures applied in one country carry the same meaning in another.

1268. Salkind NJ, Kojima K, Zelniker T: Cognitive tempo in American, Japanese, and Israeli children. Child Development 49:1024–27, 1978.

American, Japanese, and Israeli children all tend to be characterized by highly similar developmental trends for both errors and latency, as well as a synchrony within each group between peak latency and asymptotic error scores. Younger Japanese children make fewer errors than the other children until eight years of age, when their level of accuracy approaches that of ten-to-twelve-year-old American and Israeli children.

1269. Salvendy JT: Psychiatry in the Soviet Union today. Canadian Psychiatric Assn J 20:229–36, 1975.

There are several basic differences between North American and Soviet Union psychiatry. The introduction and maintenance of treatment methods and facilities in the Soviet Union usually are made independently of the community and citizen groups. The immobility of the Soviet population is another crucial variable. Simple transplantation of the Soviet system of psychiatric care delivery would have deleterious effects in a different environment.

1270. Samouilidis L: Psychoanalytic vicissitudes in working with Greek patients. Amer J Psychoanalysis 38:223–33, 1978.

In Greek patients psychoanalysis proceeds smoothly with few stormy periods and relatively fast resolutions of conflicts. The deepening and broadening of feelings are limited, and the analysis stays at a relatively superficial level. In areas where conflicts cannot be resolved, the patient acquires a readily accepting attitude. Greek patients generally favor a gradual rather than an abrupt termination.

1271. Samuda RJ: Psychological Testing of American Minorities. New York, Dodd, Mead, 1975.

The use of psychological tests in educational and occupational personnel decisions is a social injustice.

1272. Sanada T, Norbeck E: Prophecy continues to fail: a Japanese sect. J Cross-Cultural Psychology 6:331–45, 1975.

If someone holds a firm belief, he cannot discard it despite the failure of a prophecy on it, although he cannot ignore the fact that his belief has been disconfirmed. Under such circumstances, the most convenient cognition conceivable for him is the fact that others share his belief.

1273. Sand EA: Specialized mental health services for children and adolescents in France, Belgium, and French-speaking Switzerland. Intl J Mental Health 7:75–89, 1978.

Despite social and economic conditions that are very similar, and despite mental health problems that are comparable from many points of view, the organization of health care varies significantly from one European country to another.

1274. Sandoval M: Santeria: Afrocuban concepts of disease and its treatment in Miami. J Operational Psychiatry 8(2):52–63, 1977.

Santeria, the most evolved and influential of Afro-Cuban religious forms, has successfully adjusted to the new environment that Cuban nationals find in Florida. The Santeros—priests and priestesses of Santeria—and modern physicians are equally used by Cubans to treat their illnesses, the former especially for psychosomatic disorders or tensions not treatable by modern medicine.

1275. Sandoval MC: Santeria as a mental health care system: an historical overview. Social Sciences Medicine 13B(2):137–51, 1979.

Santeria is an Afro-Cuban religious system that has an essentially African world view and rituals. Santeria's intrinsic flexibility, eclecticism, and heterogeneity have allowed for functional, dogmatic, and ritual changes that enable it to meet the different needs of its many followers.

1276. Sanjek R: A network method and its uses in urban ethnograph. Human Organization 37:257–68, 1978.

The problem of urban dispersal that arises once a unit of study has been selected can be overcome with network-serial data. Neither holism nor a commitment to intensive personal investigation need be abandoned in urban ethnography if a method is used to identify the parts and show how they fit together.

1277. Sanua VD: Psychological intervention in the Arab world: a review of folk treatment. Transcult Psych Res Review 16:205–8, 1979.

Dynamic psychiatry and psychology have not influenced the Arab world. Madness is objectionable because of uncontrollable behavior or individual violence. Hallucinations and delusions may not necessarily reflect psychopathology but rather religious practices and beliefs. Since the stresses of life are attributed to the will of God, suicide is very rare. To cure both physical and mental illness, Arabs may resort to folk healers who use procedures akin to witchcraft.

1278. Sanua VD: Familial and sociocultural antecedents of psychopathology. In Handbook of Cross-Cultural Psychology, edited by HC Triandis and JG Draguns, 6:175–236. Boston, Allyn and Bacon, 1980.

In order to avoid erroneous conclusions, it is necessary to study normal behavior before recognizing pathology in specific groups. These errors are due in part to the fact that psychiatrists and psychologists are not usually exposed to social scientists in other disciplines, people who can provide them with a wider scope of concepts and techniques for assessing psychopathology.

1279. Sarason SB: Work, Aging and Social Change. New York, Free Press, 1977.

Aging, as exemplified in a study of professionals, is affected by lifelong work, education, and social values.

1280. Sartorius NS, Jablensky A, Shapiro R: Cross-cultural differences in the short-term prognosis of schizophrenic psychoses. Schizophrenia Bull 4:102–13, 1978.

Results of the international pilot study of schizophrenia (WHO 1973) indicate that patients diagnosed as schizophrenic demonstrate very marked variations of course and outcome. Schizophrenic patients in developing countries have a considerably better prognosis and outcome than patients in developed countries. Part of the variation of course and outcome is related to sociodemographic (e.g., type of onset and precipitating factors) predictors.

1281. Sata LS: A profile of Asian-American psychiatrists. Amer J Psychiatry 135:448–51, 1978.

Asian psychiatrists are the largest visible multiethnic minority group within American psychiatry. Increased attention to the special needs of this group will lead to its more appropriate utilization in this country.

1282. Sata LS, Lin KM: A comparative study of Asian FMG and USMG psychiatrists. Hosp Community Psychiatry 30:332–34, 1979.

Asian FMG psychiatrists shoulder much of the responsibility for treating minority patients in the United States. Without special training in both cultural and professional areas, they may be ill equipped for this task.

1283. Savage JE, Adair AW, Friedman P: Community-social variables related to black parent-absent families. J Marriage Family 40:779–86, 1978.

In order to cope with parent absence, significant role adjustments are made by different members of the black family. In addition, a variety of community-social variables affect the attitudes and behaviors of these families.

1284. Scheff TF: The distancing of emotion in ritual. Current Anthropology 18:483–505, 1977.

Effective ritual is the solution to a seemingly insoluble problem, the management of collectively held, otherwise unmanageable distress. Ritual is unique in that it meets individual and collective needs simultaneously, allowing individuals to discharge accumulated distress and creating social solidarity in the process.

1285. Scheper-Hughes N: Saints, scholars and schizophrenics—madness and badness in western Ireland. Med Anthropology 2:59–93, 1978.

Ireland's high mental hospitalization rates may be merely a reflection of a centuries-old Irish tendency to "search for asylum." Mental hospital patients if not diseased in a medical sense are dis-eased in a sociological sense, and sexual disturbances as well as community exclusion are often present.

1286. Scheper-Hughes N: Saints, Scholars, and Schizophrenics. Berkeley, U. of California Press, 1979.

The high prevalence of schizophrenia in rural Ireland is closely associated with cultural factors.

1287. Schlegel A (ed): Sexual Stratification: A Cross-Cultural View. New York, Columbia U. Press, 1977.

Theories of sexual inequality are divided into two broad categories: those that explain inequality as an historical product of specific material conditions, and those that link universal male dominance to differences in biological and reproductive roles.

1288. Schlegel A, Barry H: Adolescent initiation ceremonies: a cross-cultural code. Ethnology 18:199–210, 1979.

In societies having ceremonies for both sexes, boys are significantly more likely than girls to undergo painful procedures other than genital operations and to have ceremonies that result in familiar independence and focus on responsibility, while girls are significantly more likely to have ceremonies that focus on fertility and sexuality.

1289. Schleifer SJ, Schwartz AH, Thorton JC, Rosenberg SL: A study of American immigrants to Israel utilizing the SSRQ. J Psychosomatic Research 23:247–52, 1979.

Migration to a new country is an event entailing a major life change and has been associated with an increased prevalence of psychological disturbance.

1290. Schmidt K, Hill L, Guthrie G: Running amok. Intl J Social Psychiatry 23:264–74, 1977.

Amok is a dramatic behavior aberration found almost exclusively among Malayan men.

1291. Schmidt W, Popham RE: Impressions of Jewish alcoholics. J Stud Alcohol 37:931–39, 1976.

Despite a long-standing interest in the causes of Jewish sobriety, the study of the exceptional cases of Jewish alcoholics has been neglected. In Jewish alcoholics, remoteness from Jewish culture is not a sufficient explanation for the drinking problems of the group. Orthodox Jews deny the problem of alcoholism; nonorthodox Jews accept the diagnosis but deny their affiliation with the Jewish community. A third group admits to being both Jewish and alcoholic but denies the validity of the notion of Jewish sobriety.

1292. Schneider D: American Kinship. 2d ed. Chicago, U. of Chicago Press, 1980.

In American culture the relative in nature is at one extreme, the relative in law is at the other extreme. The first is a relationship of nature while the second is a set of artificial rules or regulations for conduct.

1293. Schneider I: Images of the mind: psychiatry in the commercial film. Amer J Psychiatry 134:613–20, 1977.

There are many striking temporal and cultural parallels in the development of commercial films and psychiatry. Psychiatrists have been depicted in widely varying ways, from being a madman to being a powerful force for tinkering with the soul and a wonder worker who cures patients by uncovering a single traumatic event. Postwar films dealt with emerging social issues. Contemporary films focus on madness as a metaphor or on the struggle of seemingly normal, successful people to find fulfillment.

1294. Schneider R, Sangsingkeo P, Panpanya B, Tumrongrachaniti S, Witayarut C: Incidence of daily drug use as reported by a population of Thai partners working near United States military installations: a preliminary study. Intl J Addictions 2:175–85, 1976.

Fifteen percent of Thai women who have American partners on United States military installations use drugs and/or alcohol daily. There is neither a great deal of drug use by Americans induced by interpersonal relationships with Thai women, nor can a great deal of Thai drug use be directly attributed to the influence of American soldiers.

1295. Schneider RJ, Sangsingkeo P, Punnahitanond S: A survey of Thai students' use of illicit drugs. Intl J Addictions 12:227–39, 1977.

Prevalence and patterns of drug use among Thai and American students are remarkably similar. Easy availability of drugs of abuse does not necessarily lead to endemic or epidemic use.

1296. Schoenberg B, Gerber I, Wrener A, Kutscher AH, Peretz D, Carr AC (eds): Bereavement: Its Psychosocial Aspect. New York, Columbia U. Press, 1975.

A prospective study of families reveals that the number of deaths, major hospitalizations, and psychiatric decompensations did not increase following bereavement. Ethnographers must be aware of the possibility that self-fulfilling prophecy may lead to the adoption of suboptimal practices related to grief and mourning.

1297. Schottstaedt MF, Bjork JW: Inhalant abuse in an Indian boarding school. Amer J Psychiatry 134:1290–93, 1977.

Inhalant abuse is common among Indian boarding-school children. Such abuse can be controlled by improving the moral and child-management skills of existing staff and by introducing new attitudes and ideas.

1298. Schultes RE, Hofmann A: Plants of the Gods. New York, McGraw-Hill, 1979.

Plant hallucinogens permit man in primitive societies to communicate with the supernatural realms.

1299. Schulz CH: Death-anxiety reduction through the success-achievement cultural core value: a middle-class American community case study. J Psychol Anthropology 1:321–39, 1978.

Culturally derived and reinforced ways of affirming the self, such as the desire to achieve and the actual realization of success goals, act to shield the individual in American culture from death anxiety by repressing conscious death awareness.

1300. Schwab JJ, Bell RA, Warheit GJ, Schwab RB: Social Order and Mental Health. New York, Brunner/Mazel, 1979.

An epidemiological study in Alachua County, Florida, examines the relationships among mental illness, culture change, social mobility, aspirations, and geographic mobility.

1301. Schwab JJ, Schwab ME: Sociocultural Roots of Mental Illness. New York, Plenum, 1978.

The epidemiological and cultural foundations of psychiatry are reviewed.

1302. Schwab ME: A study of reported hallucinations in a southeastern county. Mental Health Society 4:344–54, 1977.

In the general population of a county in north-central Florida, hallucinations are more commonly reported by the young, by blacks, by members of the lower socioeconomic class, and by those belonging to certain church types. These data are discussed from complementing and contrasting psychiatric and anthropologic viewpoints.

1303. Schwartz W: Degradation, accreditation, and rites of passage. Psychiatry 42:138–46, 1979.

The structures of certain classes of performative rites of passage, specifically degradation and accreditation ceremonies, can be useful in work with certain people seeking psychotherapy.

1304. Schwartzmann HB: Transformations: The Anthropology of Children's Play. New York, Plenum, 1978.

The study of play requires that researchers adapt themselves to the character of their subjects, and not the reverse. Play is absolutely central and not peripheral to human behavior. Play is an activity in which participants communicate to create a shared reality. It gives shape as well as expression to individual and societal affective and cognitive systems.

1305. Schwarz R: Beschreibung einer ambulanten psychiatrischen patientespopulation in der groben kabylei (Nordalgerien): epidemiologische und klinische aspekte. Social Psychiatry 12:207–18, 1977.

Male psychiatric patients in Algeria seek psychiatric treatment approximately twice as often as do female patients.

1306. Schweitzer RD, Buhrmann MV: An existential-phenomenological interpretation of Thwasa among the Xhosa. Psychotherapia 4:15–18, 1978.

In order to become a mental healer (or iggira) among the Xhosa (South Africa), a person has to experience a calling from his dead ancestors and a three-to-five-year period of mental instability called Thwasa, followed by a gradual process of reintegration.

1307. Scotton BW: Relating the work of Carlos Castaneda to psychiatry. Bull Menninger Clinic 42:223–38, 1978.

Castaneda implies that evaluating a patient's reality in terms of its utility in permitting growth, rather than in terms of its congruence with a given reality, is a healthier approach to the patient.

1308. Seeman MV: Name and identity. Canadian J Psychiatry 25:129–37, 1980.

Identity can be encoded in a name. A name bears the stamp of the namer's traditions and his hopes for his children. The interface between names and personal identity is illustrated clinically in syndromes of transsexualism and multiple personality, in twinning, and in the development of the ego-ideal.

1309. Segal BM: Soviet approaches to involuntary hospitalization. Intl J Social Psychiatry 23:94–102, 1977.

The misuse of psychiatry is a natural consequence of the use of psychiatry as a method to protect the state. Despite the unquestionably negative implications of these phenomena, one may hope that under pressure of public opinion, government control over Soviet psychiatry will be eventually diminished to some extent.

1310. Seiden AM: Overview: research on the psychology of women. Part 1: Gender differences and sexual and reproductive life. Amer J Psychiatry 133:995–1007, 1976.

The recent and rapid increase in research on women's issues is unequaled currently in other psychiatric fields. Recent research on gender differences in behavior and on the sexual and reproductive lives of women is reviewed.

1311. Seixas FA (ed): Currents in Alcoholism, Vol. 4: Social Aspects of Alcoholism. New York, Plenum, 1976.

Topics discussed include alcohol use in tribal societies (M Bacon), anthropological perspectives on the social biology of alcohol (DB Heath),

and drinking behavior and drinking problems in the United States (D Cahalan and I Asin).

1312. Seltzer A: Acculturation and mental disorder in the Inuit. Canadian J Psychiatry 25:173–81, 1980.

Eskimo adolescent and young adult males are especially susceptible to the anxiety generated by the process of acculturation. The interaction of acculturation stress with the biopsychosocial characteristics of the individual within his ecological group leads to an increased incidence of mental disorder. Modified supportive therapy and continuity of care aimed at increasing self-esteem through sublimation, identification, reduction of dependency, and encouragement of growth and autonomy are measures aimed at primary prevention.

1313. Sena-Rivera J: Extended kinship in the United States: competing models and the case of la familia Chicana. J Marriage Family 41:121–30, 1979.

The form and structure of the Chicano familia is not one of development within American industrial society, but rather one of transference from Mexico with antecedents traceable to pre-Columbian history. The isolated nuclear family model is not a viable hypothesis for Chicanos, nor is the "classic" extended family as posited by Parsons. The modified extended family as tested by Litwab and Sussman more closely approximates the case for Chicano households.

1314. Serpell R: Culture's Influence on Behavior. London, Methuen, 1976.

Attempts to relate a whole culture to personality patterns are overambitious. Language is an important mediator in the interaction between culture and behavior. Cross-cultural research on cognitive development and on pictorial perception suggests that not all data are amenable to an ecological interpretation.

1315. Sethi BB, Gupta SC, Lal N: The theory and practice of psychiatry in India. Amer J Psychotherapy 31:43–65, 1977.

The past, present, and future status of the concept and practice of psychiatry in India is reviewed, with the hypothesis being made that with increased sociocultural stresses brought on by rapid industrialization, a greater occurrence of emotional disorders may result.

1316. Setyonegoro RK: Social psychiatric implications of population control in Indonesia. Mental Health Society 3:194–96, 1976.

In family planning for developing countries, the ignorant masses have to be motivated not only to make use of the services but also to learn to appreciate more intense and deeper human relationships. The illiterate have also to be motivated to utilize services for parents and children and to conceive that they also share the responsibility to create a "new generation" and a "new culture."

1317. Seward JP, Seward GH: Sex Differences: Mental and Temperamental. Lexington, Mass., Lexington, 1980.

Each person should be allowed to choose his or her own male or female role according to individual need.

1318. Seymour S: Caste/class and child-rearing in a changing Indian town. Amer Ethnologist 3:783–96, 1976.

Because of a greater need for responsible and cooperative behavior, children's behavior at the lower end of the socioeconomic hierarchy more nearly approaches that of a kin-oriented, subsistence gardening society than does the behavior of middle- and upper-class children.

1319. Shapero M: The Sociobiology of Homo Sapiens. Kansas City, Pincrest Fund, 1978.

Behavior and its products are explained by adaption. The test of sociobiology is to tell the tale of how and why a metaphysical version is or is not adaptive, or was, or would be adaptive.

1320. Shapiro T: Clinical Psycholinguistics. New York, Plenum, 1979.

Topics discussed include the relationships between language structure and communication between patient and therapist.

1321. Sharma BP: Cannabis and its users in Nepal. Brit J Psychiatry 127:550–52, 1975.

Cannabis users in Nepal have a poor work record, poor social and family relationships, a lack of interest in sex, and a general loss of initiative and efficiency. There is no difference in the crime rate between cannabis users and nonusers.

1322. Sharma KN: Institutions, Networks, and Social Change. Simla, India, Indian Inst. of Advanced Study, 1975.

Traditional collectivities such as the joint family, the kindred and caste, and the jajmani system do not provide Indian villagers with sufficient social support to face demographic, economic, and social changes.

1323. Sharma SD, Gopalakrishna R: Suicide—a retrospective study in a culturally distinct community in India. Intl J Social Psychiatry 24:13–18, 1978.

Cultural and religious factors continue to play an important role in suicidal behavior in India. The rate among Hindus is higher than among Christians. More people commit suicide in their own birthplace and near their own homes.

1324. Sharon D: Wizard of the Four Winds. Wellesley Hills, Mass., Lee, 1978.

A Peruvian curandero utilizes the hallucinogenic San Pedro cactus and participates in a functional modern magicoreligious system that combines Catholic and aboriginal elements.

1325. Shatan CF: Bogus manhood, bogus honor: surrender and transfiguration in the United States Marine Corps. Psychoanalytic Review 64:585–610, 1977.

Marines are allowed to feel potent only as a collective unit. As power appendages of the commander who has stolen their masculinity, they are permitted to deck themselves in spurious virility trappings. Beneath this bogus manliness, the true business of the Corps is to make boys into killers, not "men out of boys."

1326. Shaver P, Lenauer M, Sudd S: Religiousness, conversion, and subjective well-being: the "healthy-minded" religion of modern American woman. Amer J Psychiatry 137:1563–68, 1980.

Certainty of religious beliefs rather than ambivalence is associated with better mental and physical health. Converts are different from nonconverts in religious background, childhood happiness, and authoritarian tendencies. Health-mindedness is more descriptive of nonconverts.

1327. Shephard RJ, Itoh S (eds): Circumpolar Health. Toronto, U. of Toronto Press, 1976.

Topics discussed include Eskimo mental health, personality and society, acculturative stress in northern Canada, adaptation to an extreme environment, influence of environment on the physical and psychic development of Skolt Lapp children and the adaptation of these children to cultural change, criminal homicide and alcohol problems in Greenland, psychiatric consultation in Arctic communities, and a model for psychiatric education in the North.

1328. Shepherd WC: Paradoxes about ego in the Western tradition. J Psychol Anthropology 2:323–36, 1979.

In Western society the Christian ideal of self-denial as a means of nurturing the intellectual and rational life coexists with a capitalist ego that is individualistic and manipulative. In order to maintain a fixed point for ego and identity amid the fluid nature of modern society, these two extremes of Western tradition must be forsaken for a realization of the protean nature of our identities.

1329. Sherwood R: The Psychodynamics of Race. Atlantic Highlands, N.J., Humanities, 1980.
Interviews with a native English and immigrant West Indian (Barbados) and Indian (Punjabi) families uncover the psychodynamics of racial tensions to show that interracial conflicts are related to personal identity conflicts.

1330. Shimano ET, Douglas DB: On research in Zen. Amer J Psychiatry 132:1300–1302, 1975.
Several aspects of Zen, such as psychophysiological effects of meditation and the impact of enlightenment, are potentially fruitful areas of research. True understanding of Zen can only come by practicing the discipline.

1331. Shimrat N: Sociocultural and psychodynamic characteristics of ultraorthodox psychiatric Jewish patients. Intl J Social Psychiatry 25:157–66, 1979.
There is a tendency to minimize these patients' pathology by attributing their bizarre behavior to their cultural background. However, it is imperative to remember that those who come to the hospital are no longer adjusted or adapted to their own milieu and that they deviate considerably from the norms of their own subculture.

1332. Shoham SG: Social Deviance. New York, Gardner, 1976.
Deviance is a form of and an expression of social conflict.

1333. Sholberg SC: Social desirability responses in Jewish and Arab children in Israel. J Cross-Cultural Psychology 7:301–14, 1976.
Although both Arabs and Jews have a relatively high social desirability level, it should be emphasized that within each culture social desirability tendencies are related to a specific psychological and sociocultural background.

1334. Shore JH: American Indian suicide—fact and fantasy. Psychiatry 38:86–91, 1975.
The profile of completed suicide among American Indian subjects most commonly is that of a single or separated male who hangs or shoots himself in his own home or in jail on the reservation. Alcohol abuse or solvent sniffing is involved

in 75 percent of the cases of completed suicide. Attempts at suicide are most often by a young female via a drug overdose at home following a quarrel with a relative or friend. These are impulsive acts associated with the use of alcohol in 44 percent of all cases. The suicide group could be differentiated from the control population by several factors, all of which relate to an unstable home environment.

1335. Shore JH, Nicholls WM: Indian children and tribal group homes: new interpretations of the whipper man. Amer J Psychiatry 132:454–56, 1975.
The community child care of the Plateau Indians accepts extended family and community responsibility for child care. Family stability is essential for primary prevention in community mental health.

1336. Shriver D: Medicine and Religion. Pittsburgh, U. of Pittsburgh Press, 1980.
Physicians and clergy can work together to develop strategies of care for suffering and troubled persons.

1337. Shuman MK: Culture and deafness in a Maya Indian village. Psychiatry 43:359–70, 1980.
Several factors facilitate the psychosocial adjustment of the deaf Maya Indians of southeastern Mexico to the community as a whole. These include a supportive family environment; the world view of the culture in which they live; the use of sign language to facilitate communications; and the fact that even though they are economically disadvantaged within their culture, they are able to perform meaningful and valued work. The imprecisions of the gesture language, however, make enculturation for the deaf difficult and perhaps impossible.

1338. Sievers ML, Cynamon MH, Bittker TE: Intentional isoniazid overdosage among southwestern American Indians. Amer J Psychiatry 132:662–65, 1975.
The vulnerability of southwestern American Indians to self-destructive behavior is shown in the frequency of isoniazid overdose in tuberculosis therapy. Patients should be given smaller amounts of INH at shorter intervals with compliance closely monitored to inhibit abuse.

1339. Siikala AL: The Rite Techniques of the Siberian Shaman. Helsinki, Suomalainen Triedeakakmis, Academia Scientiarum Fennica, 1978.
The shaman's role is that of a creator of a state

of interaction between this world and the other world.

1340. Silk JB: Adoption and kinship in Oceania. Amer Anthropologist 84:799–817, 1980.

Adoption in Oceania provides a means of adjusting family size in response to economic needs, a finding consistent with predictions derived from sociobiology.

1341. Simenauer E: A double helix: some determinants of the self-perpetuation of Naziism. Psychoanalytic Study Child 33:411–25, 1978.

In the face of total defeat and the complete breakdown of their ideology and convictions, the older generation in Germany initially reacted with stunned helplessness and largely hypocritical adaptations to new conditions. The younger generation, even though they are critical of their parents' past crimes, nevertheless do not want to or cannot believe that their parents passively or actively contributed to the genocide of the Jews. Thus, the current anti-Israel attitude among the young represents one means by which they rebel against and revenge themselves on their parents.

1342. Simeon G: Illness and Curing in a Guatemalan Village. Honolulu, U. of Hawaii School of Public Health, 1977.

Three local informants describe folk medical practices in their village.

1343. Simmons WS: Powerlessness, exploitation, and the soul-eating witch: an analysis of Badyaranke witchcraft. Amer Ethnologist 7:447–65, 1980.

In one Senegalese West African community, traditional witchcraft beliefs provide an idiom for interpreting conflict with the representatives of external structures as if this conflict were attributable to persons within the village. Thus, when one villager accuses another of witchcraft, he or she can be displacing grievances against the state and other outside institutions.

1344. Simoes M, Binder J: A socio-psychiatric field study among Portuguese emigrants in Switzerland. Social Psychiatry 15:1–7, 1980.

Migrating workers show no "latent traits" or symptoms that are normally considered to be typical for migrant workers, but obsessionality appears to be a characteristic psychological trait.

1345. Simon B: Mind and Madness in Ancient Greece. Ithaca, N.Y., Cornell U. Press, 1978.

Ancient Greek poets, philosophers, and physicians each had differing views about the origins and treatment of mental illness. The poets emphasized external forces and curative public rituals; philosophers emphasized interpersonal psychological conflicts and curative self-knowledge; physicians emphasized physiological processes, curative medication, and other physical treatments.

1346. Simon J: Creativity and altered states of consciousness. Amer J Psychoanalysis 37:3–12, 1977.

The separate camps of analysis and altered states of consciousness are not so far apart. Altered states of consciousness occur within the analytic or therapeutic situation in many forms.

1347. Simons RC: The resolution of the latah paradox. J Nerv Ment Disease 168:195–206, 1980.

New data show that the various forms of latah are culture-specific exploitations of a neurophysiological potential shared by humans and other mammals. Latah provides a revealing example of the complex ways in which neurophysiological, experiential, and cultural variables interact to produce a strongly marked social phenomenon.

1348. Singer K: Psychiatric aspects of abortion in Hong Kong. Intl J Social Psychiatry 21:303–6, 1975.

The medical profession faces an abortion law in Hong Kong, and in many other parts of the world, which has enmeshed social, economic, moral, and psychological problems with the physical. The law raises crucial issues for the medical professions; namely, the extent to which the profession should regard social and related problems as within its province, and its competence in dealing with such problems.

1349. Singer K, Lieh-Mak F, Ng ML: Physique, personality and mental illness in southern Chinese women. Brit J Psychiatry 129:243–47, 1976.

The intercorrelation among body build, personality, and type of mental illness in Chinese women is on the whole similar to that reported for Caucasians.

1350. Singer K, Ney PG, Lieh-Mak F: A cultural perspective on child psychiatric disorders. Comp Psychiatry 19:533–40, 1978.

Awareness of the possible role of cultural factors is of value in broadening perspectives on child psychiatric disorders and improving approaches to their management. The similarities of psychosocial factors that generate abnormal behavior and the manifestations of such behavior in Oriental and Western cultures provide the basis for the development of a universally valid approach in child psychiatry.

1351. Singer M: The function of sobriety among black Hebrews. J Operational Psychiatry 11:162–68, 1980.

While anxiety reduction is an important function of alcohol consumption, the black Hebrew community, in order to maintain anxiety, prohibits drunkenness. Anxiety serves to maintain internal cohesion in the face of internal and external threat.

1352. Singer P (ed): Traditional Healing: New Science or New Colonialism? New York, Conch, 1977.

As evidenced by essays about Nigerians, Kenyans, Mexicans, and Puerto Ricans, an emphasis on traditional healing and on witch doctors is part of a medical and anthropological conspiracy that denies the masses access to modern medicine.

1353. Singh G, Lal B: Culture and alcohol—cultural traditions and alcohol consumption in India. Comp Med East West 6:229–36, 1978.

No definite cultural tradition exists in India that could be described as being clearly and unequivocally against the use of alcohol in any form and under all circumstances. Although alcohol is frequently referred to as an evil, it is at the same time socially accepted and glamorized by its use among the ruling classes.

1354. Singh G, Verma HC: Murder in Punjab. Indian J Psychiatry 18:243–51, 1976.

According to Hindu mythology, both women and earth represent a common "mother" archetypal image. It is a matter of pride and honor for an Indian male to fight fiercely—even to commit murder—to preserve both women and land as sacred, pure objects.

1355. Singh SN: Caste differences and adjustment problems. Psychologia 18:134–41, 1975.

Evidence from responses of Hindu children to Mooney's Problem Check-list indicates that in urban and rural areas caste restrictions are losing their grip and social distance is being reduced.

1356. Slaples R, Mirande A: Racial and cultural variations among American families: a decennial review of the literature on minority families. J Marriage Family 42:887–904, 1980.

Review and assessment of the past decade's literature on Asian-American, black, Chicano,

and Native American families indicate that prior to 1970 minority families were subject to negative stereotypes that were not empirically supported. In the case of blacks and Chicanos, the family literature of the 1970s represented an improvement, depicting a positive aspect of their family life. Theory and research on Asian- and Native-American families is too limited to make any generalizations about their lifestyles.

1357. Sluzki CE: Migration and family conflict. Family Process 18:379–90, 1979.

The process of migration—both across cultures and across regions within cultures—presents outstanding regularities. A model of the migratory process that is relatively "culture free" can be developed by concentrating on patterns instead of content.

1358. Sluzki CE, Ransom D (eds): Double Bind. New York, Grune and Stratton, 1976.

Understanding of the double bind theory is a foundation of the communicational approach to the family.

1359. Smiley CW: The flower children of Ontario. Amer J Psychoanalysis 35:279–83, 1975.

A hippie group in Ontario, Canada, consisted of a large number of deeply disturbed people for whom the camaraderie and outer symbols and rituals of the hippie movement was a materialization of their fantasy life. Their rebellion was an attempt to achieve a sense of identity, a sense of integrity, and a sense of firmness of self and outlook. They considered things in the present but did not attempt to deal with issues of the future.

1360. Smith A: Powers of Mind. New York, Random House, 1975.

Faith healing, mysticism, and universal symbols are among topics of interest to the loosely defined consciousness movement.

1361. Smith CG, King JA: Mental Hospitals. Lexington, Mass., D.C. Heath, 1975.

With proper use of both organizational and administrative processes a truly therapeutic community can be realized.

1362. Smith KC, Schooler C: Women as mothers in Japan: the effects of social structure and culture on values and behavior. J Marriage Family 40:612–20, 1978.

In Japanese women, maternal role is considered central and is emphasized at the expense of a conjugal role, fostering a high degree of interdependence with their children. In Japan, as in the United States, environmental complexity produces individualistic values, reducing adherence to traditional values.

1363. Smither R, Rodriguez-Giegling M: Marginality, modernity, and anxiety in Indochinese refugees. J Cross-Cultural Psychology 10:469–78, 1979.

Although younger Americans feel more marginal than older Americans, marginality among Laotians increases with age. Cultural differences on modernity may not be the source of anxiety within refugee groups.

1364. Snow LF: Sorcerers, saints and charlatans: black folk healers in urban America. Culture Medicine Psychiatry 2:69–106, 1978.

Black Americans may forsake orthodox medical regimens for folk healers in seeking a remedy for their ills. Some find legitimate help, others are exploited.

1365. Sobel DS: Ways of Health. New York, Harcourt Brace Jovanovich, 1979.

Holistic medicine offers an alternative to physiochemical reductionism and to body-mind dualism. Areas studied include Navaho medicine, shamanism, and Yogic therapy.

1366. Sobo S: Narcissism as a function of culture. Psychoanalytic Study Child 32:155–72, 1977.

The superego needs consistent reinforcement in adolescent and adult experience. When this is lacking, regression to preoedipal narcissistic dynamics occurs even without major trauma. Although some people have suffered from narcissistic difficulties regardless of social circumstances, many others have been reasonably protected from the temptations of their unconscious in different times when society acted in its usual role as a reinforcer of the superego.

1367. Sofue T: Aspects of the personality of Japanese, Americans, Italians, and Eskimos: comparisons using the Sentence Completion Test. J Psychol Anthropology 2:11–52, 1979.

Among the traits demonstrated in using the Sentence Completion Test were strong dependency on mother and emphasis of family ties with parents by Japanese; no maternal dependence shown by Americans, especially by white females; strong positive attitudes toward parents, and particularly strong ties with mother by Italians; and positive and warm attitudes toward mother by Eskimos.

1368. Sohlberg SC: Social desirability responses in Jewish and Arab children in Israel. J Cross-Cultural Psychology 7:301–14, 1976.

Although both Arabs and Jews have a relatively high social desirability level, it should be emphasized that *within* each culture social desirability tendencies are related to a specific psychological and sociocultural background.

1369. Sokolovsky J, Cohen C, Berger D, Geiger J: Personal networks of ex-mental patients in a Manhattan SRO hotel. Human Organization 37:5–15, 1978.

Schizophrenic individuals who have small, nonmultiplex networks with a low degree of connectedness will exhibit higher rates of rehospitalization than schizophrenics with more extensive networks.

1370. Soler EG, Dammann G: Women in crisis: drug use and abuse. J Addictions Health 1:227–41, 1980.

One-third of subjects in the women-in-crisis project identified themselves as alcohol abusers, while almost another third identified themselves as drug abusers (tranquilizers). Psychiatric drugs may trigger or exacerbate a crisis interaction or may be used as a means of coping with stress.

1371. Soliday GL (ed): History of the Family and Kinship: A Select International Bibliography. Milwood, N.Y., Kraus Intl., 1980.

A bibliography listing 6,200 entries on ethnology, sociology, psychology, demography, and social history pertaining to kinsmen and their familial constructs.

1372. Sondhi PR: Issues and priorities in services in developing countries. Intl J Mental Health 7:102–5, 1978.

Despite more pressing problems and a paucity of trained personnel, it is necessary to make a beginning in the provision of psychiatric services in the developing countries because their economic growth and increasing urbanization are bound to produce a greater need than ever before.

1373. Sow I: Anthropological Structures of Madness in Black Africa. New York, Intl. Universities Press, 1980.

From a psychoanalytic perspective it is possible to delineate themes that unite African nosology, healing, cosmology, and myth.

1374. Spanos NP, Gottlieb J: Demonic possession, mesmerism, and hysteria: a social psychological perspective on their historical interrelations. J Abnormal Psychology 88:527–46, 1979.

Social psychological interpretations of the interrelations among demonic possession, mesmerism, and hysteria are discussed. The use of hysteria as a modern explanatory concept in histories of possession and mesmerism is criticized.

1375. Spanos NP, Hewitt EC: Glossolalia: a test of the "trance" and psychopathology hypotheses. J Abnormal Psychology 88(4):427–34, 1979.

Glossolalia is a pattern of vocal behavior that can be acquired by almost anyone who possesses the requisite motivation and who is exposed regularly to social environments that encourage such utterances. There is no support for the notion that glossolalia results from a trance, is related to hypnotic susceptability, or is symptomatic of psychopathology.

1376. Spencer J: The mental health of Jehovah's Witnesses. Brit J Psychiatry 126:556–59, 1975.

Jehovah's Witnesses in western Australia are more likely to be admitted to a psychiatric hospital than the general population. Followers of this sect are three times more likely to be diagnosed as suffering from schizophrenia and nearly four times more likely from paranoid schizophrenia than the rest of the population at risk.

1377. Spiegel JP: Cultural aspects of transference and counter transference revisited. J Amer Acad Psychoanalysis 4:447–68, 1976.

Distortion arising from unconscious childhood object relations and fantasies as manifested in transference or countertransference responses can only be detected when played against a fixed point of reference, in respect to which they appear bizarre or out of place.

1378. Spielberger CD, Diaz-Guerrero R (eds): Cross-Cultural Anxiety. Washington, D.C., Hemisphere, 1976.

In addition to general cross-cultural studies of anxiety in Greece, Italy, Mexico, Canada, and Sweden, the validity of the State-Trait Anxiety Inventory is examined in patients from Portugal, France, Turkey, and Spain.

1379. Spindler G (ed): The Making of Psychological Anthropology. Berkeley, U. of California Press, 1978.

Some of the most well known psychological anthropologists discuss their work in such areas as field work, culture change, cognition, psycho-cultural research, the Japanese, and the Ojibwa.

1380. Spiro ME: Gender and Culture: Kibbutz Women Revisited. Durham, N.C., Duke U. Press, 1979.

Women on a kibbutz in Israel are revolting against defamilization and now spend time with their own children and spouse as a nuclear family.

1381. Spiro ME: Whatever happened to the id? Amer Anthropologist 81:5–13, 1979.

Even when cultural beliefs, myths, or rituals are explicitly and preponderantly sexual or aggressive in content, they are typically interpreted by anthropologists as metaphors for social-structural themes. A Bororo myth is interpreted differently by structuralists and psychoanalysts.

1382. Spitzer RL, Gibbon M, Skodol A, Williams JBW, Hyler S: The heavenly vision of a poor woman: a down-to-earth discussion of the DSM-III differential diagnosis. J Operational Psychiatry 11:169–72, 1980.

While hysterical psychosis does not appear in DSM-III, two categories—brief reactive psychosis and factitious disorder with psychological symptoms—are roughly equivalent to it and may be applied to the case under consideration.

1383. Stack S: The effects of interstate migration on suicide. Intl J Social Psychiatry 26:17–25, 1980.

Stress, frustration, and feelings of uprootedness often associated with long-distance migration contribute not only to suicide among international migrants, but also among interstate migrants.

1384. Stankov L: Some experiences with the F-scale in Yugoslavia. Brit J Social Clinical Psychology 16:111–21, 1977.

Use of the F-scale in Yugoslavia delivers results that are more culturally based than politically based.

1385. Staples F, Yamamoto J, Wollson F, Kline F, Burgoyne R, Hattem J, Rice R: Cultural problems in psychiatric therapy: 9 years later. Comp Med East West 6:137–42, 1978.

Minority patients tend to receive the same type of treatment as Caucasians and to show equal benefit from it in the judgment of their therapist.

1386. Steadman HJ, Cocozza JJ: Public perceptions of the criminally insane. Hosp Community Psychiatry 29:457–59, 1978.

The criminally insane are generally considered dangerous, harmful, and violent, and as a class they are feared and rejected by society far more than are the mentally ill.

1387. Stearns BC, Penner LA, Kimmel EK: Sexism among psychotherapists: a case not yet proven. J Consulting Clin Psychology 48:548–50, 1980.

There is little support for many of the widely held assumptions about sexism in psychotherapeutic practice.

1388. Steele RL: Dying, death, and bereavement among the Maya Indians of Mesoamerica: a study in anthropological psychology. Amer Psychologist 32:1060–68, 1977.

Death, dying, and bereavement are complex psychological and biosocial problems of twentieth-century Western civilization. Some earlier cultures and societies responded successfully to the phenomena of dying and death and the intense emotions attendant upon them. In the classical Maya civilization, the primary cultural controls over death, dying, and bereavement were myths and rituals that were accepted as truth.

1389. Steer RA, Shaw BF, Beck AT, Fine EW: Structure of depression in black alcoholic men. Psychological Reports 41:1235–41, 1977.

The dimensions of depression in black alcoholic men are similar to the dimensions of patients carrying primary diagnoses of depression.

1390. Stein HF: A dialectical model of health and illness attitudes and behavior among Slovak-Americans. Intl J Mental Health 5:117–37, 1976.

The role of "health" appears to be a culturally constituted defense cluster against the role and associated conflicts of "illness." The health-illness model is a single expression of the relation between norm and deviance, with each culture having its own markers or categories.

1391. Stein HF: Aging and death among Slovak-Americans: a study in the thematic unity of the life cycle. J Psychol Anthropology 1:297–320, 1978.

Aging, death, and coping with another's death among Slovak-Americans are symptomatic of the culture-specific conflict care embedded in the life cycle.

1392. Stein HF: The Slovak-American "swaddling ethos": homeostat for family dynamics and cultural continuity. Family Process 17:31–45, 1978.

The core of the swaddling ethos is a dependency-security complex that attaches the individual to an extended family network of obligation, indebtedness, and reciprocity, induces rebellion against outside attachment, and undermines efforts toward separation-individuation, resulting in the perpetuation of an ethnic tradition.

1393. Stein HF: The salience of ethno-psychology for medical education and practice. Social Science Medicine 13B(3):199–210, 1979.

Ethnopsychology, as one expression of community-psychology, cannot *a priori* be assumed to be either a vital or an inconsequential variable in a given patient. The social sciences could be taught with greater clinical effectiveness if the issues of ethnopsychology were to be explored in relation to the students' and practitioners' own lives, and, dialectically, as the student and practitioner experience and attempt to understand their patients' experiences.

1394. Stein SP, Holzman S, Karasu TB, Chair ES: Mid-adult development and psychotherapy. Amer J Psychiatry 135:676–81, 1978.

Significant differences exist between groups of psychiatric patients and nonpatients at specific ages in the areas of sense of self, feelings about careers and sex, and relationship to parents, children, and friends. Clinical evaluation and treatment planning based on traditional psychiatric symptom clusters and characterological assessments do not address the issues of continuing development, which are critical in arriving at a better-integrated understanding of patients.

1395. Steinglass P: Assessing families in their own homes. Amer J Psychiatry 137:1523–29, 1980.

Assessment of the family in its own home provides important information about the family's style of regulating its internal environment. The Home Observation Assessment Method measures dimensions of family behavior associated with routines of daily living that are highly correlative with traditional clinical measures of psychiatric symptomatology, severity of alcoholism, and family boundaries.

1396. Steinmetz SK: Women and violence: victims and perpetrators. Amer J Psychotherapy 34:334–50, 1980.

While women have been perpetrators of crime,

throughout history they have overwhelmingly been the victims. Female children are subjected to sexual abuse much more than males, and all forms of domestic violence have a greater impact on females, demonstrating the need to take into account the severity of the physical injury and emotional trauma suffered in the assessment of victimization.

1397. Stephens RC, McBride DC: Becoming a street addict. Human Organization 35:87–93, 1976.

Street addiction affects youngsters who not only grow up in a milieu where drug addicts are perceived as a distinct group, but also come to relate to this group when friends of theirs become addicted.

1398. Stephenson PH: Hutterite belief in evil eye: beyond paranoia and towards a general theory of invidia. Culture Medicine Psychiatry 3:247–65, 1979.

A general theory of invidia (envy) must confront the idea that envy may be a causal factor in human suffering and not merely an outcome of economic disenfranchisement. Invidia (envy) may be regarded as a disease and evil eye only one of its potential avenues for expression in various cultures. The connection between invidia and paranoia can be questioned by the analysis of Hutterian beliefs in evil eye in social interaction rather than retroductive explanation. In the case of the Hutterites, it is envy itself that is feared and linked to high anxiety levels and sometimes to anxiety attacks or depression.

1399. Stephenson PS, Walker GA: The psychiatrist-woman patient relationship. Canadian J Psychiatry 24:5–27, 1979.

The psychiatrist-woman patient relationship is affected by a number of powerful, yet often subtle, pressures. Any woman referred to a male psychiatrist is likely (1) to receive a psychiatric diagnosis that categorizes her problems as individual and intrapsychic, (2) to have the societal obstacles she faces ignored or minimized, and (3) to receive treatment geared to help her adapt to traditional expectations.

1400. Stevenson HW, Parker T, Wilkinson A, Bonnvaux B, Gonzalez M: Schooling, environment, and cognitive development: a cross-cultural study. Part 3. Results: Levels of performance of Peruvian children. Monographs Society Research Child Development 43:28–46, 1978.

Attendance at school is related to improvement in performance on tests of cognitive ability. Improvement is equivalent for both Lima and Lamas, Peru, for both Quechua Indians and mestizos of mixed Spanish-Indian background, and for each socioeconomic class.

1401. Stevenson HW, Parker T, Wilkinson A, Bonnvaux B, Gonzalez M: Schooling, environment, and cognitive development: a cross-cultural study. Part 4. Results: Patterns of performance in Peruvian children. Monographs Society Research Child Development 43:47–56, 1978.

Children who attend school in comparison to those who do not show (1) an elevation in average level of performance across a variety of memory and cognitive tasks, (2) somewhat reduced within-group variability on many of the tasks, and (3) increased within-child variability in performance across both memory and cognitive tasks.

1402. Stevenson I: Cases of the Reincarnation Type, Vol. 1. Charlottesville, U. Press of Virginia, 1975.

Ten possible cases of reincarnation in India are presented.

1403. Stevenson I: Cases of the Reincarnation Type, Vol. 2. Charlottesville, U. Press of Virginia, 1978.

Ten cases of possible reincarnation in Sri Lanka are presented.

1404. Stevenson IN: Colerina: reactions to emotional stress in the Peruvian Andes. Social Science Medicine 11:303–7, 1977.

Colerina is a culturally patterned response to intolerable emotion that evokes a therapeutic reaction from the local society.

1405. Stinner WF: Modernization and family extension in the Philippines: a social demographic analysis. J Marriage Family 41:161–70, 1979.

Modernization is positively associated with overall nonnuclear membership size but is differentially related to family components (spouse of child of head, grandchild of head, and parent of head and other relatives). Nonnuclear membership components have a differential impact on nonnuclear membership size and are differentially associated with each other. The effects of modernization on nonnuclear membership size are differentially transmitted across the respective components.

1406. Stoller RJ: A contribution to the study of gender identity: follow-up. Intl J Psychoanalysis 60:433–41, 1979.

A hermaphroditic male, who was reared as a female due to his female-appearing genitals but who behaved in a masculine manner from infancy, readily switched to a male role successfully when diagnosed as a genetic and physiologic male at the age of fourteen. A rare sex hormone enzyme defect had caused the anatomic hermaphroditism but allowed the prenatal androgen priming of the brain to occur.

1407. Stone L: The Family, Sex, and Marriage in England: 1500–1800. New York, Harper and Row, 1977.

The evolution of family structure, patterns of sexual behavior, mating arrangements, and child-rearing practices is traced. The emotionally bonded, sexually liberated, child-oriented family type of current times may be no more permanent than the many family types that preceded it.

1408. Stones CR: A Jesus community in South Africa: self-actualization or need for security? Psychological Reports 46:287–90, 1980.

Members of the Jesus movement in South Africa are usually other-directed and sociocentric. Although they report themselves as having changed from being inner-directed and individualistic prior to joining the movement, the reported changes may be the effect of rising expectations.

1409. Stones CR, Philbrick JL: Purpose in life in South Africa: a comparison of American and South African beliefs. Psychological Reports 47:739–42, 1980.

South African young people have a lesser sense of meaning in their lives prior to joining a religious group than do their American counterparts.

1410. Strassman RJ, Galanter M: The Abhidharma: a cross-cultural model for the psychiatric application of meditation. Intl J Social Psychiatry 26:293–99, 1980.

An empirically derived system dealing with the experimental phenomena of meditation has heuristic value for development of clinical application of consciousness-altering techniques.

1411. Stuart IR, Murgatroyd D, Denmark FL: Perceptual style, locus of control and personality variables among East Indians and blacks in Trinidad. Intl J Social Psychiatry 24:26–32, 1978.

The patterns of needs expressed by both groups may be traced to the history of the East Indians and blacks in Trinidad. Black interests in social activities tend to be related to their history as slaves. East Indian needs tend toward higher aggression, achievement, and endurance.

1412. Stubbe H: Zur ethnopsychiatrie in Brasilien. Social Psychiatry 14:187–95, 1979.

Although official psychiatry has hitherto maintained a distinctly negative attitude toward worship-oriented therapies of native Brazilian cults, a growing interest in these phenomena has developed in recent years, marking a trend toward the development of a transcultural, anthropologically based psychiatry.

1413. Studlar DT: Racial attitudes in Britain: a causal analysis. Ethnicity 6:107–22, 1979.

British beliefs about immigrants are acquired through social processes. Once one is able to identify the complexities of how individuals arrive at their attitudes toward immigrants, then it should be possible to discover the sources of those beliefs, and whether they are learned relatively early in life as has been suggested or whether they are largely the product of later experiences.

1414. Sue S, McKinney H: Asian Americans in the community mental health care system. Amer J Orthopsychiatry 45:111–18, 1975.

Far fewer Chinese, Filipinos, and Japanese utilize American community mental health facilities as compared to white patients in proportion to their numbers in the community. Asian-American patients are older, less educated, and have a higher proportion of individuals with a diagnosis of psychosis. The dropout rate for Asian patients is extremely high (52 percent), and they average a smaller number of treatment sessions.

1415. Sue S, Zane N, Ito J: Alcohol drinking patterns among Asian and Caucasian Americans. J Cross-Cultural Psychology 10:41–56, 1979.

Chinese and Japanese students report less alcohol consumption than do Caucasians.

1416. Sugarman AA, Tarter RE (eds): Expanding Dimensions of Consciousness. New York, Springer, 1978.

Topics discussed include hallucinogenic drugs, the electroencephalogram of ecstasy, oriental and occidental paths of enlightenment, bio-feedback and meditation as an adjunct to psychotherapy, hypnosis, and mysticism.

1417. Sutker PB, Archer RP, Allain AN: Psychopathology of drug abusers: sex and ethnic considerations. Intl J Addictions 15:605–13, 1980.

There are important very general differences in personality, motivation, drug use, and value-system characteristics between black and white drug abusers.

1418. Suwanlert S, Gates D: Epidemic koro in Thailand—clinical and social aspects. Transcult Psych Res Review 16:64–66, 1979.

Koro is a stereotyped response pattern, and the syndrome is similar in individual cases and in epidemic form. The same psychodynamic concerns may operate in both men and women. The syndrome can be induced in the absence of prior psychological conditioning or concerns about potency.

1419. Swantz ML: Community and healing among the Zaramo in Tanzania. Social Science Medicine 13B(3):169–73, 1979.

The Zaramo are an ethnic group in and around Dar-Es-Salaam (Tanzania) whose life-patterns have been affected by constant intercommunication between the city and the surrounding rural areas. The healers in rural areas still diagnose various illnesses and consequently prescribe communal forms of healing, while their city counterparts look for causes in terms of horizontal social relationships and resort to individualized treatment.

1420. Szapocynik J (ed): Mental Health, Drug and Alcohol Abuse: An Hispanic Assessment of Present and Future Challenges. Washington, D.C., COSSMHO, 1979.

Topics discussed include drug abuse and occupational alcoholism among Hispanics, and cultural barriers to the utilization of alcohol prorams by Hispanics in the United States.

1421. Szasz T: The Myth of Psychotherapy. Garden City, N.Y., Anchor, 1978.

Psychotherapy is merely a combination of religion, rhetoric, and repression.

1422. Taggart JM: Men's changing image of women in Nahuat oral tradition. Amer Ethnologist 6(4):723–41, 1979.

Comparison of cognate folk tales from two Sierra Nahuat communities in Mexico shows that storytellers alter competence and sexuality of their female characters when women improve their position in a male-dominant family system.

1423. Takahashi T: Adolescent symbiotic psychopathology: a cultural comparison of American and Japanese patterns and resolutions. Bull Menninger Clinic 44:272–88, 1980.

Cultural differences between Japan and the United States are derived from the different ways each culture has of outgrowing the stage of symbiosis, especially during the separation-individuation phase.

1424. Takano R: Anthropophobia and Japanese performance. Psychiatry 40:259–69, 1977.

Japanese mental disturbances have the same dynamic structure and, to some degree, exhibit the symptoms of anthropophobia (concern about one's appearance in the eyes of others). Japanese anthropophobia has its origin deep within Japanese culture and needs to be considered in the psychotherapy of Japanese mental patients.

1425. Tambiah SJ: The cosmological and performative significance of a Thai cult of healing through meditation. Culture Medicine Psychiatry 1:97–132, 1977.

Healing ritual acts cannot be fully understood except as part of a larger frame of cultural presuppositions and beliefs. Rituals also have a distinctive patterning and structure that enhances communication and the construction and experience of cultural and social reality.

1426. Tan ES: Mental health services for children in the Southeast Asian and Western Pacific regions. Intl J Mental Health 7:96–101, 1978.

Although in the more developed countries of this region, such as Australia and New Zealand, mental health services for children do exist, it can be said that such services are confined largely to the urban areas and are difficult to come by in the more outlying, rural areas.

1427. Tanaka-Matsumi J: Taijin kyofusho: diagnostic and cultural issues in Japanese psychiatry. Culture Medicine Psychiatry 3:231–45, 1979.

Examination by American mental health professionals of the diagnostic status of the Japanese syndrome of taijin kyofusho suggests symptoms associated with this syndrome are highly heterogeneous. The assertion in Japanese psychiatry that taijin kyofusho is a culture-specific syndrome needs further clarification to enhance cross-cultural understanding of these behaviors.

The prevailing concept of culture-bound disorders, which focuses predominantly on classification of symptoms, does not give us needed information about various sociocultural contexts of psychological problems.

1428. Tanaka-Matsumi J, Marsella AJ: Cross-cultural variations in the phenomenological experience of depression. Part 1: World association studies. J Cross-Cultural Psychology 7:379–96, 1976.

The differences in the response to the word "depression" by Japanese-nationals, Japanese-Americans, and Caucasian-Americans can be attributed to variations in the self-structure that mediates the subjective experience of depression in the different cultures.

1429. Tarighati S: An exploratory study on depression in Iranian addicts. Intl J Social Psychiatry 26:196–99, 1980.

Depression is one of the clinical symptoms of drug addiction in Iran.

1430. Taylor G: Demoniacal possession and psychoanalytic theory. Brit J Med Psychology 51:53–60, 1978.

Current trends in psychoanalysis recognize the deeper psychotic core behind many apparently neurotic illnesses and apply modified psychoanalytic treatment to borderline and psychotic patients. The phenomenon of demoniacal possession contributes much to the understanding of borderline and psychotic states.

1431. Taylor RL: Psychosocial development among black children and youth: a reexamination. Amer J Orthopsychiatry 46:4–19, 1976.

Review of the literature reveals that the fundamental assumptions and empirical evidence upon which conventional views of the nature and meaning of black self-esteem are based are not supported. More recent sophisticated studies indicate that there are no demonstrable differences in self-esteem between blacks and whites.

1432. Tcheng-Laroche F, Prince RH: Middle income, divorced female heads of families. Canadian J Psychiatry 24:35–42, 1979.

The role of head of family is perfectly acceptable for many economically viable women. Women as head of family enjoy good health and normal stress levels and are generally positive about being head of the family. On the negative side, loneliness, absence of the father, and limited social lives are most often problems.

1433. Teja JS: Mental illness and the family in America and India. Intl J Social Psychiatry 24:225–31, 1978.

The American cultural emphasis on individuation and role adequacy is reflected in a much higher incidence of adjustment reactions and personality disorders among American patients than among Indian patients.

1434. Teoh J, Soewondo S, Sidharta M: Epidemic hysteria in Malaysian schools: an illustrative episode. Psychiatry 38:258–68, 1975.

Epidemic hysteria has been endemic in predominantly rural Malay schools in Malaysia from time immemorial. A complex interweaving of psychological, religious, cultural, and sociological factors are involved in the precipitation of an outbreak.

1435. Teplin LA: A comparison of racial/ethnic preferences among Anglo, black, and Latino children. Amer J Orthopsychiatry 46:702–9, 1976.

Black and Anglo children prefer photographs of their own group children, but Latinos prefer photographs of Anglo children over their own. The present-day Latino child can be viewed as being similar to the black of ten years ago.

1436. Terechek R: The psychoanalytic basis of Gandhi's politics. Psychoanalytic Review 62:225–37, 1975.

Gandhi's political relevance is directly related to the viability of his psychological theories. If man's psyche is invariably characterized by some need to express aggression, then the politics of coercion and violence is necessary. But Gandhi reminds us that if man is best understood as a being who seeks a sense of worth and positive interpersonal relations, then coercion is an inappropriate modality of politics.

1437. Terrace HS: Nim. New York, Alfred Knopf, 1979.

Although the findings are ambiguous, great effort was spent in attempting to teach a chimpanzee to communicate and to form sentences.

1438. Thacore VR, Gupta SC: Faith healing in a north Indian city. Intl J Social Psychiatry 24:235–40, 1978.

The primitive belief that illness and misfortunes result from infringement of taboos or from intervention of supernatural forces exists even today in many cultures. Consequently, in order to guard against and vitiate such influences, magic, sorcery, and rituals are resorted to with the help of native healers.

1439. Thacore VR, Gupta SC, Suraiya M: Psychiatric mobility in a north Indian community. Brit J Psychiatry 126:364–69, 1975.

In a north Indian urban community, mental illness is significantly higher in the age group twenty-six to sixty-five years among the married compared to unmarried, and among those holding semiskilled and unskilled jobs. Most patients suffer from neurosis, alcoholism, mental retardation, and nocturnal enuresis.

1440. Thanaphum S: Social psychiatric implications of population control in Thailand. Mental Health Society 3:190–93, 1976.

Contraceptive services can be a significant addition to preventive psychiatric services in the areas of poverty, overpopulation, premarital pregnancy, and illegitimacy. Psychiatrists and other mental health personnel should be available as consultants and encourage group members to become interested in the need for population control.

1441. Thernstrom S (ed): Harvard Encyclopedia of American Ethnic Groups. Cambridge, Mass., Harvard U. Press, 1980.

American ethnic groups are described and characterized by geographic origin; migratory states; race; language or dialect; religion; ties that transcend kinship, neighborhood, and community boundaries; shared traditions, values, and symbols; literature, folklore, and music; food preferences; settlement and employment patterns; political interests; institutions; and internal sense of distinctiveness.

1442. Thomas DR: Cooperation and competition among Polynesian and European children. Child Development 46:948–53, 1975.

Cook Islands children and rural New Zealand Maori children are more cooperative in problem-solving situations than European and urban Maori children. Older children and boys among these groups are more cooperative than younger children and girls.

1443. Thompson KS: A comparison of black and white adolescents' beliefs about having children. J Marriage Family 42:133–40, 1980.

Both black males and females express stronger belief than whites that having children promotes greater marital success, personal security, and approval from others. Black couples also believe that they should have as many children as they

wish. Females of both ethnic groups perceive themselves as exposed to stronger social pressures to have children than are males.

1444. Thompson RH: Ethnicity versus class: an analysis of conflict in a North American Chinese community. Ethnicity 6:306–26, 1979.

The fundamental change in social organization of Toronto's Chinese community has come about through a proliferation of new and functionally differentiated Chinese statuses and roles. In spite of modernizing processes that have reduced the scope of class conflict and confined its expression to more restricted contexts that have diminished the "revolutionary" character of classes, Marx's theory of class is essentially correct and can be usefully applied to the analysis of conflict in industrial society.

1445. Thompson SK: Gender labels and early sex role development. Child Development 46:339–47, 1975.

Three year olds, to a greater extent than children six and twelve months younger, can apply gender labels properly, are certain of their own gender, use same-sex gender labels to guide behavior, and are aware of sex-role stereotyping.

1446. Thompson WR: Cross-cultural uses of biological data and perspectives. In Handbook of Cross-Cultural Psychology, edited by HC Triandis and WW Lambert, 1:205–52. Boston, Allyn and Bacon, 1980.

Cross-cultural psychology and neo-Darwinian biology share some major commitments. The intrinsic and extrinsic mechanisms that produce evolutionary change have considerable bearing on cultural variation. Some psychological areas of particular interest in this connection are intelligence, mental illness, and color vision. Relevant work on these is discussed.

1447. Tiffany SW (ed): Women and Society. Montreal, Eden, 1979.

Ethnographic case studies of women are presented, with a focus on sex roles.

1448. Tinbergen EA, Tinbergen N: The aetiology of childhood autism: a rejoinder to criticism by Wing and Ricks. Psychological Medicine 6:545–49, 1976.

The disagreement is not so much a matter of facts per se as one of how to look at the problems. The primary aim of what we have written has been to sketch a method of approach, to illustrate its potential, and to advocate the application of this approach in child psychiatry.

1449. Titchener JL, Kapp FT: Family and character change at Buffalo Creek. Amer J Psychiatry 133:295–99, 1976.

Traumatic neurotic reactions were found in 80 percent of the survivors of the 1972 Buffalo Creek dam disaster. Two years after the disaster, the clinical picture of unresolved grief, survivor shame, and feelings of impotent rage and helplessness—the "Buffalo Creek syndrome"—persisted.

1450. Toch H: Living in Prison: The Ecology of Survival. New York, Free Press, 1978.

Interviews with inmates illustrate how they perceive their prison environment.

1451. Tolsdorf CC: Social networks, support, and coping: an exploratory study. Family Process 15:407–17, 1976.

The network model can be used to investigate the larger social system with which individuals interact. It can also be a valuable approach to the expansion of family research.

1452. Tomak AK: The Family and Sex Roles. Toronto, Holt, Rinehart & Winston of Canada, 1975.

Role learning, with special emphasis on traditional and changing female roles, is examined in Canada, Western Europe, Japan, and the Middle East.

1453. Torki MA: Validation of the MMPI MF Scale in Kuwait. Psychological Reports 47:1152–54, 1980.

Item validity with the MMPI should be studied when tests developed in one culture are to be used in another culture, since the cultures may attach different meanings to particular items.

1454. Torres-Matrullo C: Acculturation and psychopathology among Puerto Rican women in mainland United States. Amer J Orthopsychiatry 46:710–19, 1976.

A significant correlation exists between level of acculturation and education and both personality adjustment and psychopathology among Puerto Rican women in the United States. There is still respect for and adherence to traditional family-related values in Puerto Rican women.

1455. Torrey EF: Schizophrenia and Civilization. New York, Jason Aronson, 1980.

As evidenced by epidemiological and anthropological studies, schizophrenia is unevenly distributed, e.g., it is more common in India among members of higher castes, and in Papua New Guinea it is more common in areas that have had longer contact with Western civilization.

1456. Totman J: The murderess: a psychosocial study of criminal homicide. San Francisco, R & E Research Associates, 1978.

Women may murder their mates and children when their relationship with the mate or child is directly and overtly destructive to them and their sense of identity, when they cannot share their concerns and get support, when they have exhausted all other courses of action, and when they have redefined and reinterpreted their negative situation so that it calls for action not previously considered possible. An understanding of murder and female criminality includes a focus on sex roles and their relationship to social structure.

1457. Tousignant M: Espanto: a dialogue with the gods. Culture Medicine Psychiatry 3:347–61, 1979.

Espanto or susto (a folk illness in Mexico) cannot be conceived of as a syndrome in the medical sense. A semilogical analysis shows that espanto can better be described as an indigenous theory whose function is to relate illness events to other levels of reality.

1458. Townsend JM: Cultural conceptions and mental illness. J Nerv Ment Disease 160:409–21, 1975.

German patients generally agree that mental illness is a biologically determined and rather incurable condition. In contrast, American patients generally believe that the individual is partially responsible for his condition and with the proper motivation and help can improve. Institutionalization consists more in conditioning the patient to accept his status than in convincing him he is insane.

1459. Townsend JM: Cultural Conceptions and Mental Illness. Chicago, U. of Chicago Press, 1978.

The social-role approach to mental illness is contrasted with the clinical universalist approach in a study comparing German and American mental patients, mental-hospital staff, and high-school students.

1460. Townsend JM: Cultural conceptions and the role of the psychiatrist in Germany and America. Intl J Social Psychiatry 24:250–58, 1978.

The role of the psychiatrist in each culture seems to reflect basic cultural conceptions of mental disorders. Germans tend to view mental disorders as endogenous in origin, relatively incurable, and less subject to environmental influence than do Americans.

1461. Townsend JM: Stereotypes of mental illness: a comparison with ethnic stereotypes. Culture Medicine Psychiatry 3:205–29, 1979.

Popular and professional conceptions of mental illness share specific traits with ethnic stereotypes in that (1) they are exaggerated and serve to erect a qualitative boundary where none objectively exists, (2) they are maintained through selective perception, rationalization, and sanctions, (3) they help to erect the "thresholds," i.e., the criteria, for crossing or recrossing the boundary, and (4) they serve to define relations, including those of power, between groups. Because they perform these important cognitive and conative functions, they persist despite a flow of personnel across them and despite repeated demonstrations of their inaccuracy. They cannot be expected to change until the actual relations between groups change.

1462. Townsend JM, Carbone CL: Menopausal syndrome: illness or social role—a transcultural analysis. Culture Medicine Psychiatry 4:229–48, 1980.

Examination of evidence including cross-cultural and intracultural variations of "menopausal syndrome," to test the thesis that menopausal syndrome is largely a social role foisted on middle-aged women in this society, indicates that the more psychological and psychosomatic symptoms do vary with cultural role expectations.

1463. Tramer L, Boran S: Problems associated with culture contact in the psychotherapeutic setting: disparity of expectations between the Western-trained therapist and the non-Western therapist. Mental Health Society 3:182–89, 1976.

In a group of lower-class French-speaking North Africans receiving treatment at a community mental health center in Israel, there is fundamental disparity between patients' and therapists' expectations from therapy. Patients expect quick relief and regard themselves as passive recipients. Therapists expect active participation from patients and view treatment as a slow process.

1464. Trevino FM, Bruhn JG: Incidence of mental illness in a Mexican-American community. Psychiatric Annals 7(12):33–51, 1977.

The largest users of the Laredo, Texas, Community Mental Health Center are single males and females between fifteen and fifty-nine. Most male patients are diagnosed as schizophrenic, have alcohol or drug problems, or have transient situational behavioral disorders. Most female patients are diagnosed as neurotic. This profile would be helpful in assessing the need for therapeutic and preventive programs in Laredo and has applicability in other Mexican-American communities.

1465. Triandis HC (ed): Handbook of Cross-Cultural Psychology.Vol. 1: Perspectives, ed. with WW Lambert; Vol. 2: Methodology, ed. with JW Berry; Vol. 3: Basic Processes, ed. with W Lonner; Vol. 5: Social Psychology, ed. with RW Brislin; Vol. 6: Psychopathology, ed. with JG Draguns. Boston, Allyn and Bacon, 1980.

This work is a collection of articles, each of which has been entered separately in this bibliography. (Volume 4 was published in 1981).

1466. Triandis HC (ed): Variations in Black and White Perceptions of the Social Environment. Urbana, U. of Illinois Press, 1976.

The development of more effective job training and retention programs for the hardcore unemployed involves teaching white supervisors to see the world as black workers see it, and vice versa.

1467. Trost J: Attitudes toward and occurrence of cohabitation without marriage. J Marriage Family 40:393–400, 1978.

Opinion among the Swedes is that there is a higher commitment and a higher responsibility among those having been married for a long time than among those having been married for a short time. Also, there is a higher degree of commitment and responsibility among those having been married for five years than among those having been living together out of wedlock for five years.

1468. Trotter RT, Chavira JA: Curanderismo: an emic theoretical perspective of Mexican-American folk medicine. Medical Anthropology 4:423–87, 1980.

Interviews with midwives, herbalists, sobadores (persons who treat sprains and muscle aches), and curanderos reveal supernatural treatments are reserved for complex illnesses such as susto, empacho, and caida de mollera. Curanderismo has three levels of organization: material (physical manipulation and home remedies), spiritual, and mental (focusing of mental vibrations). The concept of energy is central to the diagnosis and treatment of all illness. Rituals include the barrida, sahumerio, sorfilegios, and velaciones.

1469. Trumback R: The Rise of the Egalitarian Family. New York, Academic, 1978.

Between 1690 and 1780 romantic love was increasingly accepted as justification for marriage in England. Women returned to breast-feeding their own children, and more attention was paid to child health.

1470. Tseng WS: The nature of somatic complaints among psychiatric patients: the Chinese case. Comp Psychiatry 16:237–45, 1975.

It is very important for the psychiatrist to be aware of and therapeutically oriented toward the deeper meaning of the patient's somatic complaints, rather than remaining confined to the literal problems as presented by the patient. Most Chinese patients may use less differentiated patterns of expressing affective problems. Such somatic ways of expressing problems can be understood variously from a sociocultural point of view.

1471. Tseng WS, Hsu J: Minor psychological disturbances of everyday life. In Handbook of Cross-Cultural Psychology, edited by HC Triandis and JG Draguns, 6:61–97. Boston, Allyn and Bacon, 1980.

Severe clinical psychopathology manifested in psychoses is caused by multiple factors with a great deal of biological influence, which makes the study of the cultural contribution relatively difficult. By contrast, the minor pathologies observed in daily life are more closely related to the psychological aspect, as well as the sociological aspect, and such behavior is worth studying as a projection of cultural traits.

1472. Tseng WS, McDermott JF: Psychotherapy: historical roots, universal elements and cultural variations. Amer J Psychiatry 132:378–84, 1975.

The development of psychotherapy is traced from the supernatural world to the natural world to the physical person and then to the psychological person. The various forms of psychotherapy share fundamental elements of treatments, modified by cultural factors.

1473. Tseng WS, McDermott JF, Maretzki T: Adjustment in Intercultural Marriage. Honolulu, U. Press of Hawaii, 1977.

Marriage between persons from different cultural backgrounds may result in adjustment problems. Therapists must be aware of cultural stereotypes, value systems, nonverbal communication, and differences in male-female roles.

1474. Tsoi WF, Kok LP, Long FY: Male transsexualism in Singapore: a description of 56 cases. Brit J Psychiatry 131:405–9, 1977.

Male transsexualism in Singapore does not refer to the same condition as described by different authors. Etiologically these cases are not determined by early childhood experiences.

1475. Tsunoda T: Difference in the mechanism of emotion in Japanese and Westerner. Psychotherapy Psychosomatics 31:367–72, 1979.

Cerebral hemisphere dominance of steady-state vowels and human emotional and natural sounds differs between Japanese and Westerners, with the Japanese showing a verbal hemisphere dominance, while the Westerner shows a nonverbal hemisphere dominance. The theory of mental structure and vowels states that such a difference in the brain is related to emotional activities and forms the starting point of mental structure and culture. The emotional stimulation of human olfaction is used to confirm this theory.

1476. Turiel E, Edwards CP, Kohlberg L: Moral development in Turkish children, adolescents, and young adults. J Cross-Cultural Psychology 9:75–86, 1978.

The stage sequence of development for all three Turkish groups is the same as has been previously found for other Western and non-Western groups.

1477. Turner V: Revelation and Divination in Ndembu Ritual. Ithaca, N.Y., Cornell U. Press, 1975.

Ndembu diviners, in order to discover the causes of death, illness, or other misfortune, interrogate involved persons and make use of divining icons. Chihamba is a cult of affliction; in a ritual of this cult, a male demigod is revealed to the patients, who are eventually declared healed.

1478. Tutt N (ed): Violence. London, Her Majesty's Stationery Office, 1976.

Topics discussed include historical perspectives of violence, violence in the home and family, aggression in the community, and social values of aggression.

1479. Tyhurst L: Psychosocial first aid for refugees. Mental Health Society 4:319–43, 1977.

The social dynamics that occur in each of the refugee entry situations in Canada and that form the background of the social displacement syndrome are discussed. A specific project of direct aid to incoming refugees designed and carried out by consultant social psychiatrists is outlined, as are generalizations concerning the principles of "psychosocial first aid" for refugees.

1480. Udai P, Venkateswara RT: Cross-cultural surveys and interviewing. In Handbook of Cross-Cultural Psychology, edited by HC Triandis and JW Berry, 2:127–79. Boston, Allyn and Bacon, 1980.

Two main problems in the use of surveys are those of comparability and proper sampling design. Interviewing will continue to be the most-used research method since in several cultures people are not literate enough to answer mail questionnaires and such questionnaires are alien to these cultures.

1481. Uecker AE, Boutilier LR, Richardson EH: "Indianism" and MMPI scores of men alcoholics. J Stud Alcohol 41:357–62, 1980.

Indians with at least as severe addiction as whites show slightly less evidence of psychiatric disorders on the MMPI. The psychopathology that Indians do reveal indicates neuroticism primarily. Indians who identify more strongly with their own culture experience more conflict between their need to retain their Indian identity and their need to adjust to the dominant culture, thus producing neurotic symptoms. Caution is advised in using the MMPI in the diagnosis of Indians' psychiatric problems.

1482. Umbenhauer SL, DeWitte LL: Patient race and social class: attitudes and decisions among three groups of mental health professionals. Comp Psychiatry 19:509–15, 1978.

Social class bias continues to be a pervasive phenomenon among psychiatrists, psychologists, and social workers. Neither racial nor social class biases are greater at later stages of professional training than at earlier stages or for those who have completed training than for those still in training.

1483. Ungerleider JT, Wellisch DK: Coercive persuasion (brainwashing), religious cults, and deprogramming. Amer J Psychiatry 136:279–82, 1979.

Cult members who strayed or dropped out after deprogramming were found to be legally competent. Forceable removal from any group that they have belonged to for more than one year is exceedingly difficult. People who continue to be cult members have difficulty with impulse control and use cults as an externalized superego. Those who leave the cult have trouble with social and emotional alienation and lack of ego mastery.

1484. Ungerleider JT, Wellisch DK: Cultism, thought control and deprogramming: observations on a phenomenon. Psychiatric Opinion 16:10–15, 1979.

Psychological assessment of young cult members who are abducted and resist deprogramming indicates that these people have difficulty with management of aggressive impulses, have strong dependency needs, and have histories of difficulties in social relations. Group membership supplies formalized external controls and interpersonal constancy and approval.

1485. Uzoka AF: Willingness of Nigerian university students to accept psychological treatment. Social Psychiatry 15:123–26, 1980.

There is a need to be cognizant of the possible impact of a stated or implied treatment goal on the acceptance of psychological treatment among university-educated patients in Africa.

1486. Vaillant GE: Natural history of male psychological health. Part 3: Empirical dimensions of mental health. Arch Gen Psychiatry 32:420–26, 1975.

Relatively objective items such as length of vacation, divorce, heavy use of mood-altering drugs, career dissatisfaction, and visits to medical physicians can—as a cluster—statistically identify the abstract concept of mental health. Mental health may be defined as a continuum.

1487. Vaillant GE: Natural history of male psychological health. Part 5: The relation of choice of ego mechanisms of defense to adult adjustment. Arch Gen Psychiatry 33:535–45, 1976.

In order to conceptualize the continuum that underlies mental health, identification of a person's dominant defensive styles may be superior to the current scheme of static unitary diagnoses.

1488. Vaillant GE: Natural history of male psychological health. Part 6: Correlates of successful marriage and fatherhood. Amer J Psychiatry 135:653–59, 1978.

Objective measures of good object relations are reliable among raters, stable over time, and powerfully correlated with alternative measures of mental health and maturity. The capacity for object relations exists as an autonomous personality dimension, akin to intelligence or music talent. Capacity to love is as strongly associated with subsequent physical as with subsequent mental health.

1489. Valentine CA, Valentine B: Brain damage and the intellectual defense of inequality. Current Anthropology 16:117–50, 1975.

The learned debate about the nature of inequality in class and ethnically stratified societies is a spurious controversy. One key underlying idea shared among seemingly opposed experts is that the position of the oppressed stems from their own weaknesses. There is grave danger that this orthodoxy will be employed to justify extreme oppression ranging from mass drug programs to psychosurgery for controlling rebellious groups.

1490. van den Berghe P: Human Family Systems: An Evolutionary View. New York, Elsevier, 1979.

Cross-cultural variations in systems of kinship and marriage are based on sociobiology.

1491. van den Berghe P, Barash DP: Inclusive fitness and human family structure. Amer Anthropologist 79:809–23, 1977.

Kin-selection theory provides a model to formulate testable hypotheses predicting cooperation and conflict for categories of kinsmen. It also suggests an alternative way of looking at incest, endogamy, exogamy, rules of descent, and type of marriage.

1492. Vandewiele M: How Senegalese secondary school students feel about Euro-African mixed marriage. Psychological Reports 46:789–90, 1980.

An accommodating attitude toward interracial marriage is present among young Senegalese, with about a third of those interviewed being in favor of such a marriage.

1493. Vandewiele M: Wishes of Senegalese secondary school students. Psychological Reports 46:256–58, 1980.

The wishes of high school students in Senegal are basically related to the socioeconomic and cultural environment of their country. The traditional ethics of mutual solidarity and responsibility toward the parents constrains the youth's desire for more independence and an individual destiny.

1494. Van Wormer KS: Sex Role Behavior in a Women's Prison: An Ethological Analysis. San Francisco, R & E Research Associates, 1978.

Observation of interaction among female inmates in a prison classroom reveals a wide range of masculine and feminine behavior with a heavy leaning on the feminine end of the continuum. The observations call into question recent claims that male and female behavior is actually very similar. The implication of the study is that if females in a prison classroom manifest such striking personality differences, how much greater would the difference be in a group composed of men as well as women?

1495. Vassiliou G: Problems in Greece—and the world over. Psychiatric Opinion 12(7):6–13, 1975.

A comparison of Greek psychiatrists' experience with other psychiatrists from countries undergoing a similar phase of the "modernization" process indicates more or less parallel attitudes and problems. The "comparative" enumeration of cases labeled as schizophrenia and so on, with statistics that largely compare entities not amenable to comparisons, becomes meaningless. If psychosocial functioning and malfunctioning are the outcome of the transaction of all processes operating in each milieu, then it is this transaction that we have to learn to regulate in ways enhancing functioning and reducing malfunctioning.

1496. Vayda AP: War in Ecological Perspective. New York, Plenum, 1976.

As exemplified by the Maring of New Guinea, the Maori of New Zealand, and the Iban of Borneo, a pattern of violent conflict —regardless of the nature of the original injuries to which the offended group responds —is an adaptive mechanism that ensures the exploitation of needed resources by an expanding population.

1497. Veith I: Psychiatric foundations in the Far East. Psychiatric Annals 8(6):12–41, 1978.

In China, group therapy takes place not necessarily as a treatment of choice but rather because there still are not enough specialists to take care of each patient, despite the proliferation of psychiatry in China.

1498. Velimirovic B (ed): Modern Medicine and Medical Anthropology in the U.S.-Mexico Border Population. Pan Amer Health Organ Scientific Pub #359, 1978.

Topics discussed include susto, curanderismo, espiritismo, new models for alcohol counseling, lay healing and mental health, and the integration of indigenous and Western medicine.

1499. Verdonk A: Migration and mental illness. Intl J Social Psychiatry 25:295–305, 1979.

The rate of population admissions with a specific diagnosis is often higher for certain groups of immigrants than for the native people.

1500. Verinis JS: Maternal and child pathology in an urban ghetto. J Clin Psychology 32:13–15, 1976.

There is no relationship between maternal pathology and child disturbance for black middle- and working-class families.

1501. Vignes AJ, Hall RCW: Adjustment of a group of Vietnamese people to the United States. Amer J Psychiatry 136:442–44, 1979.

Vietnamese refugees have generally adjusted well without losing their cultural identity. The major sociological stresses in people who have difficulty in adjusting are loss of role identity and self-esteem, prejudice, and suspicion of helping agencies and the United States government.

1502. Vincent MO: Christianity and psychiatry: rivals or allies. Canadian Psychiatric Assn J 20:527–32, 1975.

The science of man and Christian faith are complimentary rather than competitive. Human thinking, feeling, and acting may be described at many levels—psychological, social, physical, or theological. An exhaustive description on one level does not preclude meaningful descriptions on other levels.

1503. Visher JS, Visher EB: Impressions of psychiatric problems and their management: China 1977. Amer J Psychiatry 136:29–32, 1979.

Mental illness in China is effectively treated in large mental hospitals with a mixture of Western psychotropic medications, traditional Chinese medicine, and group therapy. Personal, political, and cultural stresses continue to be responsible for emotional conflicts and symptoms in spite of the success of the Chinese social experiment.

1504. Viukari M, Elosuo R, Tierala R: Mental health services for the elderly living in the community in Finland. Intl J Mental Health 8:76–100, 1979–1980.

There are problems and shortcomings in mental health services for the elderly in Fin-

land, as almost everywhere. A lack of coordination and understanding among agencies has left serious gaps in services and resulted in inappropriate use of existing facilities for the aged.

1505. Vizedom MB: An encounter as a rite of passage. Amer Anthropologist 78:897–98, 1976.

A series of sensitivity or encounter sessions for the staff of a residential treatment center for disturbed boys can be regarded as a rite of passage.

1506. Vlassoff C: Unmarried adolescent females in rural India: a study of the social impact of education. J Marriage Family 42:427–36, 1980.

While education is linked to more modern attitudes and greater knowledge, considerable traditionalism prevails even among the most educated adolescents in rural India. The present rural school system is of limited relevance to female adolescents in India.

1507. Volkan V: Cyprus—War and Adaptation. Charlottesville, U. of Virginia Press, 1979.

Psychoanalytic theory, particularly that of internalized object relations as it relates to group conflict, sheds light on the struggles between Greeks and Turks on Cyprus.

1508. Volkan VD: Symptom formations and character changes due to upheavals of war: examples from Cyprus. Amer J Psychotherapy 33:239–62, 1979.

Aggression paradoxically increases self-esteem, and hostility between groups can be traced to the perception that the survival of the self or self-esteem is threatened. The development of group narcissism to compensate for the hurt that developed after the 1974 war on Cyprus illustrates this.

1509. VonElm B, Hirschman C: Age at first marriage in Peninsular Malaysia. J Marriage Family 41:877–91, 1979.

The average age at marriage in Peninsular Malaysia has risen from 18.5 years in 1947 to 22.3 years in 1970. Substantial differentials in age at first marriage are associated with ethnicity, years of formal schooling, and premarital work experience, while lesser differences are observed for social and geographic origins.

1510. Waddell JO: For individual power and social credit: the use of alcohol among Tucson Papagos. Human Organization 34:9–15, 1975.

Drinking among the Papagos serves both to maintain a system of social credit and egalitarian economics and to provide a means whereby individuals can attain personal power in an otherwise egalitarian social system.

1511. Walker KN, MacBride A, Vachon MLS: Social support networks and the crisis of bereavement. Social Science Medicine 11:35–41, 1977.

There is often a lack of fit between the social and psychological needs of the individual in crisis and the individual's social support network. Unless the person experiencing bereavement or other crisis is severely stressed and in need of intensive treatment, the mental health professional may be most effective by adjusting the fit between individual needs and network support structure.

1512. Walls PD, Walls LH, Langsley DG: Psychiatric training and practice in the People's Republic of China. Amer J Psychiatry 132:121–28, 1975.

The history of psychiatric treatment in China is traced, with emphasis on the years after 1949. Chinese psychiatric theory emphasizes sociopolitical factors, merging the patient's ego with the collective ego.

1513. Walsh B, Walsh D, Whelan B: Suicide in Dublin. Part 2: The influence of some social and medical factors on coroners' verdicts. Brit J Psychiatry 126:309–12, 1975.

Coroners' verdicts on cases of suicides in Ireland are based upon evidence of intent of self-inflicted death. Those who died by cutting, hanging, drugs, or gas are significantly more likely to receive a suicide verdict than those whose deaths are due to drowning, jumping, shooting, or poisoning.

1514. Walsh N: Psychiatry in the People's Republic of China. Psychiatric Annals 8(6):42–63, 1978.

Chinese society does provide a high degree of consensus and creates homogeneous social attitudes. Despite this, patients do become seriously ill and require hospitalization. However, the small number of psychiatrists and beds in relation to the vast population suggests that the Chinese have developed community care to a successful degree.

1515. Walstedt JJ: Reform of women's roles and family structures in the recent history of China. J Marriage Family 40:379–92, 1978.

Although the People's Republic of China has fallen far short of its own goal of a classless society in which women are equal with men, the general thrust over the years has been in the direction of improving women's status. Full equality in marriage and in the larger society will not come in China until many more women have a voice in their own destiny.

1516. Walters WE: Community psychiatry in Tutuila, American Samoa. Amer J Psychiatry 134:917–19, 1977.

Underreporting of mental illness in Tutuila is due to a social system that cures mental disorders by family group process and shamanistic rituals, making such disorders less disruptive and absolving the affected individual of personal guilt.

1517. Wanberg K, Lewis R, Foster FM: Alcoholism and ethnicity: a comparative study of alcohol use patterns across ethnic groups. Intl J Addictions 13:1245–62, 1978.

American Indian, black, Hispanic, and Anglo groups all appear to be experiencing significant disruption in social and vocational areas, with the American Indian group revealing greater social and alcohol symptom disruption than the other three groups.

1518. Ward C: Therapeutic aspects of exorcism. Transcult Psych Res Review 16:82–83, 1979.

Exorcism among Pentecostals in Trinidad functions primarily as a placebo providing some relief for the individual and catharsis for the congregation as a whole.

1519. Ward C, Beaubrun M: Trance induction and hallucination in spiritualist Baptist mourning. J Psychol Anthropology 2:479–88, 1979.

Spiritual Baptist mourning rites differ from many altered states of consciousness in that they are naturally occurring, self-induced, and used to achieve spiritual fulfillment. The encounters offer social and therapeutic advantages, with increased prestige in the church and short-term tension release and anxiety reduction.

1520. Ward JA, Fox J: A suicide epidemic on an Indian reserve. Canadian Psychiatric Assn J 22:423–26, 1977.

The social conditions of acculturation, cultural conflict, negative self-image, loss of extended family, and alcohol misuse creating a state of anomie can cause an epidemic of suicide in an Indian community.

1521. Ware H: Polygyny: women's views in a transitional society, Nigeria 1975. J Marriage Family 41:185–95, 1979.

In Nigeria there are no clear-cut divisions

between monogynous and polygynous marriages, possibly because nearly all marriages are potentially polygynous. Wives in polygynous marriages may have greater autonomy because they have less invested in the marriage and because, in losing part of their husbands' economic and moral support, they also gain independence. Many Yoruba women do not value their husbands very highly.

1522. Warner R: Deception in shamanism and psychiatry. Transnational Mental Health Res Newsletter 18:2, 6–12, 1976.

As exemplified by a visit to a Huichol Indian shaman, native healers often practice deception (such as hiding objects in their mouths that they then pretend to suck out of the patient) in order to impress and to cure patients. Some of these deceptive practices resemble those practiced by psychiatrists.

1523. Warner R: Witchcraft and soul loss: implications for community psychiatry. Hosp Community Psychiatry 28:686–90, 1977.

Mental health centers can be made more relevant to Chicanos by providing such services as home visits and family therapy.

1524. Warner R: Racial and sexual bias in psychiatric diagnosis, psychiatrists and other mental health professionals compared by race, sex, and discipline. J Nerv Ment Disease 167(5):303–10, 1979.

Minimal racial bias is observed among mental health professionals in psychiatric diagnosis. Hysterical and antisocial personality disorders are sex-biased diagnoses; race of the therapist also influences diagnosis. Therapists are more likely to make judgments biased against patients who are of the same race and sex as themselves.

1525. Warner R: Deception and self-deception in shamanism and psychiatry. Intl J Social Psychiatry 26:41–52, 1980.

Both shamans and psychiatrists are obliged to use a degree of self-deception in assuming their roles. The shaman must rationalize his use of trickery to impress his patients, and the psychiatrist deceives himself that his psychotherapeutic techniques have specific healing properties in the face of evidence that suggests that he often merely mobilizes the general effects of placebo and suggestion.

1526. Warnes H: Cultural factors in Irish psychiatry. Transcult Psych Res Review 16:100–103, 1979.

Irish society resembles Lewis's "culture of poverty." For Irish persons self-disclosure is more likely to be accepted in the confessional or in a pub than in a psychiatrist's office. An authoritarian doctor-patient relationship is desired but often leads to pseudocompliance and to acute crises that arouse shame, helplessness, injury to pride, anger, and mistrust.

1527. Warren DM: The interpretation of change in a Ghanaian ethnomedical study. Human Organization 37:73–77, 1978.

Change among the Bono of Ghana is a process of accommodation of ideas and institutions introduced into the indigenous cultural structure rather than a process of conflict between the traditional and modern elements of the population.

1528. Warren MA: The Nature of Woman. Point Reyes, Calif., Edgepress, 1980.

Women's issues are discussed as encyclopedia entries, and an extensive guide to the literature is presented.

1529. Warren N (ed): Studies in Cross-Cultural Psychology, Vol. 1. New York, Academic, 1977.

(A) Hologeistic studies specifically designed to test relevant hypotheses could still provide a sound source of evidence for the validity of Freudian theory. (B) Both malnutrition and socioeconomic factors affect mental development in Guatemala. (C) The effect of all culture-contact situations that evoke in individuals the need to cope with an unfamiliar culture can be analyzed in terms of the development of new coping repertoires and of the use of new cognitive, dynamic, and performance mechanisms.

1530. Warwick DP: The politics and ethics of cross-cultural research. In Handbook of Cross-Cultural Psychology, edited by HC Triandis and WW Lambert, 1:319–71. Boston, Allyn and Bacon, 1980.

Politics and ethics must be taken seriously in cross-cultural research as the studies can be affected in their perception, reception, and success within a given culture. Examples are given to show how politics and ethics may influence cross-cultural studies. There needs to be a greater and more candid discussion of ethical and political questions in cross-cultural research.

1531. Wasson RG, Cowan G, Cowan F, Rhodes W: Maria Sabina and Her Mazatec Mushroom Velada. New York, Harcourt Brace Jovanovich, 1975.

A Mazatec shamaness, with the assistance of a plant hallucinogen, attempts to cure a young man whose spirit double has been eaten by a puma.

1532. Watkins D, Astilla E: Stability of self-esteem of Filipino girls. Psychological Reports 45:993–94, 1979.

While young Filipinas have only moderately stable self-esteem, the relative instability of their scores on the Coopersmith Self-Esteem Inventory cannot be explained in terms of level of self-esteem or field-dependence/independence.

1533. Watts FN, Bennett DH: Social deviance in a day hospital. Brit J Psychiatry 132:455–62, 1978.

Violence and poor social integration have no relation to outcome in a day hospital program. There is no basis for excluding patients from day hospitals on the assumption that they are less likely to be helped than other nonpsychotic patients.

1534. Waxler NE: The normality of deviance: an alternate explanation of schizophrenia in the family. Schizophrenia Bull 14:38–47, 1975.

Erikson's theory of deviant behavior alerts family researchers not to consider families that have a member with symptoms of schizophrenia as special or uniquely structured groups, or as special or unique sets of personalities, but instead as "normal" groups whose deviant members may serve the same "normal" purposes as any deviant in any society.

1535. Waxler N: Is mental illness cured in traditional societies? Culture Medicine Psychiatry 1:233–53, 1977.

In traditional societies, people think of mental illness as brief, easily cured, and nonrecurrent. The mentally ill person is rapidly reintroduced through treatment into a normal position in society with stigma. The course of mental illness is greatly affected by these conceptual and behavioral reactions on the part of patients, healers, and society in general.

1536. Waxler NE: Is outcome for schizophrenia better in nonindustrial societies? The case of Sri Lanka. J Nerv Ment Disease 167(3):144–58, 1979.

The prognosis of schizophrenia is much better in nonindustrial societies. The good outcome cannot be explained by artifacts of sampling, by diagnostic methods, by type of treatment, or by the family's willingness to tolerate deviance. The good prognosis can be attributed to cultural factors such as the traditional system of beliefs, structure of treatment systems, and family norms.

1537. Webber DL: Mental health problems amongst Aboriginal children of northern Australia. Intl J Social Psychiatry 26:118–23, 1978.

Many needs of the mentally ill Aboriginal children of Australia are met by the child guidance center there. However, further efforts will be necessary to coordinate mental health and educational processes toward reducing the difficulties that tribally oriented children experience with schooling.

1538. Weidman HH: Falling-out: a diagnostic and treatment problem viewed from a transcultural perspective. Social Science Medicine 13B(2):95–112, 1979.

Falling-out is a state in which the individual collapses without warning, occasionally with some degree of salivation but without convulsions, tongue-biting, or bowel or bladder incontinence. The condition is a significant health problem for black Americans, Bahamians, and probably for Haitians.

1539. Weil A: The Marriage of the Sun and the Moon. Boston, Houghton Mifflin, 1980.

Humans are born with a drive to experience diverse modes of awareness. The sun and the moon are symbolic of the mind; not only do they represent the dualism of consciousness but also they are actual expressions of that dualism, e.g., people in the path of a total eclipse of the sun may experience dramatic alterations in consciousness. The concept of the solar mind and the lunar mind helps to explain alterations in consciousness induced by such means as sweat lodges, drugs, and plants such as datura, yogé, and certain mushrooms.

1540. Weiner BP, Marvit RC: Schizophrenia in Hawaii: analysis of cohort mortality risk in a multi-ethnic population. Brit J Psychiatry 131:497–503, 1977.

Schizophrenia in Hawaii is diagnosed in the second or third decades of life; males are admitted to treatment at a younger age than females, and most continue in treatment after ten years. The prevalence of schizophrenia in Caucasians in Hawaii is comparable to that on the mainland. This rate is below that found for other ethnic groups. Higher rates of suicide in schizophrenics are culture related, depending on acceptance or rejection of the mentally ill, as all ethnic groups do not have a high rate.

1541. Weinstein L: Alcoholism as a political problem in Chile. Mental Health Society 3:72–76, 1976.

Chile has a very serious alcohol problem. During Allende's government, there was an increasing concern for the national patterns of drinking. Persons addicted to alcohol formed part of an "alcohol culture" that, in the context of the situation in Chile in 1972, was ideologically opposed to the revolutionary process.

1542. Weisenberg M, Kreindler ML, Schachat R, Werboff J: Pain: anxiety and attitudes in black, white and Puerto Rican patients. Psychosomatic Medicine 37:123–35, 1975.

Puerto Ricans have the highest level of Trait Anxiety, whites the lowest, and blacks are in the middle. On Dental Anxiety Scale, Puerto Ricans score highest, blacks lowest, and whites in between. In attitudinal differences reflecting a relative willingness to deny, get rid of, or avoid dealing with the pain, Puerto Ricans score highest, whites lowest, and blacks in between.

1543. Weisfeld GE: An ethological view of human adolescence. J Nerv Ment Disease 167(1):38–55, 1979.

Applying an evolutionary analysis from ethology to human adolescence, reproductive maturation and gaining independence from parents seem to be the two basic developmental functions. Morphological, behavioral, and cultural factors complement each other in attaining these developmental functions. An ethological understanding of adolescence is important to offer a useful perspective on the problems of American youth.

1544. Weisner TS, Gallimore R: My brother's keeper: child and sibling caretaking. Current Anthropology 18:169–90, 1977.

Child caretaking has an important role in the consideration of alternatives to maternal caretaking. There is certainly no evidence that children suffer when cared for in part by older children as opposed to by their parents.

1545. Weiss JMA, Perry ME: Transcultural attitudes toward antisocial behavior: the "worst" crimes. Social Science Medicine 10:541–45, 1976.

In regard to crime prevention and enforcement activities, the public sees a need for greater emphasis on taking action with respect to those antisocial behaviors clearly viewed as most threatening: homicide and other forms of violence against the person, theft, exploitation, and public dishonesty.

1546. Weiss JMA, Perry ME: Transcultural attitudes toward antisocial behavior: opinions of mental health professionals. Amer J Psychiatry 134:1036–38, 1977.

In ranking the "most serious crimes," mental health professionals are most concerned about crimes of violence, theft, exploitation, and public dishonesty. In perceived strategies for social control of crime, mental health professionals tend toward a strong emphasis on an organized problem-solving approach, including research, programs of prevention and defense, and treatment and rehabilitation.

1547. Weiss JMA, Weiss JA: Assessment of social class in transcultural psychiatric research. J Operational Psychiatry 10:12–19, 1979.

Most psychiatrists use Hollingshead and Redlich's Index of Social Position to determine social class. Occupation alone is a sufficient indicator of social class.

1548. Weissman MM, Klerman GL: Sex differences and the epidemiology of depression. Arch Gen Psychiatry 34:98–111, 1977.

Sex differences in depression in Western society are real and not an artifact of reporting or health-care behavior.

1549. Weitz S: Sex Roles. Oxford and New York, Oxford U. Press, 1977.

The biological, psychological, social, and cultural foundations of sex roles are identified. In both China and Israel the social role of women has been modified.

1550. Weitz S (ed): Nonverbal Communication. 2d ed. Oxford and New York, Oxford U. Press, 1979.

The study of nonverbal communication includes facial expression and visual interaction, body movement and gesture, paralanguage, proximity behaviors (proxemics, architecture, exocrinology, touch), and multichannel communication (sentics, biological rhythms, Profile of Nonverbal Sensitivity Test).

1551. Werbin J, Hynes K: Transference and culture in a Latino therapy group. Intl J Group Psychotherapy 25:396–401, 1975.

When dealing with minority groups the focus should be more on individuals in order to avoid stereotyping both the Latino and the Anglo. There is nothing in the Latino culture per se that requires a radically different therapeutic approach. However, an awareness of the group members' differing customs, values, and ways of communication is extremely useful, particularly during the initial phases of the group.

1552. Werkman S: Bringing Up Children Overseas. New York, Basic Books, 1977.

Families with children who move to a foreign country should be aware of the nature of relationships with foreigners, of the need to change expectations and behavior, and of developmental issues related to identity formation.

1553. West SA, Macklin J (eds): The Chicano Experience. Boulder, Colo., Westview, 1979.

The immigrant lifeways, adaptation and change, and ethnic boundary maintenance of Chicanos are presented.

1554. Westermeyer J: The pro-heroin effects of anti-opium laws in Asia. Arch Gen Psychiatry 33:1135–39, 1976.

Antinarcotic laws can be effective only by changing society's attitude toward traditional drugs from ambivalence to opposition and by mobilizing resources to treat and rehabilitate all addicts within a short period of time.

1555. Westermeyer J: Cross racial foster home placement among Native American psychiatric patients. J National Med Assn 69:231–36, 1977.

Native-American children placed in white foster homes often experience alcoholism, behavioral disorders, and suicidal activity during their teenage years when they receive stereotypical racial labels and are rejected by the white culture that they have identified with.

1556. Westermeyer J: Narcotic addiction in two Asian countries. Drug Alcohol Dependence 2:273–85, 1977.

The Hmong raise the opium poppy, and thus the drug is available in their homes, while ethnic Lao purchase opium. The Hmong have more female addicts and more young opiate users and addicts and seek treatment earlier than the Lao.

1557. Westermeyer J: Indigenous and expatriate addicts in Laos: a comparison. Culture Medicine Psychiatry 2:139–50, 1978.

Narcotic addiction in Asia is primarily a behavior of early and middle adulthood rather than of adolescence or senescence. Asian addicts are not nearly so "deviant" as narcotic addicts in the United States. Narcotic availability, per capita income, and access to heroin do strongly affect narcotic use patterns. Data obtained from tribal Lao and expatriate addicts in Asia do not demonstrate specific cultural factors significant to narcotic addiction.

1558. Westermeyer J: Sex roles at the Indian-majority interface in Minnesota. Intl J Social Psychiatry 24:189–94, 1978.

In most social institutions, there are more Indian women in influential positions, with more Indian men relegated to custodial positions.

1559. Westermeyer J: The Apple Syndrome in Minnesota: a complication of racial-ethnic discontinuity. J Operational Psychiatry 10:134–40, 1979.

American Indian children with white foster parents often develop behavioral problems during adolescence because of rejection by their peers. The Apple Syndrome refers to the Indian who is red on the "outside" yet has a white ethnic identity "inside."

1560. Westermeyer J: Ethnic identity problems among ten Indian psychiatric patients. Intl J Social Psychiatry 25:188–97, 1979.

Identity problems are probably no more common among American Indian people than in the general population. However, some Indian people do have an uncommon type of identity problem: negative or ambivalent feelings regarding their own racial and ethnic identity.

1561. Westermeyer J: Folk concepts of mental disorder among the Lao: continuities with similar concepts in other cultures and in psychiatry. Culture Medicine Psychiatry 3:301–17, 1979.

In Laos folk concepts for mental disorder, while predominantly inferring etiology (e.g., spirit-caused disorder), have certain terms that also emphasize particular descriptive psychopathology or behavioral abnormality. Broad folk categories of mental disorders bear considerable similarity to some psychiatric and neurologic categories within medicine. Lao folk terms for mental disorder also closely resemble those of other Southeast Asian cultures, although illiterate tribal peoples appear to have fewer terms than literate peasant peoples.

1562. Westermeyer J: Medical and nonmedical treatment for narcotic addicts: a comparative study from Asia. J Nerv Ment Disease 167(4):205–11, 1979.

Those addicts in Laos who choose the more traditional monastery program as opposed to the medical facility are of older mean age and include a greater proportion of females and ethnic Lao people. Mortality among addicts over age sixty is considerably higher at the monastery than at the medical facility. Over time, fewer addicts chose the monastery program than the medical program.

1563. Westermeyer J: Influence of mental illness on marriage, reproduction, and parenting in a society without psychiatric services. J Nerv Ment Disease 168:614–20, 1980.

In Laos among the mentally ill, single persons have an earlier onset of mental illness as compared to those who have been married. Those who have married and produced children have a high rate of divorce from their spouses and separation from their children following onset of mental illness. Mentally ill subjects eighteen years or older are less apt to be married than opium addicts in the same population.

1564. Westermeyer J: Psychosis in a peasant society: social outcomes. Amer J Psychiatry 137:1390–94, 1980.

Social disability associated with chronic psychosis cannot be ascribed totally to diagnostic labeling or institutionalization in Laos.

1565. Westermeyer J (ed): Anthropology and Mental Health. The Hague, Mouton, 1976.

Topics discussed include witchcraft beliefs and psychosomatic illness, humoral theory and therapy in Tunisia, Japanese-American suicide, ethnic psychopathology in Hawaii, kifafa (epilepsy) among the Bantu, spiritual healers, "brainwashing" therapy among the Coast Salish, primary prevention and culture, holocultural studies, value change as a model for predicting changes in mental deviance rates in developing countries, and coalition of a Kali healer and a psychiatrist in Guyana.

1566. Westermeyer J, Kroll J: Violence and mental illness in a peasant society: characteristics of violent behaviors and "folk" use of restraints. Brit J Psychiatry 133:529–41, 1978.

In Laos people are more assaultive, pose a risk to themselves, and have to be restrained during the course of their mental illness. Those in early stages of their illness are more violent than those in their later stages. When violent or dangerous behavior occurs, there is use of restraints by "folk"; restraints are released as soon as practicable.

1567. Westermeyer J, Peng G: Opium and heroin addicts in Laos. J Nerv Ment Disease 164(5):346–50, 1977.

In Laos, heroin and opium addicts differ significantly on most demographic characteristics such as place of residence, frequency of daily use, money spent on the drugs, dose of methadone used for detoxification, and rate of deterioration following drug use. It is difficult to know whether these observed differences are due to drug factors or demographic factors.

1568. Westermeyer J, Peng G: Opium and heroin addicts in Laos. Part 2: A study of matched pairs. J Nerv Ment Disease 164(5):351–54, 1977.

In Laos, heroin addicts take more doses of drug per day, spend more money per day on narcotic drugs, require higher detoxification doses of methadone, and seek treatment much sooner than opium addicts. There is an urban distribution of heroin addicts and a mixed urban-rural residence of opium addicts. Heroin is not more "addictogenic" than opium.

1569. Westermeyer J, Rosenberg P: Role, ritual, and the grynnfluk. Amer J Orthopsychiatry 47:341–47, 1977.

Cohabitation, whatever its duration and its outcome, is on its way to becoming an established variation of our society's courtship rituals. Parents should be aware of their own reaction to the grynnfluk relationship, and therapists and counselors must be prepared to aid couples and their parents in accepting the emotional ties that attend the relationship and in dealing with the particular stress it produces.

1570. Westermeyer J, Wintrob R: "Folk" criteria for the diagnosis of mental illness in rural Laos: on being insane in sane places. Amer J Psychiatry 136:755–61, 1979.

Folk criteria for mental illness in Laos are determined primarily by the persistence of socially dysfunctional behavior. Important criteria for labeling a person insane are unprovoked assaultive or destructive behavior, social isolation, self-neglect, socially disruptive or inappropriate behavior, and inability to do productive work.

1571. Westermeyer J, Wintrob R: "Folk" explanations of mental illness in rural Laos. Amer J Psychiatry 136:901–5, 1979.

Folk explanations of mental illness in Laos are focused on supernatural causes, physical causes, social problems, and psychological states. Many self-evident factors like familial prevalence are not considered important. Responsibility for the illness is attributed to factors outside the subjects' control, thus absolving them from blame and ensuring support from the social group.

1572. Whisnant L, Brett E, Zegans L: Implicit messages concerning menstruation in commercial educational materials prepared for young adolescent girls. Amer J Psychiatry 132:815–20, 1975.
Commercial educational materials are valuable sources of information on menstruation, although emphasizing hygiene rather than menarcheal changes. More research is needed into the physical and mental changes of puberty. Parents and social institutions are obligated to provide more comprehensive information.

1573. Whisnant L, Zegans L: A study of attitudes toward menarche in white middle-class American adolescent girls. Amer J Psychiatry 132:809–14, 1975.
Menarche is an emotional event, marking the adolescent's emergence as an adult woman capable of reproduction and a new relationship with her mother. There is a need to develop appropriate substitutes for primitive rituals, to satisfy the psychological needs of young girls, and to treat menarche as more than a hygienic crisis.

1574. White GM: Conceptual universals in interpersonal language. Amer Anthropologist 82:759–81, 1980.
A comparison of models of cognitive organization of three languages (A'ara, Oriya, English) indicates that common conceptual themes underlie the meanings and uses of personality descriptors cross-culturally.

1575. Whitehead TL: Residence, kinship and mating as survival strategies: a West Indian example. J Marriage Family 40:817–28, 1978.
While nuclear domestic units bound by legal marriage between the conjugal pair are the ideal and represent stability and respectability in capitalistic economics, they are not the most adaptive family and residential structures in areas of low wage and employment opportunities. Flexibility in residence, kinship, and mating patterns offer the best opportunities for combining resources.

1576. Whiting BB, Whiting JWM: Children of Six Cultures. Washington, D.C., Howard U. Press, 1975.
Data collected from farming communities in Okinawa, India, Kenya, Mexico, the Philip-

pines, and New England may facilitate the cross-cultural testing of hypotheses pertaining to the development of human social behavior. Children in different cultures display different patterns of the same behaviors; these patterns are predictable by socioeconomic system and household structure.

1577. Whitwell FD, Barker MG: "Possession" in psychiatric patients in Britain. Brit J Med Psychology 53:287–95, 1980.
While cultural factors may exert a pathoplastic influence leading some toward "possession," the main causes of the disturbance lie within the individual.

1578. Whyte MK: Cross-cultural codes dealing with the relative status of women. Ethnology 17:211–37, 1978.
Because of the view that "the status of women" is not a meaningful concept cross-culturally, the reasons why women have higher status in some societies than in others cannot be tested.

1579. Whyte MK: The Status of Women in Preindustrial Societies. Princeton, N.J., Princeton U. Press, 1978.
No evidence exists for any general "status of women" complex that varies consistently from culture to culture. The status of women tends to vary independently from culture to culture.

1580. Wilder J: Male and female: the significance of values. Amer J Psychotherapy 31:11–18, 1977.
With the rapid technological and educational expansion of the past decades, women have been given greater opportunities and have had their values altered, but wide acceptance of these values by society has yet to be accomplished.

1581. Wilkinson DY: Black Male/White Female. Cambridge, Mass., Schenkman, 1975.
The motivations for marriage between black males and white females are studied, as are social barriers against interracial unions and the social and political implications of these unions.

1582. Williams FE: The Vailala Madness and Other Essays. Honolulu, U. Press of Hawaii, 1977.
Reprints of essays from 1920 to 1940 propose that the development of a cargo cult among the Elema of Papua New Guinea demonstrates the mental instability of the natives.

1583. Williams JE, Best DL, Boswell DA: The measurement of children's racial attitudes in the early school years. Child Development 46:494–500, 1975.

Pro-Euro/anti-Afro bias among Euro-American children reaches a peak at the second-grade level and subsequently declines. Methodologically, the Pram-II procedure is useful for the assessment of racial bias among children in the early school grades.

1584. Williams JE, Moreland JK: Race, Color, and the Young Child. Chapel Hill, U. of North Carolina Press, 1976.

The acquisition of color racial bias can be understood in a developmental context.

1585. Williams MR (ed): Psychological Anthropology. The Hague, Mouton, 1975.

Topics discussed include illness and healing, the Oedipus complex and the Bengali family, culture and the expression of emotions, and aggression in the !Ko-Bushmen.

1586. Williams TR (ed): Socialization and Communication in Primary Groups. The Hague, Mouton, 1975.

The socialization process is context-sensitive and communicative; it reflects individual creativity, society-specific structures, and universal properties.

1587. Williamson RC: Socialization, mental health, and social class: a Santiago sample. Social Psychiatry 11:69–74, 1976.

As compared to the middle class, the lower class of Santiago, Chile, disproportionately shows parental rejection, perceives parents as punitive, feels greater distance from parents, and recalls a less consistent and predictable emotional climate in the home.

1588. Wilson EO: On Human Nature. Cambridge, Mass., Harvard U. Press, 1978.

Much of human behavior, including the incest taboo, is best understood in sociobiological terms.

1589. Wilson LG: The clinical home visit in cultural psychiatry. J Operational Psychiatry 11:27–33, 1980.

The clinical home visit, when the psychiatrist is working in cross-cultural settings, allows for better case identification and more accurate assessment, a better understanding of a patient's actual milieu, a more accessible atmosphere to negotiate or mediate between conflicting family members, and a better understanding of the patient's "explanatory model" of illness.

1590. Wilson LG: Community psychiatry in Oceania: fifteen months' experience in Micronesia. Social Psychiatry 15:175–79, 1980.

When working as a psychiatrist in a developing area like Micronesia, virtually all encounters in the community can be teaching ones. The teaching and consultative aspects of community psychiatry take precedence over all other activities since these are such neglected areas.

1591. Wilson LG, Ries R, Bokan J: Transcultural psychiatry on an American psychiatric ward. Hosp Community Psychiatry 31:759–62, 1980.

Because many immigrant groups in the United States maintain their original customs and traditions, a transcultural approach may be necessary in many clinical situations.

1592. Wilson LG, Shore JH: Evaluation of a regional Indian alcohol program. Amer J Psychiatry 132:255–58, 1975.

A 44 percent improvement rate at an average of eighteen months after discharge was seen in this Northwest Indian alcohol program. There was no significant difference in response to treatment between age groups.

1593. Wilson M: For Men and Elders. New York, Africana, 1977.

The Nyakynsa-Ngonde people of Tanzania and Malawi have undergone great changes in the relations between generations and between men and women from 1875 to 1971.

1594. Wilson OM: "The normal" as a culture-related concept: historical consideration. Mental Health Society 3:57–61, 1976.

We still retain from our historical past the notion that mental or emotional illness bespeaks, if not possession by spirits, at least an irreversible condition. By modern psychiatric criteria for mental health, many creative scientists and artists would be considered abnormal. On the other hand, the concept of normalcy has recently been used to rationalize political misbehavior. Is it possible to develop a viewpoint of "normal" that is consistent with our culture and yet broad enough to encompass the uncommon?

1595. Wing JF: The social context of schizophrenia. Amer J Psychiatry 135:1333–39, 1978.

Over the past twenty-five years psychiatry has increased its understanding of the social context of schizophrenia, e.g., describing and recognizing acute and chronic syndromes, social causes of symptoms and disabilities, the relationship between social and pharmacological treatments, and rational approaches to planning and prescribing services and counseling patients and their relatives. All four areas promise to lead to further progress.

1596. Wing L, Ricks DM: The aetiology of childhood autism: a criticism of Tinbergens' ethological theory. Psychological Medicine 6:533–43, 1976.

The major problem in evaluating this theory, apart from the absence of any evidence in its favor, is the lack of precision with which the Tinbergens use the terms *autism* and *Kanner's syndrome*.

1597. Witkin HA, Berry JW: Psychological differentiation in cross-cultural perspective. J Cross-Cultural Psychology 1:4–87, 1975.

The basic tenet of differentiation theory—that manifestations of more differentiated or less differentiated functioning in various psychological domains are diverse expressions of an underlying organism-wide process of development toward greater psychological complexity—has two implications: one is that any manifestation of differentiation may be used to identify an individual's overall level of psychological differentiation; another is that the search for the sources of a given psychological characteristic during development is placed in a broad context. Thus, the differentiation framework provides both a conception and a methodology for inquiry into the role of socialization across cultures.

1598. Witt PH, Gynther MD: Another explanation for black-white MMPI differences. J Clin Psychology 31:69–70, 1975.

Differences in connotative meaning may account for some of the differences in responses of blacks and whites to the MMPI.

1599. Wittkower ED, Dubreuil G: Psychoanalysis and anthropology: some considerations. J Amer Acad Psychoanalysis 4:427–32, 1976.

Psychoanalysts and anthropologists are ill equipped to function as social engineers in the field of primary prevention. To do this requires political involvement. They are qualified to give advice on the basis of knowledge derived from individual patients. However, hasty explanations should be avoided, and hopes should not be raised that cannot be materialized.

1600. Wittkower ED, Warnes H: Transcultural

psychosomatics. Canadian Psychiatric Assn J 20:143–50, 1975.

On cross-cultural comparison there are striking differences in the rates of some psychosomatic disorders. Cardiovascular and gastrointestinal psychosomatic disorders are more frequent in the urban populations of developing countries and in the cities of Europe and America than in a rural population.

1601. Wober M: Psychology in Africa. London, Intl. African Institute, 1975.

The findings of hundreds of psychological studies (many of which use projective tests, questionnaires, and matrices) are cataloged and discussed.

1602. Wohlberg GW: A black patient with a white therapist. Intl J Psychoanal Psychotherapy 4:540–62, 1975.

A violent, antiwhite, hostile, paranoid schizophrenic patient dramatically altered her attitudes, behavior, and defenses in constructive changes with the help of a therapist who himself became aware of the need to adopt a flexible approach, to control his own aggression, to be frank, and to examine his own motivations.

1603. Wolf M, Witke R (eds): Women in Chinese Society. Stanford, Calif., Stanford U. Press, 1975.

Wide-ranging essays on Chinese women include chapters on suicide and "coming of age."

1604. Wolfe JC: Special report: community mental health in China. Comm Mental Health J 16:241–48, 1980.

Mental health treatment in China does not emphasize confidentiality as much as treatment in most Western nations does. What is of prime importance for the Chinese is the reintegration of the person into society as a functional and productive member.

1605. Wolfgang A (ed): Non-Verbal Behavior: Applications and Cultural Implications. New York, Academic, 1979.

Anthropological, ethnological, psychiatric, and (primarily) psychological studies on nonverbal behavior are presented. Specific areas include the political-ethnic adaptiveness of communication codes and the consequences of varying listening patterns during interracial interviews.

1606. Wolman RN: "Women's issues" in couples treatment—the view of the male therapist. Psychiatric Opinion 13(1):13–17, 1976.

The women's revolution has added depth and dimension to psychotherapy, especially to psychotherapy with married couples. It has promoted a reevaluation of the basic principles of therapy and of the values and the attitudes of therapists, giving them an unusual opportunity for growth.

1607. Wong N: Psychiatric education and training of Asian and Asian-American psychiatrists. Amer J Psychiatry 135:1525–29, 1978.

The Asian and Asian-American physician in a standard psychiatric residency is faced with discrimination at several levels. Special problems of professional role confusion and personal identity may create barriers to professional development and productivity. Specialized programs focusing on ethnic minority groups within a general psychiatric residency are needed to alleviate the problem.

1608. Wood CS: Human Sickness and Health: A Biocultural View. Palo Alto, Calif., Mayfield, 1979.

Human culture sets limitations on the health of a society as well as on a people's ability to accept many aspects of health care. Shamans and spiritualists are curers with social functions.

1609. Worell J: Sex roles and psychological well-being: perspectives on methodology. J Consult Clinical Psychology 46:777–91, 1978.

Current methods of examining sex roles allow for increased knowledge of the theoretical and psychometric definitions of androgyny, the relationship of sex-role typing to other aspects of interpersonal functioning, and procedures in sex-role and gender distinction.

1610. World Health Organization: Schizophrenia: An International Follow-up Study. New York, Wiley, 1979.

A two-year follow-up of patients included in the Cross-National International Pilot Study of Schizophrenia reveals that schizophrenic patients from developing countries improved significantly more than those from developed countries.

1611. Wright GN, Phillips LD, Whalley PC, Choo GT, Ng K, Tan I, Wisudha A: Cultural differences in probablistic thinking. J Cross-Cultural Psychology 9:285–99, 1978.

The British adopt a more finely differentiated view of uncertainty, both verbally and numerically, than do Asians in response to uncertain situations.

1612. Wu IH, Windle C: Ethnic specificity in the relative minority use and staffing of community mental health centers. Comm Mental Health J 16:156–68, 1980.

The more members of a specific ethnic minority that a center employs, the higher the relative utilization rate for that ethnic minority will be. However, because each ethnic minority is distinct in cultural background and ethnic identification, there may be little or no relationship between the relative utilization rate of a specific minority and the relative staffing rate of other minorities.

1613. Yamamoto J: Research priorities in Asian-American mental health delivery. Amer J Psychiatry 135:457–58, 1978.

Asian-Americans underutilize mental health services. More research is needed to determine the effect of language differences, familial reactions, community education, cultural changes, cross-cultural misdiagnosis, and therapeutic methods in mental health delivery.

1614. Yamamoto J, Iga M: Japanese suicide: Yasunari Kawabata and Yukio Mishima. J Amer Acad Psychoanalysis 3:179–86, 1975.

Because of the Japanese tradition of seppuku and the cultural belief in ancestors that results in the blurring of the border between life and death, suicide for both authors seemed to be a constructive act—making a trip to another world for Kawabata and influencing social change for Mishima.

1615. Yamamoto J, Wagatsuma H: The Japanese and Japanese-Americans. J Operational Psychiatry 11:130–39, 1980.

The issues relevant in evaluating the acculturation of Japanese-Americans are discussed. There is concern about the fragmentation of the strength of the Japanese family, with its traditional emphasis on group support and interdependency, as the Japanese-Americans become more Westernized.

1616. Yanagisako SJ: Women-centered kin networks in urban bilateral kinship. Amer Ethnologist 4:207–26, 1977.

Examining the interplay of people's cultural constructs in the determination of social relationships provides a more adequate understanding of female centrality than approaches that treat the social organization of kinship as if it existed apart from the cultural system of kinship.

1617. Yanagisako SJ: Variance in American kinship: implications for cultural analysis. Amer Ethnologist 5(1):15–29, 1978.

Analysis of Japanese-American kinship strongly suggests that the symbolic meanings people attach to cultural units such as the "person," "relative," and "family" may be just as restricted in scope and context and just as tied to a particular set of social fields as are normative rules for action. Whether we can claim greater generality and detachment from specific cultural contexts for the symbolic aspects of units requires further examination. Further, we must make central to the pursuit of cultural analysis an investigation of the interpretations of cultural domains and the relationships among the levels of analysis we identify for heuristic purposes.

1618. Yaroshevosky F: Self-mutilation in Soviet prisons. Canadian Psychiatric Assn J 20:443–46, 1975.

Self-mutilation by Soviet prisoners is a form of desperate communication with both the authorities and the world at large regarding the unbearable conditions in prisons.

1619. Yassa R: A sociopsychiatric study of an Egyptian phenomenon. Amer J Psychotherapy 34:246–51, 1980.

After the 1967 Egyptian-Israeli War, the appearance of the Virgin Mary and miraculous cures were reported. The religious phenomenon was related to the loss of self-esteem suffered by the defeated Egyptians, with some cases of hysterical neurosis being cured by seeing the Virgin.

1620. Yee TT, Lee RH: Based on cultural strengths, a school primary prevention program for Asian-American youth. Comm Ment Health Journal 13:239–48, 1977.

Ethnic minorities need to rely on their own subculture for the kind of psychological and social support required for positive mental health.

1621. Young A: Magic as a "quasi-profession": the organization of magic and magical healing among Amhara. Ethnology 14:245–65, 1975.

The Debtera of the Amhara, an ecclesiastic group of the Ethiopian Orthodox Church, is a quasi profession that monopolizes a highly volatile resource—knowledge. The Debtera's public misconceives the sources of their knowledge in a way that stigmatizes the Debtera magician-

healers. The layman's misconception is exploited by those healers who, in the course of their careers, acquire the social and technological means necessary for manipulating the stigma to their own advantage.

1622. Young A: Internalizing and externalizing medical belief systems: an Ethiopian example. Social Science Medicine 10:147–56, 1976.

While ordinary Amhara people attribute generic medical powers against most sicknesses to certain clerical healers, in reality these men share no distinctive medical traditions. Their medical knowledge is mainly a compendium of herbal recipes, and their punitive generic powers are an illusion intentionally encouraged and exploited by many of the healers themselves.

1623. Young A: Some implications of medical beliefs and practices for social anthropology. Amer Anthropologist 78:5–24, 1976.

In order to explain why medical beliefs and practices persist, it is necessary to discover their practical and special meanings. It is useful to consider certain kinds of sickness episodes as a subspecies of a class of events usually associated with ritual performances.

1624. Young JC: Illness categories and action strategies in a Tarascan town. Amer Ethnologist 5(1):81–97, 1978.

Examination of a set of Mexican folk-illness terms by cluster analysis indicates that the distinctions that best explain the resulting illness categories are also among the most important considerations involved in the formulation of strategies for preventing and alleviating illness.

1625. Young JC: Medical Choice in a Mexican Village. New Brunswick, N.J., Rutgers U. Press, 1980.

Villagers in a rural Mexican community are convinced of the superiority of modern medicine over folk remedies.

1626. Young JC: A model of illness treatment decisions in a Tarascan town. Amer Ethnologist 7(1):106–31, 1980.

A model based on cognitive-ethnographic methods whereby actors use information in selecting among the viable treatment alternatives can account for 91 percent correct treatment choices made.

1627. Yu ESH: Chinese collective orientation and need for achievement. Intl J Social Psychiatry 26:178–89, 1980.

The concepts of independence and individualism, so strongly emphasized and highly valued in American culture, are alien to Chinese students socialized in the traditional manner, in which interdependence and affiliation are emphasized.

1628. Yule W, Berger M, Rutter M, Yule B: Children of West Indian immigrants: intellectual performance and reading attainment. J Child Psychol Psychiat Allied Disciplines 16:1–17, 1975.

Children from immigrant families score well below children from nonimmigrant families in tests of intellectual performance and educational attainment.

1629. Yutiao MY, Kinzie JD: Consultation with the Filipino boarding home: an after-care facility in Hawaii. Intl J Social Psychiatry 21:130–36, 1975.

Filipino boarding home operators, if provided with consultation sensitive to their values, can become even more effective in caring for elderly ex-mental hospital patients.

1630. Zahan D: The Religion, Spirituality, and Thought of Traditional Africa. Chicago, U. of Chicago Press, 1979.

Underlying African spirituality is the theme that man exists not for God but for man himself, who is the keystone of the African religious structure. A duality of the soul underlies African witchcraft, divinatory practices, and healing procedures, as exemplified especially by the Bambara (Sudan).

1631. Zak I: Structure of ethnic identity of Arab-Israeli students. Psychological Reports 38:239–46, 1976.

Despite the peculiar situation of the Arab minority in Israel, two orthogonal factors emerge, an Arab identity and an Israeli identity.

1632. Zaretsky II, Leme MP (eds): Religious Movement in Contemporary America. Princeton, N.J., Princeton U. Press, 1975.

Among the topics discussed are spiritism, cults, ritual, and healing.

1633. Zarroug ETA: The frequency of visual hallucinations in schizophrenic patients in Saudi Arabia. Brit J Psychiatry 127:553–55, 1975.

Visual hallucinations in schizophrenics are common in Saudi Arabia. It is necessary to investigate the role of culture in the occurrence of these symptoms.

1634. Zarrouk ETA: The usefulness of first-rank symptoms in the diagnosis of schizophrenia in a Saudi Arabian population. Brit J Psychiatry 132:571–73, 1978.

"Made" phenomena and "somatic passivity" are common first-rank schizophrenic symptoms in a Saudi Arabian population. The influence exercised by cultural factors on the basic symptomatology is important, and the study of transcultural psychiatry should receive adequate attention.

1635. Zavalloni M: Values. In Handbook of Cross-Cultural Psychology, edited by HC Triandis and RW Brislin, 5:73–120. Boston, Allyn and Bacon, 1980.

Literature on values from both a cross-cultural and an interdisciplinary perspective is reviewed. The results of a survey approach to the study of values point to consistent and sometimes striking differences between cultures. The problem of how to explain the underlying mechanisms that produce these differences leads to the necessity of studying the cognitive and motivational bases of values in a cross-cultural context. Values research is best seen as a part of research on social influence.

1636. Zegiob LE, Forehand R: Maternal interactive behavior as a function of race, socioeconomic status, and sex of the child. Child Development 46:564–68, 1975.

While white mothers exhibit more cooperative behavior than black mothers, the sex of the child is less critical than socioeconomic class in determining maternal interaction behavior.

1637. Zeldine G: Pour une sociologie des maladies en Nouvelle Caledonie. Circulaire d'information no. 77, Commission du Pacifique Sud, 1977.

A significant increase in the rate of psychiatric admissions among the indigenous population of New Caledonia from 1969 to 1974 is attributed to an economic boom. The increase in suicide attempts among women is the result of disruptions in family structure due to increased contact with the outside world.

1638. Zeldine G, Bourrett D: An ontological approach to mental illness with regard to the traditional etiology of mental illness in Melanesian culture. Transcult Psych Res Review 15:177–80, 1978.

There are noticeable differences in the mental illnesses reported by people in Melanesian societies. Only congenital mental disorders are truly recognized by the Melanesians as "folie." Acquired disorders are concluded to be "illnesses of the spirit." Healing of acquired illness is sought through "allies" and medicines, both of which can induce, as well as alleviate, illness.

1639. Zeldow PB: Sex differences in psychiatric evaluation and treatment: an empirical review. Arch Gen Psychiatry 35:89–93, 1978.

Research evidence concerning sex-related differences in psychiatric/psychological assessment and treatment is diverse and ambiguous.

1640. Ziemska M: Early Child Care in Poland. New York, Gordon and Breach, 1978.

Child rearing in Poland is linked with the socialistic political system of government.

1641. Ziv A, Shani A, Nebenhaus S: Adolescents educated in Israel and in the Soviet Union: differences in moral judgment. J Cross-Cultural Psychology 6:108–21, 1975.

Soviet-educated adolescents are significantly more realistically oriented in their moral judgment than are Israelis. For both Soviets and Israelis, girls are more realistically oriented than boys.

1642. Zu HJ: The Guyana incident: some psychoanalytic considerations. Bull Menninger Clinic 44:345–63, 1980.

Through narcissistic, religious, and hero images, James Jones maintained the active cooperation of his followers that led to the mass suicide in Guyana.

1643. Zurabashvili ZD, Nanershvili BR: Psychiatry in Georgia, USSR. Psychiatric Annals 8(6):66–73, 1978.

Work therapy constitutes one of the essential rehabilitation methods of modern psychiatry in Georgia in the Soviet Union.

Secondary Author Index

Subject Index